Behavioral Dentistry

Edited by

David I. Mostofsky, Albert G. Forgione, and
Donald B. Giddon

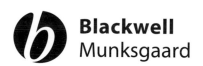
Blackwell
Munksgaard

David I. Mostofsky, PhD, earned his doctorate in experimental psychology from Boston University. He has published widely in the area of behavior as it relates to dentists and their patients. He is currently director of the Laboratory for Experimental Behavioral Medicine at Boston University, and is on the medical staff of Children's Hospital Medical Center in Boston. He is a fellow of the American Psychological Society and the International Behavioral Neuroscience Society. He is on the editorial boards of four journals, including the *Journal of Behavioral Medicine*.

Albert G. Forgione, PhD, earned his doctorate in psychology at Boston University. He is professor, chief clinical consultant, and head of the Clinical Research Section at the Gelb Craniomandibular Pain Center at Tufts University School of Dental Medicine in Boston. He is a consultant for Boeing and several other Fortune 500 companies. He is a member of Behavioral Scientists in Dentistry and the International Association of Dental Research, is on the admitting committee for Tufts University Medical Center, and is a licensed psychologist in the Commonwealth of Massachusetts.

Donald B. Giddon, DMD, PhD, is founder and former president of the Behavioral Sciences and Health Services Research Group. He currently serves as clinical professor of psychology at the University of Illinois College of Dentistry and clinical professor of community health at the Brown University Medical School. He is also on the faculties of Harvard University and New York University. At NYU, he has served as professor and dean of the School of Dentistry.

© 2006 by Blackwell Munksgaard,
published by Blackwell Publishing,
a Blackwell Publishing Company

Blackwell Publishing Professional
2121 State Avenue, Ames, Iowa 50014-8300, USA
Tel: +1 515 292 0140

Blackwell Wissenschafts Verlag, Kurfürstendamm 57,
10707 Berlin, Germany
Tel: +49 (0)30 32 79 060

Editorial Offices:
9600 Garsington Road, Oxford OX4 2DQ, UK
Tel: 01865 776868

Blackwell Publishing Asia Pty Ltd
550 Swanston Street, Carlton South,
Victoria 3053, Australia
Tel: +61 (0)3 9347 0300

Library of Congress Cataloging-in-Publication Data

Behavioral dentistry / edited by D.I. Mostofsky, A.G. Forgione,
    and D.B. Giddon.
        p. ; cm.
    Includes bibliographical references and index.
    ISBN-13: 978-0-8138-1213-7 (alk. paper)
    ISBN-10: 0-8138-1213-5 (alk. paper)
    1. Dentistry—Psychological aspects. I. Mostofsky, David I.
    II. Forgione, Albert G. III. Giddon, Donald B., 1930-   .
    [DNLM: 1. Dental Care—psychology. 2. Health Behavior.
    3. Physician-Patient Relations. 4. Practice Management, Dental.
    WU 29 B419 2006]
    RK53.B36 2006
    617.690199—dc22
                                        2005013347

For further information on Blackwell Publishing's dental publications, visit our Dentistry Subject Site:
www.dentistry.blackwellmunksgaard.com

The last digit is the print number: 9 8 7 6 5 4

Contents

Contributors   vii

Preface   xi

Part I   Biobehavioral Processes

1   **The Oral and Craniofacial Area and Interpersonal
     Attraction**   3
     Donald B. Giddon and Nina K. Anderson

2   **Oral Health and Quality of Life**   19
     Marita R. Inglehart

3   **Stress and Inflammation: A Bidirectional Relationship**   29
     Salomon Amar

4   **Saliva in Health and Disease**   37
     Mahvash Navazesh

5   **Biofeedback in the Treatment of Myofascial Pain
     Disorder and Temporomandibular Joint Pain**   51
     A. G. Forgione and Bruce L. Mehler

6   **Hypnosis in Dentistry**   65
     Bruce Peltier

Part II   Anxiety, Fear, and Pain

**7   Emotional and Environmental Determinants of
          Dental Pain**   **79**
          Daniel W. McNeil, John T. Sorrell, and Kevin E. Vowles

8   Chronic Orofacial Pain: Biobehavioral Perspectives   **99**
          Samuel F. Dworkin and Jeffrey Sherman

9   Chairside Techniques for Reducing Dental Fear   **115**
          Ronald W. Botto

10   Bruxism   **127**
          Alan G. Glaros

11   Stress, Coping, and Periodontal Disease   **139**
          Gernot Wimmer and Rudolf O. Bratschko

12   Health Behavior and Helping Patients Change   **149**
          Anne Koerber

Part III   Changing Behaviors

13   Behavior Management in Dentistry: Thumb Sucking   **163**
          Raymond G. Miltenberger and John T. Rapp

**14   Management of Children's Disruptive Behavior
          During Dental Treatment**   **175**
          Keith D. Allen

**15   Nonpharmacological Approaches to Managing
          Pain and Anxiety**   **189**
          Eugene Hittelman and Saul Bahn

16   Self-Efficacy Perceptions in Oral Health Behavior   **203**
          Anna-Maija Syrjälä

17   Behavioral Issues in Geriatric Dentistry   **213**
          Joseph L. Riley III

Part IV   Professional Practice

18   Oral Health Promotion with People with Special Needs   **231**
          Paul Glassman

19   Health Behavior and Dental Care of Diabetics   **243**
          Mirka C. Niskanen and Matti L. E. Knuuttila

20   Interpersonal Communication Training in Dental Education   **255**
          Toshiko Yoshida and Kazuhiko Fujisaki

21   Community Health Promotion   **265**
          Ray Croucher, Wagner Marcenes, and Allan Pau

Index   **277**

Contributors

Keith D. Allen, PhD Munroe-Meyer Institute for Genetics and Rehabilitation, University of Nebraska Medical Center, 985450 Nebraska Medical Center, Omaha, NE 68198-5450.

Salomon Amar, DMD, PhD Department of Periodontology and Oral Biology, Boston University Medical Center, 700 Albany Street, W-201E, Boston, MA 02118.

Nina K. Anderson, PhD Clinical Instructor, Department of Oral and Developmental Biology, Harvard University, School of Dental Medicine.

Saul Bahn, DMD, MSD Professor, Division of Biological Science, Medicine and Surgery, Department of Oral and Maxillofacial Surgery, New York University College of Dentistry, 345 East 24th Street, New York, New York 10010-4086.

Ronald W. Botto, PhD Director of Clinical Behavioral Science, Department of Pediatric Dentistry, College of Dentistry, University of Illinois at Chicago.

Rudolf O. Bratschko School of Dentistry, Department of Prosthodontics, Auenbruggerplatz 12, A-8036 Graz, Austria.

Ray Croucher Institute of Dentistry, Barts and The London, Queen Mary's School of Medicine and Dentistry, Queen Mary (University of London), London, UK.

Samuel F. Dworkin, DDS, PhD University of Washington, Department of Oral Medicine, Box 356370, Seattle, WA 98195-6370.

A.G. Forgione, PhD Craniofacial Pain Center, Tufts University School of Dental Medicine, One Kneeland Street, 6th Floor, Boston, MA 02111.

Kazuhiko Fujisaki Gifu University School of Medicine, Medical Education on Development Center Gifu University School of Medicine, 1-1, Yanagido, Gifu City, Gifu, Japan 501-1112.

Donald B. Giddon, DMD, PhD Clinical Professor, Department of Oral and Developmental Biology, Harvard University, School of Dental Medicine.

Alan G. Glaros, PhD Associate Dean and Professor, Kansas City University of Medicine and Biosciences, 1750 Independence Ave, Kansas City, MO 64106.

Paul Glassman, DDS, MA, MBA Professor of Dental Practice, Associate Dean for Information and Educational Technology, Director of the AEGD Program, University of the Pacific, Arthur A. Dugoni School of Dentistry, 2155 Webster St., San Francisco, CA 94115.

Eugene Hittelman, EdD Associate Professor, Department of Epidemiology and Health Promotion, New York University College of Dentistry, 345 East 24th Street, New York, New York 10010-4086.

Marita R. Inglehart, PhD Department of Perio/Prevention/Geriatrics, School of Dentistry, University of Michigan, Ann Arbor, MI 48109-1078.

Matti L. E. Knuuttila Professor, Department of Periodontology and Geriatric Dentistry, Institute of Dentistry, University of Oulu, and Oral and Maxillofacial Department, Oulu University Hospital, Finland.

Anne Koerber, DDS, PhD Director of Behavioral Science, Department of Pediatric Dentistry MC 850, University of Illinois at Chicago College of Dentistry, 801 South Paulina, Chicago, IL 60612.

Wagner Marcenes Institute of Dentistry, Barts and The London, Queen Mary's School of Medicine and Dentistry, Queen Mary (University of London), London UK.

Daniel W. McNeil, PhD Professor of Psychology, Department of Dental Practice and Rural Health, West Virginia University School of Dentistry, Morgantown, WV 26506-9415.

Bruce L. Mehler, MA NeuroDyne Medical, 52 New Street, Cambridge MA 02138.

Raymond G. Miltenberger, PhD   North Dakota State University, Department of Psychology, 115 Minard Hall, Fargo, ND 58105.

Mahvash Navazesh, DMD   Associate Professor and Chair, Division of Diagnostic Sciences, University of Southern California, School of Dentistry, 925 West 34th Street, Room 4320, Los Angeles, CA 90089-0641.

Mirka C. Niskanen, DDS, PhD   Oral and Maxillofacial Department, Department of Otorhinology, Keski-Pohjanmaa Central Hospital, Finland.

Allan Pau   Institute of Dentistry, Barts and The London, Queen Mary's School of Medicine and Dentistry, Queen Mary (University of London), London, UK.

Bruce Peltier, PhD, MBA   Professor of Psychology and Ethics, Arthur A. Dugoni School of Dentistry, 2155 Webster Street, University of the Pacific, San Francisco, CA 94115.

John T. Rapp, PhD   Texana MHMR Center, BTTC, 1818 Collins Road, Richmond TX 77469.

Joseph L. Riley III, PhD   University of Florida College of Dentistry, Public Health Service and Research, 1600 SW Archer Road, PO Box 100404, Gainesville, FL 32610.

Jeffrey J. Sherman, PhD   University of Washington School of Dentistry, Department of Oral Medicine, Box 356370, Seattle, WA 98195.

John T. Sorrell, PhD   VA Palo Alto Health Care System, San Mateo County Medical Center, Center for Health Care Evaluation, 795 Willow Rd. (152-MPD), Menlo Park, CA 94025.

Anna-Maija Syrjälä, PhD   Department of Periodontology, Institute of Dentistry, P.O. BOX 5281, FIN-90014, University of Oulu, Finland.

Kevin E. Vowles, PhD   University of Virginia Health System, Department of Anesthesiology, Division of Pain Management, Charlottesville, VA 22908-1008.

Gernot Wimmer   Medical University Graz, Dental School, Department of Prosthetics, Restorative Dentistry and Periodontology, Medizinische Universität Graz, Universitätsklinik für Zahn-, Mund- und Kieferheilkunde, Abteilung für Zahnersatzkunde, Auenbruggerplatz 12, A-8036 Graz, Austria.

Toshiko Yoshida   Behavioral Pediatric Dentistry, Okayama University Graduate School of Medicine and Dentistry, 2-5-1, Shikata-cho, Okayama City, Okayama, Japan 700-8525.

Preface

The importance of social science in the world of dentistry has been duly recognized and is reflected in the curriculum and accreditation requirements for dental schools. The professional responsibilities of the dentist, in both general dentistry and its specializations, involve more than mastery of technical skills. The social sciences, and psychology in particular, had much to say about the dynamics of applied dental medicine, including, but not limited to, interactions between patients and dental professionals, coping with the stress of dental pain, special considerations for examining and treating the very young and the very old, and compliance with recommended oral health practice.

In the recent past, a more mature and refined body of psychological theory and technology has become available for specific applications to health professions. In addition to specialties such as health psychology, the emergence of behavioral medicine as an interdisciplinary collaboration within health science and practice provides its distinct flavor of adapting nondrug and nonsurgical options for use in interventions and treatment. As an added component in the armamentarium of the frontline clinician, it reflects the advantages that derive from translational research. Since dentistry is based on empirical research, it is quite natural to extend to dentistry the advances that have already proven themselves in other areas of medicine and health.

For the practicing dentist and dental professional, as well as for the psychologist and others with an interest in dental medicine, the opportunities for effectively managing many potentially troubling yet routine concerns will be highly appreciated. The problems associated with managing the difficult patient, needle phobia, community programs for establishing and maintaining oral health practice, and designing optimal dental training curricula are among the common concerns that require the attention of the dental profession and that have been recognized for quite some time. Recent developments point to the role of stress in inflammatory processes and oral health and behavioral strategies for their management; behavioral interventions for dealing with orofacial pain; special behavioral considerations for diabetic, geriatric, and handicapped patients; behavioral control of bruxism; and the list continues. Less familiar to many in the dental community is an appreciation of the importance of some of the existing techniques, such as behavior modification, biofeedback, and hypnosis, as they may be applied to the practice of dentistry.

Currently, few if any books are available in the area of behavioral dentistry. To be sure, numerous sections and chapters on behavioral dentistry appear in general purpose monographs and texts of health psychology and behavioral medicine. We expect that a dedicated volume that is targeted for dental professionals (both practitioners and students) will be a valued addition to training and continuing education in the dental community. We also expect that a variety of health specialists with an interest in dentistry-related topics, whose primary discipline may be from dentistry, psychology, medicine, public health, and the allied health sciences, will find this volume instructive as they plan to utilize behavior technologies in the care and management of dental patients. We do not claim that our volume will provide a definitive or encyclopedic statement for each of the separate topics to be discussed. We do hope this book will provide an entry to the impressive literature on behavioral dentistry, will motivate the serious reader and student to consider the message of the volume as s/he proceeds in a dental career, and will offer practical solutions that can be implemented without burdensome cost or effort to both the dental team and the patient.

The contributors to this volume make up a roster of international experts in many of the subspecialties that define behavioral dentistry, and many of our authors serve in leadership roles in national dental organizations and societies.

A key priority in designing our table of contents was to go beyond a social psychology primer on interpersonal behavior or discussion of psychosocial aspects of dental practice. We considered it crucial to mention some of the recent developments that are important in treatment, including, for example, an understanding of the psychobiology of stress, behavioral techniques for managing pain, bruxism, disruptive patients, diabetic patients, and geriatric issues.

Although we attempted to throw a wide net and present the range of issues and techniques that can be expected from a closer union with behavior sciences, because of page restrictions we were not able to include many important topics or to invite a number of prominent experts to discuss their work. It is our hope that succeeding editions will enable us to better approach that goal with success.

Biobehavioral Processes

The Oral and Craniofacial Area and Interpersonal Attraction

Donald B. Giddon and Nina K. Anderson

Introduction

"One's eyes are what one is, one's mouth what one becomes." Galsworthy's words (1932) eloquently describe the contribution of the face and mouth to the individual and society. In this chapter, evidence will be presented demonstrating the importance of the craniofacial areas for interpersonal attraction. In other words, what role do the structure and function of the cranial and orofacial areas play in the perception of attraction of one individual for another? Such information is vitally important to the understanding of the motivation of patients to seek oral health care and satisfaction with treatment outcomes.

The importance of the mouth may be conceptualized into three sequential levels, varying in biological and social significance: survival, socialization, and self-actualization. Survival needs must be met before attention can be turned toward socialization and subsequently self-actualization (Maslow, 1970). Until these basic needs are met, the organism can devote little energy to socialization, except as the relation to others is important to satisfying basic survival or procreative needs.

In addition to serving the hierarchy of needs, the mouth becomes the child's first emotional contact with the world. When milk is not forthcoming, the child is provided with the first prototype of pain. Following the discomfort of teething, the teeth, together with the facial muscles, provide a major means for communicating the emotions or how one feels about the words fear or anger, as well as providing the organism with the actual means for defensive *or* aggressive behavior necessary for survival. With the development of speech, communication becomes more efficient, thereby facilitating cooperative behavior necessary for survival.

Relative to the survival and social functions of the mouth, there are some interesting studies indicating that there is a basic need for oral activity such as chewing and smoking (Friedman & Fisher, 1967), as well as the sometimes fatal consequences of oral erotic behavior (Giddon, 1999). Clinical and experimental observations have indicated that quantity and quality of sucking influence later behaviors of infants and puppies (Levy, 1934). Moreover, it was found that while men showed positive correlations between sucking and manual strength, vital capacity, and age-related personality variables, women only had a negative correlation between sucking and repression (Bergman, Malasky, & Zahn, 1967), suggesting embarrassment by the sucking task and possibly explaining the reluctance of patients with petechial hemorrhages of the soft palate to discuss their likely oral sexual etiology (Giddon, 1999).

Socialization involving the face and mouth begins with their role in perceptual differentiation of the self from others. The child quickly learns that while it can take in milk, it cannot devour the mother's breast, the entire mother, or its own hand or foot. By confrontation then with its own oral cavity, the child learns to see itself apart from the rest of the world. Following such differentiation, the child learns the importance of cooperative interaction and the role of the orofacial areas in communication with other individuals to attain its goals.

Less well recognized are the parafunctional displays of the tongue by all races and primates (Smith, Chase, & Lieblich, 1974). Toddlers tend to show their tongues when engrossed in difficult tasks such as finger painting or climbing over obstacles, or in awkward social situations such as being scolded. Similarly, adults show the tongue during tasks requiring intense concentration, as when making a tricky shot at pool or backing into a small parking space, or in a socially threatening situation such as being interrupted in conversation. Simians in close quarters also were found to exhibit the tongue during complex tasks such as peeling bananas or during unpleasant confrontations (Smith et al., 1974). Biting the tongue may also displace aggression or reduce tension, similar to chewing gum or squeezing a rubber ball.

The face, mouth, and related structures involved in facial expression can also be traced historically, primarily through drawings and other forms of art. Signs and symbols for the teeth are seen in drawings of the earliest civilizations and often are given mystical significance. The ancient cultures in Mexico and Central America prominently display the teeth in many designs. In an ancient stone head of Amenemhet III, carved around 2000 BC, one can see "not only the warrior and the ruler, but the individual man. . . . In the strong mouth, the dropping lines about the nose and eyes, and the shadowing brows, we discern a man who, though still powerful, has lost faith" (Gardner, 1936).

Biologically, the great significance of the mouth and face may well be due in part to the disproportionately large representation of the somatic, sensory, and motor cerebral cortices (Penfield & Rasmussen, 1978) and partly related to sharing an area in the limbic system responsible for eliciting genital and aggressive behavior, including biting (MacLean, 1973).

Olfactory and Gustatory System

In addition to its role in consumatory and sexual behavior in mammals, the olfactory sense is important to other facets of socialization. As an example, mouth odors communicate information about personal habits, behavior, ethnicity, and physical health (Largey & Watson, 1972). Although oral malodor may have other sources than the mouth itself, the dentists or hygienists are usually the first health professionals to recognize, treat, and/or refer patients to other specialists such as a gastroenterologist. As with other human perceptions, emotional as well as cognitive variables influence the patient's response to this interpersonally disabling condition, which may not be assessed objectively. Eli et al. (2001) found that patient's self-rating of oral odor was significantly higher than the evaluation of an objective "odor judge." Moreover, individuals with exaggerated fears of offending others ("halitophobia") may engage in social avoidance behaviors similar to those with an unattractive dentofacial appearance by covering the mouth while talking or laughing, talking out of the side of their mouths, or keeping at a "safe" distance. In extreme cases, halitophobics may behave similarly to patients with body dysmorphic disorder and isolate themselves or commit suicide (Yaegaki, 1995). Even dental health professionals may have difficulty communicating with some patients about malodor, unless the patient specifically asks them to discuss the relation of halitosis to clinically observed signs of oral disease (e.g., gingival or periodontal inflammation).

The actual act of consuming food is also influenced by social factors. Compared to persons with natural dentition, denture wearers are relatively handicapped in the ability to appreciate subtle differences in taste of solid food, taking more than twice as long as subjects with natural dentitions to render an accurate judgment of different concentrations of sucrose in solid food (Giddon et al., 1954). Thus, denture wearers not wishing to appear different in the presence of persons with natural dentitions may attempt to chew the food faster than allows for perception of subtle differences in flavor.

Visual Perception and Interpersonal Attraction

Perception, which is simply defined as the organization and interpretation of sensory input, can be influenced by a variety of physical, physiological, psychological, and social factors (Hochberg, 1988). Even with the results of new imaging technologies, however, debate continues about the relative contribution of genetic and environmental factors to perception and whether face perception is feature or configuration based (e.g., Gestalt) (Giddon, 1995).

For example, physical factors associated with visual perception include stimulus characteristics of frequency and wave length leading to judgments of the color attributes hue, saturation, brightness, and so on. In addition to the obvious neurophysiological role of the visual pathways, there may be higher-order neurons that respond selectively to curves (Dobbins, Zucker, & Cynader, 1987; Hubel & Wiesel, 1965). Physiologically based needs also affect perception; for example, individuals deprived of food or sex will perceive ambiguous stimuli presented as projective tests as representing food or sex, respectively (Murray, 1938).

The role of psychological factors in perception is exemplified in loved ones being perceived as more beautiful, or conversely, as noted by Cash and others (Archer & Cash, 1985; Pruzinsky, 1990), in depressed individuals viewing themselves more negatively than nondepressed individuals despite the fact that there are no differences between judgments of the same individuals by others. Except to note the use of camouflage techniques by dentists and plastic surgeons to create illusions of an improved physical appearance, further discussion of perceptual theory is beyond the scope of this chapter.

The appearance of the face has been used as an indicator of health, wealth, personality, and other psychological characteristics for thousands of years. While most literature on physiognomy and phrenology (Spurzheim, 1908) is not scientifically rigorous, there are a number of documented studies on the significance of facial appearance and the positive and negative social consequences of impressions and stereotypes based upon perception of facial appearance (Alley & Hildebrandt, 1988; Giddon, Schack, & Anderson, 2004; Zebrowitz, 1997). Some stereotypes are based on the following assumptions:

1. Similarities between human and animal faces indicate similar psychological qualities (e.g., a person with a sharp pointed face resembling a fox was sharp and cunning).
2. Prognathic individuals are always angry or aggressive.
3. A stranger whose face resembles a familiar individual or group must share the same characteristics, or "halo effect."

Physical appearance provides cues of fitness, fecundity, age, gender, and emotional states with significant implications for educational and employment opportunities, social affiliations, mate selection, and mental health (Adams & Crossman, 1978; Albino et al., 1990; Alley & Hildebrandt, 1988; Berscheid & Gangestad, 1982; Buss, 1994; Cunningham, 1986; Hatfield & Sprecher, 1995; Iliffe, 1960; Rhodes et al., 2001; Thornhill & Gangestad, 1993; Thornhill & Grammer, 1999; Udry, 1965).

The importance of facial symmetry was first noted as the balance between masculine and paternal left side or yang and the female and maternal right side or yin (Spurzheim, 1908). According to evolutionary psychobiologists, who promulgate the "good genes theory," symmetrical people may also be genetically superior in physical and intellectual abilities essential for survival in an adverse society (Berscheid & Gangestad, 1982; Buss, 1994; Kodric-Brown & Brown, 1985). Dentofacial asymmetry may also detract from attractiveness. For example, as has been demonstrated by Kokich, Kiyak, and Shapiro (1999) and others, who found that discrepancies between the dental and facial midlines adversely affected perceptions of what was considered to be an attractive smile. Such variations in judgments may be related to the significant differences in the threshold of detection of discrepancies among orthodontic, dental, and layperson judge groups (Giddon, 1995; Mejia-Maidelet al., 2005).

There are also important differences between the right and left sides of the face in the information displayed. In studies using facial chimeras or half faces, most subjects judge chimeras made from the right half of the original face to most closely resemble the person as a whole, while the left face chimera is judged as expressing more emotion (pronounced smiling, etc.) than the right (Heller, Nitschke, & Miller, 1998). Using facial chimerics, Reis and Zaidel (2001) found that right-right composites were judged significantly healthier than left-left composites for women but not men.

Based on the inherent asymmetry of the face (Ferrario et al., 1994), and the clinical importance of the profile for orthodontists in treatment planning and assessment of treatment outcomes, as well as the possibility that cerebral lateralization may influence facial perception, a study of lateralization of perception was undertaken by the Giddon group (Friedman, 2003). Right and left color digitized profile images were taken of forty-nine male and female subjects in natural head position flipped horizontally to create unaltered right, unaltered left, a mirror unaltered right, and mirror unaltered left. Additional extreme protrusive and retrusive mandibular positions for the four profiles resulted in twelve images for determination of accuracy of self-perception and preference for right or left images. The most significant findings were that:

1. Subjects were less accurate in choosing their own left-facing than right-facing profiles.
2. Familiarity with the Hebrew language (read from right to left) appeared to be directly related to preference for right-facing profiles. One may speculate that when subjects view right facing profiles of themselves, their ability to recognize these images is reduced because the most salient facial features are transmitted to the subjects' left hemisphere, which is less specialized than the right hemisphere for self facial recognition (Fridlund, 1994).

Although philosophers, artists, plastic surgeons, and orthodontists have long argued over the merits of one or more features in the attraction of the face and body, the first experimental study dates back to 1921. Perrin found that the mouth and face were high on the list of attributes that were used to distinguish the most attractive from the most "repulsive" women on the University of Texas campus (Perrin, 1921).

As noted by Patzer (1985), Cunningham (1986), and Cunningham et al. (1995), there is a hierarchy among components of the total body in judging attractiveness, with the face being the most important. Within the face, the mouth and eyes are primary in these judgments of attractiveness, as well as personality, temperament, social class, and intelligence. Evidence from fMRI, PET, and other imaging techniques (Aharon et al., 2001; Haxby, Hoffman, & Gobbini, 2002; Johnston & Franklin, 1993; Nakamura et al., 1998) has in fact confirmed the hypotheses of Lorenz and others (Lorenz, 1937) that such preferences are innate or imprinted. O'Doherty et al. (2003) found that attractive faces activated the medial orbitofrontal cortex, a region involved in representing stimulus-reward value. Responses in this region were further enhanced by a smiling facial expression.

Other authors have attempted to rank or classify faces on the basis of attractiveness, finding considerable agreement among judges in various societies (Iliffe, 1960; Jones & Hill, 1993; Perrett, May, & Yoshikawa, 1994). In addition to the cross-cultural studies of Jones and Hill (1993), further evidence that beauty is not necessarily in the eyes of the beholder was recently demonstrated by Johnston and Franklin (1993), who found that given 17 billion combinations of facial features from which to select the most attractive face, essentially the same face was generated by all subjects. Such judgments obviously may be influenced by psychosocial and cultural factors, including the role of the advertising, cosmetics, hair style, fashion, movie, and TV industries (Englis & Ashmore, 1994; Giddon, 1985), as well as professional judgments of orthodontists, dentists, and plastic surgeons. Although many segments of society may try to deprecate the value of physical attractiveness, most studies continue to support its importance for self-esteem. Whatever the society, however, there is a preference for some ideal facial and/or body characteristic in mating behavior. Conversely, institutionalized criminals and mentally ill individuals have been found to be less attractive than the average population (Archer & Cash, 1985; Kohn, 1988; Napoleon, Chassin, & Young, 1980).

Historically, plastic and reconstructive surgeons, orthodontists, and dentists have struggled with the paradox of diagnosis and treatment of dysmorphic appearance and malocclusion being based on morphological and functional considerations, while patient decisions are based on the esthetic outcome of the treatment. That is, 80% percent of those adults seeking orthodontic care for themselves or their children are motivated by a desire for improved appearance regardless of structural or functional considerations (Baldwin, 1980; Giddon, 1983). One of the major reasons for this apparent paradox is that the same objective anthropometric information is perceived differently by clinician and patient (Miner, Anderson, & Giddon, 2001), with most people tending to err in estimation of the size of their own features in the direction of the perceived norm (Thompson & Smolak, 2001). Not until the late 1960s did orthodontists begin to acknowledge the role of subjective factors in the perception of appearance or esthetic satisfaction in determining patient behaviors relating to motivation, compliance, and satisfaction with treatment outcomes (Giddon, 1995).

Consequently, a number of new orthodontic indices were developed which included perceptions of attractiveness by self and others. The Eastman Esthetic Index was developed by Howitt and Stricker (Howitt, Stricker, & Henderson, 1967) and was validated by correlation with other measures of children's self-esteem. Tedesco and Albino then developed a dental-facial attractiveness rating (DFA) (Tedesco, Albino, Cunat, Green et al., 1983; Tedesco, Albino, Cunat, Slakter, & Waltz, 1983) as the measure of a child's perception of his or her occlusion. The most inclusive index, the Dental Aesthetic Index (DAI) developed by Jenny, Cons, and Kohout in 1983, incorporated social and psychological factors in addition to traditional measures of malocclusion. The major difference from most previous indices was the inclusion of the general public's esthetic rating of 200 representative occlusal conditions found in a population of 500,000 people. Klages, Bruckner, and Zenter (2004), found an interaction between the Aesthetic Component of the Index of Orthodontic Treatment Need (IOTN) with self-consciousness scores and social appearance concerns; that is, the impact of dental aesthetics on social appearance concern was stronger in subjects with high private and public self-consciousness than subjects with low self-consciousness. Furthermore, Eli et al. (2001) found that the appearance of the dentition had a significant impact on first impressions. Prahl-Anderson, Boersma, van der Linden, and Moore (1979) further noted that motivation for orthodontic treatment is a function of three factors: objective signs, subjective symptoms, and social sufficiency. Objective signs are deviations from an established norm, such as various indices of malocclusion; subjective symptoms include cognitive variables, such as recognition by the patient of a problem requiring treatment; and social sufficiency, which varies according to the Zeitgeist, is recognition by society that malocclusion creates a problem for the patient.

Similarly, Maxwell and Kiyak (1991) found that self-perceptions of the face were not associated with cephalometric measures. Even though the patient has little idea of his or her own profile, unless there is a perceived dysmorphia (Hershon & Giddon, 1980), Bell et al. (1985) concluded that the profile is more important than frontal views for patient motivation to undergo orthodontic treatment. Regardless, then, of clinically determined structural or functional deviation, it is the self-perception of appearance that seems to be the best predictor of the patient's decision to undergo orthodontic and/or surgical correction (Perrett et al., 1994; Udry, 1965) and subsequently post-treatment satisfaction (Dongieux & Sassouni, 1980; Jones & Hill, 1993). Using cephalometric and other anthropometric measures with the various classification schemes, the anatomical bases of these differing perceptions or preferences of patients and clinicians can now be determined and compared (Giddon, 1995; Miner et al., 2001).

Many studies have documented the importance of the face, and the mouth in particular, to perceived physical attractiveness and self-concept. First impressions are also based in part on facial appearance and what is expressed by the face, for it is upon the face that the entire gamut of human needs, intentions, and emotions is reflected. Therefore, it is not surprising that such great significance is attached to the deformity or defect of the mouth or related structure, and, conversely, that the results of esthetic restorations, orthodontics, maxillofacial surgery, and prosthodontics not to mention cosmetics and hairstyle become important to both physical and mental health.

Outside the range of "normal" attractiveness are patients with craniofacial anomalies (CFAs). Oral clefts including cleft lip, cleft palate, and the combined cleft lip and palate (CLP) represent one of the most common congenital malformations with approximately one for every eight hundred to a thousand live births each year in the United States (Shulman et al., 1993). There is definite laterality with left-sided clefts being twice as common as right-sided ones (Abyholm, 1978). Moreover, individuals with craniofacial anomalies such as CLP have structurally different faces from "normal" individuals (Eder, 1995) and may be judged on a qualitatively different aesthetic scale: that is, they may evoke different perceptual processes from those to "normal" but unattractive individuals (Reis & Hodgins, 1995).

The influence of facial attractiveness on the development of self-concept may also differ qualitatively between CFA and "normal" individuals. For example, an 11-year-old child who is genetically endowed with attractive features may well develop a better self-concept than a child who underwent surgical reconstruction.

Many craniofacially deformed individuals also have communication difficulties and develop compensatory speech patterns, hypernasality, resonance, and articulation problems, which make them difficult to understand. Such individuals may also have restricted muscular movement or scarring in the orofacial areas, which interfere with normal signaling patterns (Robinson, Rumsey, & Partridge, 1996) or the ability to encode emotion, such as pain, happiness, fear, anger (Ekman, 1992a, 1992b). Infants use facial expressions as signals to induce caretakers, particularly their mothers, to pay attention and in the development of mother infant attachments. Anomaly related perturbations in the facial musculature and subsequent facial expressions may lead mothers to misinterpret cues, which may adversely affect the development of secure attachments essential for the development of self-awareness and self-esteem.

Facial Expression and Nonverbal Communication

Perhaps the most important role of the face, and mouth as its central feature, involves the visual and auditory systems in interpersonal attraction and both verbal and nonverbal communication (Fridlund, 1994). The listener focuses attention on the speaker's face, while the speaker focuses on the face of the listener. Thus, the orofacial area, including the posture of the head, is of great importance as a powerful source of nonverbal signals. Perception of the visual and auditory signals from the craniofacial area helps the observer understand the stimulus person better and in return the observer is also understood (Smith et al., 1974). To know that one is understood both by content and affect is absolutely essential to successful interpersonal communication.

Following the cross-cultural observations of Darwin suggesting that emotional expressions were innate, Ekman and Oster (1979) and others (Eibl-Eibesfeldt, 1970; Izard, 1977) concluded that across cultures, genders, and individuals born deaf and blind, facial expressions of fear, happiness, anger, and sadness are recognized universally.

Facial expression is an essential component of nonverbal communication (Ekman & Friesen, 1978; Fridlund, 1994) and is made possible by action of the muscles that are attached to the cranial vault. There are over one hundred functionally distinct muscles including those controlling facial expression in the head (Duchenne, 1859; Ekman & Friesen, 1978; Huber, 1931). Control of the lower facial muscles is predominantly contralateral, while the upper facial muscles are innervated bilaterally (Borod & Koff, 1990). As may be seen in figure 1.1, Kontsevich and Tyler (2004) found that the mouth, in particular the position of the chelions, are essential to judgments of facial expressions as sad or happy. It was also found that the left side of the mouth moved more than the right side during spontaneous smiles, but not posed smiles (Wylie & Goodale, 1988) in left-handed females and right-handed males.

Similarly, using the Facial Action Coding System (FACS), Ekman and Friesen (1978) have found that the dominating facial area differs across emotions, with happiness and disgust best predicted from the mouth region, while fear and sadness involve the eye and brow region (see fig. 1.2).

The ability to use facial expression efficiently can also be compromised in

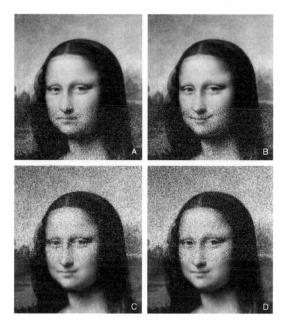

Fig. 1.1. Importance of chelions in perception of facial expression.

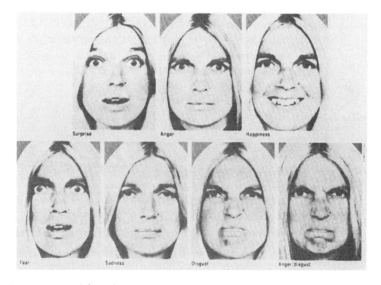

Fig. 1.2. Universal facial expressions.

patients with problems ranging from simple toothache, ill-fitting dentures, oral or sinus infections, cancer, even orthodontic appliances, to the more complex neuromuscular disorders and craniofacial anomalies (Robinson et al., 1996). Various physical disorders and mental illness of orofacial origin can also seriously impact upon the speech and hearing apparatus. For example, in a study by Tuz, Onder, and Kisnisci (2003), 78% of patients with temporomandibular joint disease had at least one otologic complaint, such as otalgia, tinnitus, vertigo, or hearing loss resulting from impingement on the auditory canal and surrounding structures (i.e., Costen's Syndrome [Michael, 1997]).

A number of diseases, syndromes, and even orthodontic treatment, as noted earlier, can adversely affect both verbal and nonverbal communication. For example, mandibulofacial dysostosis and possibly velocardiofacial syndrome are conditions in which speech disorders relating to resonance, voice quality, and articulation have been noted (Gray, Smith, & Schneider, 1996; Vallino-Napoli, 2002). A specific problem of speech articulation has also been noted for patients with implants or prostheses, such as difficulty in pronouncing "s" or "z," which may also be related to age or hearing (Manders et al., 2003). For the parents or caregivers who are most eager to interact with their CL or CLP children, the dysmorphology or dysfunction of the speech apparatus often involving the muscles of facial expression makes it difficult to meet the expectancies of meaningful or understandable responses of the child (Endriga & Speltz, 1997; Field & Vega-Lahr, 1984).

Given the wealth of literature that indicates differences across cultures in the nuances of speech content and affect related in part to facial expressions, it is essential that the clinicians be aware of the subtle differences between normal and abnormal functioning of the speech and hearing apparatuses essential to communication and interpersonal attraction.

Acknowledging then the biopsychological basis for the significance of the oral and craniofacial area, it is no wonder that in contrast to other parts of the body, pain and suffering relating to the oral cavity in particular are often much out of proportion to the actual stimulus. Clinically, this is noted by the following comments:

1. "When I get this tooth out, I'm going to have them all out."
2. "I hate this more than anything else." (Sosnow, 1962)
3. As Cervantes is reported to have said through Don Quixote, "I'd rather lose my thumb than a molar tooth."

Conversely, one should not overlook the fact that the mouth is not only the source of so much suffering and pleasure but may be the target as well. By virtue of their already established channel for expression of aggression, the oral tissues are subject to the ravages of stress and tension mediated through the voluntary motor system, as in bruxism, or through the involuntary neuroendocrine system, as in psychosomatic diseases (Giddon, 1966).

Whether right or wrong, the physical, mental, and dental health consequences of society's pernicious attitudes toward this information are significant and pervasive (Giddon, 1985). Thus, it is not surprising that the appearance of the orofacial area is relatively more important than function as reasons for seeking orthodontic or dental care.

Summary

In summary, the contributions of the various components of the craniofacial area to interpersonal attraction have been described in terms of their sources of objective and subjective information provided to the observer and the observed. Part of the problem of doctor-patient relationships may well be due to the failure of the clinician to appreciate the significance of the craniofacial area to an individual patient and the extreme distress caused by any perception of unacceptable facial appearance or even a speech impediment. Cash and others (Archer & Cash, 1985) note, for example, that depressed patients are more likely than nondepressed patients to request cosmetic surgery, and that patients with hypochondriasis and body dysmorphia seek out dentists, plastic surgeons, dermatologists, and other specialists who may alleviate their body image concerns. Often, the most disturbing complications to surgeons and patients are psychological rather than physical. Ineffective communication and management of psychological complications of surgery can have profound consequences, resulting in delay in recuperation and return to work, poor patient compliance, dissatisfaction with the surgical outcome, and hostility toward clinicians.

References

Abyholm, F. E. (1978). Cleft lip and palate in Norway: registration, incidence and early mortality in infants with CLP. *Scandinavian Journal of Plastic and Reconstructive Surgery, 12*, 29–34.

Adams, G. R., & Crossman, S. M. (1978). *Physical Attractiveness: A Cultural Imperative.* Roslyn Heights, New York: Libra Press.

Aharon, I., Etcoff, N., Ariely, D., Chabris, C. F., O'Connor, E., & Breiter, H. C. (2001). Beautiful faces have variable reward value: fMRI and behavioral evidence. *Neuron, 32*(3), 537–51.

Albino, J. E., Alley, T. R., Tedesco, L. A., Tobiasen, J. A., Kiyak, H. A., & Lawrence, S. D. (1990). Esthetic issues in behavioral dentistry. *Annals of Behavioral Medicine, 12*(4), 148–55.

Alley, T. R., & Hildebrandt, K. A. (1988). Determinants and consequences of facial aesthetics. In T. R. Alley (ed.), *Social and Applied Aspects of Perceiving Faces* (pp. 101–40). Hillsdale, NJ: Lawrence Erlbaum.

Archer, R. P., & Cash, T. F. (1985). Physical attractiveness and maladjustment among psychiatric inpatients. *Journal of Social and Clinical Psychology, 3*(2), 170–80.

Baldwin, D. C. (1980). Appearance and aesthetics in oral health. *Community Dentistry Oral Epidemiology, 9*, 244–56.

Bell, R., Kiyak, H. A., Joondeph, D. R., McNeill, R. W., & Wallen, T. R. (1985). Perceptions of facial profile and their influence on the decision to undergo orthognathic surgery. *American Journal of Orthodontics, 88*, 323–32.

Bergman, P., Malasky, C., & Zahn, T. P. (1967). Relation of sucking strength to personality variables. *Journal of Consulting Psychology, 31*(4), 426–28.

Berscheid, E., & Gangestad, S. (1982). The social psychological implications of facial physical attractiveness. *Clinics in Plastic Surgery, 9*, 289–96.

Borod, J. C., & Koff, E. (1990). Lateralization for facial emotional behavior: a methodological perspective. *International Journal of Psychology, 25*, 157–77.

Buss, D. M. (1994). The strategies of human mating. *American Scientist, 82*, 238–49.

Cunningham, M. R. (1986). Measuring the physical in physical attractiveness: quasi-experiments on the sociobiology of female facial beauty. *Journal of Personality and Social Psychology, 50*(5), 925–35.

Cunningham, M. R., Roberts, A. R., Barbee, A. P., Druen, P. B., & Wu, C. H. (1995). "Their ideas of beauty are, on the whole, the same as ours": consistency and variability in the cross-cultural perception of female physical attractiveness. *Journal of Personality and Social Psychology, 68*(2), 261–79.

Dobbins, A., Zucker, S. W., & Cynader, M. S. (1987). Endstopped neurons in the visual cortex as a substrate for calculating curvature. *Nature, 329*(6138), 438–41.

Dongieux, J., & Sassouni, V. (1980). The contribution of mandibular positioned variation to facial esthetics. *Angle Orthodontist, 50*, 334–39.

Duchenne, G. B. A. (1859). *The Mechanism of Human Facial Expression*. New York: Cambridge University Press.

Eder, R. A. (1995). *Craniofacial Anomalies: Psychological Perspectives*. New York: Springer Verlag.

Eibl-Eibesfeldt, I. (1970). *Ethology: The Biology of Behavior*. New York: Holt, Rinehart and Winston.

Ekman, P. (1992a). Facial expressions of emotion: an old controversy and new findings. *Philosophical Transactions Royal Society London B, 335*, 63–69.

——. (1992b). Facial expressions of emotion: new findings, new questions. *Psychological Science, 3*(1), 34–38.

Ekman, P., & Friesen, W. V. (1978). *The Facial Action Coding System*. Palo Alto, CA: Consulting Psychologists Press.

Ekman, P., & Oster, H. (1979). Facial expressions of emotion. *Annual Review of Psychology, 30*, 527–54.

Eli, I., Baht, R., Koriat, H., & Rosenberg, M. (2001). Self-perception of breath odor. *Journal of the American Dental Association, 132*(5), 621–26.

Endriga, M. C., & Speltz, M. L. (1997). Face-to-face interaction between infants with orofacial clefts and their mothers. *Journal of Pediatric Psychology, 22*(4), 439–53.

Englis, B. G., & Ashmore, R. (1994). Beauty before the eyes of beholders: the cultural encoding of beauty types in magazine advertising and music television. *Journal of Advertising, 23*(3), 49–64.

Ferrario, V. G., Sforza, C., Poggio, C. E., & Tartaglia, G. (1994). Distance from symmetry: a three-dimensional evaluation of facial asymmetry. *Journal of Oral and Maxillofacial Surgery, 52*, 1126–132.

Field, T. M., & Vega-Lahr, N. (1984). Early interactions between infants with craniofacial anomalies and their mothers. *Infant Behavior and Development, 7*, 527–30.

Fridlund, A. J. (1994). *Human Facial Expression*. New York: Academic Press.

Friedman, L. M. (2003). *Self-perception of right- versus left-facing facial profiles*. Unpublished M.Med.Sci. Thesis, Harvard School of Dental Medicine, Boston, MA.

Friedman, S., & Fisher, C. (1967). On the presence of a rhythmic, diurnal, oral instinctual drive cycle in man: a preliminary report. *Journal of the American Psychoanalytic Association, 15*(2), 317–43.

Galsworthy, J. (1932). Flowering wilderness. In J. Bartlett (ed.), *Familiar Quotations* (13th ed., p. 838a). Boston: Little, Brown.

Gardner, H. (1936). *Art Through the Ages: An Introduction to Its History and Significance*. New York: Harcourt, Brace, and Co.

Giddon, D. B. (1966). Psychophysiology of the oral cavity. *Journal of Dental Research, 45*, 1627–636.

——. (1983). Through the looking glasses of physician, dentists and patients. *Perspectives in Biology and Medicine, 26*(3), 451–58.

——. (1985). Ethical considerations for the fashion industry. In M. R. Solomon (ed.), *The Psychology of Fashion* (pp. 225–32). Lexington, MA: DC Heath Company.

——. (1995). Orthodontic applications of psychological and perceptual studies of facial esthetics. *Seminars in Orthodontics, 1*(?), 82–93.

——. (1999). Mental-dental interface: window to the psyche and soma. *Perspectives in Biology and Medicine, 43*(1), 84–97.

Giddon, D. B., Dreisbach, M. E., Pfaffman, C., & Manly, R. S. (1954). Relative abilities of natural and artificial dentition patients for judging the sweetness of solid foods. *Journal of Prosthetic Dentistry, 4*(2), 263–68.

Giddon, D. B., Schack, K., & Anderson, N. K. (2004). Craniofacial anthropometrics and perceived personality attributes. *Journal of Dental Research* 83(Spec Iss A): Abstract #1315, (www.dentalresearch.org).

Gray, S. D., Smith, M. E., & Schneider, H. (1996). Voice disorders in children. *Pediatric Clinics of North America, 43*(6), 1357–384.

Hatfield, E., & Sprecher, S. (1995). Men's and women's preferences in marital partners in the United States, Russia and Japan. *Journal of Cross-Cultural Psychology, 26*(6), 728–50.

Haxby, J. B., Hoffman, E. A., & Gobbini, M. I. (2002). Human neural systems for face recognition and social communication [review]. *Biological Psychiatry, 51*(1), 59–67.

Heller, W., Nitschke, J. B., & Miller, G. A. (1998). Lateralization in emotion and emotional disorders. *Current Directions in Psychological Science, 1,* 26–31.

Hershon, L. E., & Giddon, D. B. (1980). Determinants of facial profile self-perception. *American Journal of Orthodontics, 78,* 279–95.

Hochberg, J. (1988). Visual perception. In R. C. Atkinson, R. J. Herrnstein, G. Lindzey, & R. D. Luce (eds.), *Stevens' Handbook of Experimental Psychology* (2d ed., vol. 1, pp. 195–276). New York: John Wiley & Sons.

Howitt, J., Stricker, G., & Henderson, R. (1967). Eastman esthetic index. *New York State Dental Journal, 33,* 215–20.

Hubel, D. H., & Wiesel, T. N. (1965). Receptive fields and functional architecture in two nonstriate visual areas (18 and 19) of the cat. *Journal of Neurophysiology, 28,* 229–89.

Huber, E. (1931). *Evolution of Facial Musculature and Facial Expression.* Baltimore: John Hopkins Press

Iliffe, A. H. (1960). A study of preferences in feminine beauty. *British Journal of Psychology, 51*(3), 267–73.

Izard, C. E. (1977). *Human Emotions.* New York: Plenum.

Jenny, J., Cons, N. C., & Kohout, F. J. (1983). Comparison of SASOC; a measure of Dental Aesthetic Index, with three orthodontic indices and orthodontic judgment. *Community Dentistry Oral Epidemiology, 11,* 236–41.

Johnston, V., & Franklin, M. (1993). Is beauty in the eye of the beholder? *Ethology and Sociobiology, 14,* 183–99.

Jones, D., & Hill, K. (1993). Criteria of facial attractiveness in five populations. *Human Nature, 4*(3), 271–96.

Klages, U., Bruckner, A., & Zenter, A. (2004). Dental esthetics, self awareness and oral health related quality of life in young adults. *European Journal of Orthodontics, 26*(5), 507–14.

Kodric-Brown, A., & Brown, J. H. (1985). Why the fittest are prettiest. *The Sciences, Sept./Oct.,* 26–33.

Kohn, A. (1988). You know what they say . . . are proverbs nuggets of truth or fool's gold? *Psychology Today, 22*(4), 36–41.

Kokich, V. O., Jr., Kiyak, H. A., & Shapiro, P. A. (1999). Comparing the perception of dentists and lay people to altered dental esthetics. *Esthetic Dentistry, 11*(6), 311–24.

Kontsevich, L. L., & Tyler, C. W. (2004). What makes Mona Lisa smile? *Vision Research, 44,* 1493–498.

Largey, G. P., & Watson, D. R. (1972). The sociology of odors. *American Journal of Sociology, 77*(6), 1021–34.

Levy, D. M. (1934). Experiments on the sucking reflex and social behavior of dogs. *American Journal of Orthopsychiatry, 4,* 203–24.

Lorenz, K. (1937). The companion in the bird's world. *Auk, 54*, 247–73.

MacLean, P. D. (1973). The brain's generation gap: some human implications. *Zygon, 8*, 113–27.

Manders, E., Jacobs, R., Nackaerts, O., Van Looy, C., & Lembrechts, D. (2003). The influence of oral implant-supported prostheses on articulation and myofunction. *Acta oto-rhino-laryngologica belgica, 57*(1), 73–77.

Maslow, A. (1970). *Motivation and Personality* (2d ed.). New York: Harper & Row, Inc.

Maxwell, R., & Kiyak, H. A. (1991). Dentofacial appearance: a comparison of patient self-assessment techniques. *International Journal of Adult Orthodontics and Orthognathic Surgery, 6*, 123–31.

Mejia-Maidel, M., Evans, C. A., Viana, G., Anderson, N. K., & Giddon, D. B. (2005). Preferences for Mexican facial profiles between Mexican Americans and Caucasians. *Angle Orthodontist, 75*(6), 763–68.

Michael, L. A. (1997). Jaws revisited: Costen's syndrome. *The Annals of Otology, Rhinology, and Laryngology, 106*(10 Pt 1), 820–22.

Miner, R. M., Anderson, N. K., & Giddon, D. B. (2001). *Comparison of children's computer-imaged profiles as perceived by patient, parent and clinician.* Paper presented at the American Association of Orthodontists 101st Annual Session, May 5, 2001, On-Site Program, p. 62, #59, Ontario, Canada.

Murray, H. A. (1938). *Explorations in Personality.* New York: Oxford University Press.

Nakamura, K., Kawashima, R., Nagumo, S., Ito, K., Sugiura, M., Kato, T., et al. (1998). Neuroanatomical correlates of the assessment of facial attractiveness. *Neuroreport, 9*(4), 753–57.

Napoleon, T., Chassin, L., & Young, R. D. (1980). A replication and extension of "physical attractiveness and mental illness." *Journal of Abnormal Psychology, 89*(2), 250–53.

O'Doherty, J., Critchley, H., Deichmann, R., & Dolan, R. J. (2003). Dissociating valence of outcome from behavioral control in human orbital and ventral prefrontal cortices. *Journal of Neuroscience, 23*(21), 7931–939.

Patzer, G. L. (1985). *The Physical Attractiveness Phenomena.* New York: Plenum Press.

Penfield, W., & Rasmussen, T. (1978). *The Cerebral Cortex of Man: A Clinical Study of Localization of Function.* New York: Macmillan Publishing Co.

Perrett, D. I., May, K. A., & Yoshikawa, S. (1994). Facial shape and judgments of female attractiveness. *Nature, 368*(6468), 239–42.

Perrin, F. A. C. (1921). Physical attractiveness and repulsiveness. *Journal of Experimental Psychology, 4*, 203–17.

Prahl-Anderson, B., Boersma, H., van der Linden, F. P. G. M., & Moore, A. W. (1979). Perceptions of dentofacial morphology by laypersons, general dentists, and orthodontists. *Journal of the American Dental Association, 98*, 209–12.

Pruzinsky, T. (1990). Psychopathology of body experience: expanded perspectives. In T. F. Cash & T. Pruzinsky (eds.), *Body Images: Development, Deviance and Change* (pp. 170–90). New York: Guilford Press.

Reis, H. T., & Hodgins, H. S. (1995). Reactions to craniofacial disfigurement: lessons from the physical attractiveness and stigma literature. In R. A. Eder (ed.), *Craniofacial Anomalies: Psychological Perspectives* (pp. 177–200). New York: Springer Verlag.

Reis, V. A., & Zaidel, D. W. (2001). Brain and face: communicating signals of health in the left and right sides of the face. *Brain Cognition, 46*(1–2), 240–44.

Rhodes, G., Yoshikawa, S., Clark, A., Lee, K., McKay, R., & Akamatsu, S. (2001). Attractiveness of facial averageness and symmetry in non-western cultures: in search of biologically based standards of beauty. *Perception, 30*(5), 611–25.

Robinson, E., Rumsey, N., & Partridge, J. (1996). An evaluation of the impact of social interaction skills training for facially disfigured people. *British Journal of Plastic Surgery, 49*, 281–89.

Shulman, J., Edmonds, L. D., McClearn, A. B., Jensvold, N., & Shaw, G. M. (1993). Surveillance for and comparison of birth defect prevalences in two geographic areas, United States, 1983–88. *MMWR 42, No. SS1-11-5.*

Smith, J. W., Chase, J., & Lieblich, A. K. (1974). Tongue showing: a facial display of humans and other primate species. *Semiotica, 11*, 201–46.

Sosnow, I. (1962). The emotional significance of the loss of teeth. In L. R. Borland & P. W. Vinton (eds.), *Dental Clinics of North America: Symposia on I. Psychology in Dentistry, II. Removable Partial Dentures* (pp. 637–50). Philadelphia: Saunders.

Spurzheim, J. G. (1908). *Phrenology or the Doctrine of the Mental Phenomena* (Revised edition from the second American ed.). Philadelphia & London: J. B. Lippincott Company.

Tedesco, L. A., Albino, J. E., Cunat, J. J., Green, L. J., Lewis, E. A., & Slakter, M. J. (1983). A dental-facial attractiveness scale part I: reliability and validity. *American Journal of Orthodontics*(4), 38–43.

Tedesco, L. A., Albino, J. E., Cunat, J. J., Slakter, M. J., & Waltz, K. J. (1983). A dental-facial attractiveness scale part II: consistency of perception. *American Journal of Orthodontics, 8*(1), 44–46.

Thompson, J. K., & Smolak, L. (2001). *Body Image, Eating Disorders, and Obesity in Youth: Assessment, Prevention and Treatment.* Washington, DC: American Psychological Association.

Thornhill, R., & Gangestad, S. W. (1993). Human facial beauty: averageness, symmetry, and parasite resistance. *Journal of Human Nature, 4*(3), 237–69.

Thornhill, R., & Grammer, K. (1999). The body and face of woman: one ornament that signals quality. *Evolution and Human Behavior, 20*, 71–76.

Tuz, H. H., Onder, E. M., & Kisnisci, R. S. (2003). Prevalence of otologic complaints in patients with temporomandibular disorder. *American Journal of Orthodontics and Dentofacial Orthopedics, 123*(6), 620–23.

Udry, J. R. (1965). Structural correlates of feminine beauty preferences in Britain and the United States: a comparison. *Sociology and Social Research, 49*, 330.

Vallino-Napoli, L. D. (2002). A profile of the features and speech in patients with mandibulofacial dysostosis. *Cleft Palate and Craniofacial Journal, 39*(6), 623–34.

Wylie, D. R., & Goodale, M. A. (1988). Left-sided oral asymmetries in spontaneous but not posed smiles. *Neuropsychologia, 26*(6), 823–32.

Yaegaki, K. (1995). Oral malodor and periodontal disease. In M. Rosenberg (ed.), *Bad Breath: Research Perspectives* (pp. 87–108). Tel Aviv: Ramot Publishing.

Zebrowitz, L. A. (1997). The bases of reading faces. In *Reading Faces*. Boulder, CO: Westview Press.

Oral Health and Quality of Life

Marita R. Inglehart

Oral-health-related quality of life is a concept that was originally conceptualized by Giddon in 1978 in his discussion of the relationship between the mouth and patients' quality of life (see also Giddon, 1987). However, this concept was not empirically explored until the late 1980s. Oral-health-related quality of life (OHRQoL) is defined as that part of a person's quality of life that is affected by this person's oral health. Specifically, OHRQoL considers how oral health affects the person's functioning (biting, chewing, speaking), sensations of pain/discomfort, and psychological (appearance, self-esteem) as well as social well-being. OHRQoL is usually assessed by either asking patients or research subjects questions concerning these four aspects of their quality of life, or having close relatives or caregivers answer these questions for the patients (proxy measurement). OHRQoL focuses clinicians' attention on the patient as a whole, and thus fosters truly patient-centered care.

It can remind basic and clinical researchers in the oral health sciences that the ultimate outcome of any intervention or treatment should be an improvement of a person's quality of life; and it can support dental and dental hygiene educators in their efforts to train patient-centered, culturally sensitive, future health care providers. Communicating OHRQoL concerns to the public can be a successful way to advocate for patients in need of dental care and/or without access to dental care. It is a powerful behavioral concept that can unite clinicians, researchers, and educators in their ultimate goal of improving patients' lives and public health in general.

In the year 2000, the first-ever Surgeon General's Report on Oral Health was published in the United States (U.S. Department of Health and Human

Services, 2000). In her foreword to this report, the secretary of the U.S. Department of Health and Human Services, Donna E. Shalala, wrote, "oral health problems can lead to needless pain and suffering, causing devastating complications to an individual's well-being, with financial and social costs that significantly diminish quality of life and burden American society" (U.S. Department of Health and Human Services, 2000, p.7). Shalala's focus on the relevance of dental health for a person's quality of life reflects a programmatic shift away from viewing oral health and disease merely as the number of decayed, missing, and filled teeth due to caries, or in terms of attachment loss or pocket depth due to periodontal disease to a truly patient-centered perspective of oral health. In some sense, this sentence applied the more than a half-century-old World Health Organization's definition of health as "a state of complete physical, mental and social well-being and not merely the absence of disease and infirmity" to oral health (World Health Organization, 1948), by directing the attention from the oral cavity to the person as a whole.

This chapter will describe why and how the concept of oral-health-related quality of life was introduced into the oral health sciences, how the development of valid and reliable measurement scales opened the door to demonstrating its significance in research, and how the findings of this research can be used by clinicians, researchers, and dental educators to take a new look at the objectives of their professional lives.

Having a chapter on OHRQoL in this volume on behavioral science contributions to dentistry can show how a behavioral science concept can enrich and refocus research in the oral health sciences, how it can contribute to making clinicians more patient centered, and how it can provide guidance to dental/dental hygiene educators in their efforts to educate patient-centered and culturally sensitive future providers who see the value of working in interdisciplinary teams including behavioral scientists.

Oral-Health-Related Quality of Life—Definition and Historical Reflection

Oral-health-related quality of life can be defined as a person's assessment of how (1) functional factors (such as being able to chew, bite, swallow, or speak), (2) psychological factors (concerning, e.g., the person's appearance, smile, and self-esteem), and (3) social factors (such as eating or speaking in front of others) related to the oral cavity, as well as the experience of pain/discomfort affect this person's well-being and quality of life (for a more detailed discussion of the concept see Inglehart & Bagramian, 2002a).

Before OHRQoL was introduced to the scientific community in the 1980s, outcomes of clinical interactions with dental patients and of oral health-related research were likely to be measured either as the person's functional status or the degree to which caries (e.g., number of decayed, missing, or filled teeth or surfaces due to caries), or periodontal disease were present. The introduction of OHRQoL clearly widened the perspective to include considerations of how oral health/disease and the treatment of oral disease affect a person's life in general.

The shift from defining health and disease in a purely biological manner may have begun when the World Health Organization offered its programmatic definition of health as more than just physical health in the 1940s (World Health Organization, 1948). However, this perspective did not really systematically develop until the 1970s when scientists and patients alike began to consider it explicitly. In medicine, Engel (1977) introduced his now famous biopsychosocial model of health in this time period. This model stressed a holistic approach to patient care and reflected on the value of treating patients instead of "body parts." Around this same time, a change occurred in the way the term "quality of life" was used in the social sciences. Until the 1970s, quality of life had been largely used to describe societies. Starting in the 1970s, the term began to be used when analyzing individuals' well-being (Campbell, 1976; Andrews & McKennell, 1980). In psychology, wellness began to be considered as a crucial aspect of a person's life, and health psychology began to develop as an independent area of research around this time (Peterson, 2002).

While it took the research community in the United States until the 1970s to start focusing on the concept of quality of life, it seems as if patients' interactions with the health care system were always motivated by quality of life issues such as suffering from pain or not being able to function. Thinking back in the history of dentistry, it seems as if patients had been motivated to seek (or avoid) dental care because they had a toothache, or were afraid of pain, wanted to have dentures to enhance their appearance, or had functional problems since the beginning. However, quality of life issues began to be explicitly considered as factors in treatment decision making in the 1970s. In this time period, patients encountered new cancer treatments (e.g., chemotherapy) that were likely to prolong their lives but reduced the quality of their lives drastically, which led them to reflect on the cost and benefit of such treatment and to consider quality of life as a crucial factor for their decisions (Cimprich & Paterson, 2002).

In dentistry, the National Institute of Dental and Craniofacial Research (NIDCR) played a major role in introducing the concept of oral-health-related quality of life (OHRQoL) to the scientific community by funding two major conferences centered on this term and supporting significant numbers of research studies on this topic (Bryant & Kleinman, 2002). The first conference was organized by Slade in 1996 and focused on the measurement of OHRQoL (Slade, 1997a). Slade brought together the leading researchers on OHRQoL such as Atchison (Atchison & Dolan, 1990); Cohen (Cohen & Jago, 1976); Gift (Gift & Redford, 1992; Gift & Atchison, 1995); Kressin (1996); Locker (1988); Reisine (1988); Sheiham, Maizels, and Maizels (1987); and Strauss (Strauss & Hunt, 1993) for a conference in Chapel Hill, North Carolina, and collected their contributions in a book that documented the state of the art of measuring OHRQoL at that time. In May 2000, Bagramian and Inglehart organized the second conference as an interdisciplinary workshop on OHRQoL at the University of Michigan (see Inglehart & Bagramian, 2002b). This meeting had over 80 participants from as far away as Great Britain and South America who worked together with researchers from dentistry, medicine, nursing, psychology, and public health to reflect on the role of OHRQoL for clinicians, basic, clinical, and behavioral researchers as well as dental educators in the oral health sciences. These two meetings have inspired numerous research studies since then and made the term "OHRQoL" widely used, as a literature search with this term on Medline/Medsearch will show.

Oral-Health-Related Quality of Life—How Do We Assess It?

One major step in establishing a new concept in a scientific field is to develop measurement instruments. Slade (2002) provides an excellent overview of the three ways OHRQoL is assessed, namely with social indicators, global self-ratings of OHRQoL, and multiple item surveys of OHRQoL. Social indicators of OHRQoL such as the days of restricted work due to dental visits or days of work missed because of dental pain (see Reisine, 1985, for a first pioneering study; Gift, 1992) or children's restricted activity days due to dental problems or dental visits (General Accounting Office, 2000) can serve an important function by showing that oral disease has a clear impact on society as a whole.

Global self-ratings of OHRQoL usually ask respondents in surveys such as the third National Health and Nutrition Examination Survey (NHANES) of the U.S. adult population to rate their dental health on a five-point scale ranging from 1 = poor to 5 = excellent (see Gift, Atchison, & Drury, 1998). Such a global assessment can allow comparisons between different population groups in one country, or even between countries (see, e.g., the results of the International Collaborative Study; Chen et al., 1997). However, it clearly does not reflect the complexity of OHRQoL concerns. Multiple-item surveys are the instruments of choice when patients or research respondents' OHRQoL should be assessed. Slade (2002) offered an excellent overview of ten OHRQoL questionnaires for adults. He showed that these surveys not only differ in the number of dimensions of quality of life they consider, but range in the number of items from merely three items to as much as fifty-six questions.

One of the most widely used instruments is the Oral Health Impact Profile (OHIP; Slade & Spencer, 1994). It consists of forty-nine questions concerned with the respondents' functioning; pain; physical, psychological, and social disability; and handicap. The items are answered on five-point rating scales. A short version of this scale, the OHIP–14, is available as well (Slade, 1997b). In addition to these general OHRQoL scales, condition-specific scales such as the Xerostomia Related Quality of Life Scale (Henson et al., 2001) were developed as well. Recently, scales assessing children's QHRQoL were published as well (see Filstrup et al., 2003, for measuring OHRQoL from a younger age on; see Jokovic et al., 2002, for measuring OHRQoL in older children).

An interesting consideration when measuring OHRQoL in children or patients whose special needs may make it difficult to communicate, such as in patients with autism or dementia, is concerned with determining OHRQoL when the child or adult patient is unable to answer questions. In this case, proxy measurement, namely asking a significant other to evaluate the child's or adult's OHRQoL, may be a solution. One major question concerning proxy measurement is whether it is a valid way to determine OHRQoL. Research showed that parents' assessment of their child's OHRQoL correlated significantly with objective oral health indicators such as decayed, missing, and filled teeth due to caries and decayed, missing, and filled surfaces due to caries scores (see Filstrup et al., 2003), as well as with their children's self-assessments. An additional benefit of asking parents or caregivers about another person's OHRQoL may be that it could engage the patient in reflecting on the importance of oral health for his or her quality of life.

Oral-Health-Related Quality of Life—Its Role in Research

Research concerning oral health issues is amazingly diverse. It ranges from basic science research, to clinical research, behavioral research, and public health-related studies, and it addresses quite diverse topics ranging from tissue regeneration to access to care issues. OHRQoL can play an important role in all these different types of research. Concerning basic science research, Somerman (2002) made a powerful argument when she pointed to the fact that the outcome of all research endeavors is the improvement of orocraniofacial health and ultimately quality of life, and that basic science research cannot reach this outcome in isolation. She described how basic science research has to become part of an interwoven cycle of activity, where it connects with translational, clinical, behavioral, and health services research as well as with clinical practice and education to ultimately reach the goal of improving oral health. She illustrated this vision of the interconnectedness of basic science research by using one specific area of research in the oral health sciences, namely the regeneration of orocraniofacial tissues as an example. Her analysis of this research field led her to argue that while considerable progress has been made in the areas of biomimetics, biomaterials, and tissue engineering, the existing therapies based on this research have limitations. In order to develop therapies that have more predictable outcomes and truly enhance patients' oral health and quality of life, many factors such as the pain involved for the patient and esthetic concerns need to be addressed. In summary, her argument focused on breaking basic science research out of its relative isolation, by demonstrating that the ultimate goal of enhancing oral health and quality of life can only be reached in an interconnected effort with other researchers, clinicians, and educators. OHRQoL in her argument is not merely the ultimate outcome of basic research, but guides it by providing additional factors that need to be considered on the way to new therapies (Somerman, 2002).

Clinical research quite obviously needs to consider OHRQoL as one important short- and long-term outcome of certain treatments. In addition, OHRQoL can make an important argument for or against adopting a treatment approach. Henson et al. (2001) showed, for example, how preserving salivary output in head and neck cancer patients by using parotid-sparing radiotherapy affected these patients' quality of life quite significantly. Patients who had been treated with the traditional radiotherapy had significantly worse quality of life scores than patients treated with the new approach.

In other instances, quality of life concerns can provide an argument against using a new treatment approach—despite its clinical effectiveness. Flamenbaum et al. (2003) showed, for example, that chemomechanical caries removal in children may not be preferable compared to the traditional technique. These authors used a randomized controlled clinical trial to compare the clinical efficacy, operator perspective, and patient perspective of chemomechanical and traditional caries removal of twenty-two first and second occlusally cavitated deciduous molars respectively. They found that the new technique took significantly more time than the older method. This fact may explain why the operators reported significantly worse ratings of the children's behavior in the chemomechanical condition than in the traditional condition, and why the children did not respond positively to the new treatment. If effectiveness alone would have been the criteria to evaluate this new technique, it would have resulted in a quite favorable evaluation. However, the consideration of how the new technique affected the pediatric patients' quality of life can be a powerful consideration for clinicians who consider the adoption of such a new technique.

Clinical research also needs to carefully assess long-term outcomes of certain treatments. One example for OHRQoL research with this objective in mind is research on the quality of life of denture patients. Gray, Inglehart, & Sarment (2002) showed for example that quite a considerable percentage of the 120 research respondents with conventional dentures who had received their dentures between five months and nine years before they participated in the study reported either discomfort (20%) or strong discomfort (20%) caused by their dentures. Understanding what may affect whether denture patients have a positive or poor OHRQoL is therefore a crucial question (see also Heydecke et al., 2004).

Finally, public health researchers studying oral health issues can also see the benefit of considering OHRQoL indicators (Eklund & Burt, 2002). Understanding how oral health disparities and lack of access to care affect the quality of life of millions of U.S. citizens (U.S. Department of Health and Human Services, 2000) needs to be carefully documented to inform politicians and the public in general about the status quo. It also can be potentially a powerful tool for advocates who want to reduce these disparities and bring more social justice to the health care system.

In summary, the OHRQoL concept can provide the common denominator that connects researchers with different research backgrounds and research agendas, because it can bring a patient-centered focus to research in the oral health sciences.

Oral Health-Related Quality of Life and Clinical Practice

OHRQoL cannot merely offer a new perspective for researchers in the oral health sciences, it can also affirm a clinician's patient-centered approach to providing care, and thus ultimately improve patient-provider interactions. When Atchison (2002) reflected on the role of OHRQoL in clinical research and the clinical domain, she called her chapter "Understanding the 'Quality' in Quality Care and Quality of Life." This title could serve as a reminder for clinicians to reflect on the meaning of the term "quality care" and the role QHRQoL issues could play when providing quality care for all patients. From the moment patients schedule appointments to the time when they leave the dental office and return to their regimen of oral health promotion at home, OHRQoL can be of considerable importance.

Providing quality care may begin with taking a medical and dental history that includes questions concerning how oral health affects the patient's quality of life thus showing genuine interest in the patient. Understanding the relevance of a patient's chief complaint for this patient's quality of life can be crucial in getting a clear sense of the patient's expectations concerning the treatment outcome. Assuring that treatment is provided in a way that pain is avoided to the degree possible, and providing pain medication in such a way that pain is managed well are just two instances that show that a clinician considers the patient's quality of life issues. Ultimately, such a consideration will not merely benefit the patient, but will be positive for all persons involved in the clinical interaction.

A recent study with adolescent orthodontic patients showed, for example, that the best predictor of the number of missed appointments (as determined in a clinical chart review) was the pain these patients reported to have experienced during their orthodontic appointments (Khan et al., 2004). The more pain they reported to have suffered, the more missed appointments they had. This finding is just one of many research results that shows that patients' quality of life concerns can shape their seeking or avoiding dental care, and can affect their cooperation with treatment recommendations. Finally, even when providing oral hygiene instructions and health education in general, a consideration of the patient's quality of life may be one crucial factor that will ultimately determine if the patient will engage in the recommended course of action or not. In summary, OHRQoL is a concept that clinicians could use as a one guiding consideration in all patient interactions. It would assure that the care they provide is patient centered and of the highest quality.

Oral-Health-Related Quality of Life and Dental/Dental Hygiene Education

In 1995, the Institute of Medicine published an agenda-setting report on the future of dental education, which included some clear recommendations (Institute of Medicine, 1995). Some of these central recommendations were concerned with educating future health care providers in such a way that they will provide truly patient-centered care, will be culturally literate and sensitive to diversity issues, and will be able to work with an interdisciplinary perspective that sees oral health in the context of a patient's overall health. Inglehart, Tedesco, and Valacovic (2002) took these recommendations as a starting point to reflect which role OHRQoL issues could play in this situation. They started with an analysis of survey data from 1,864 respondents consisting of dental school faculty as well as directors in hospital programs, dental hygiene and dental assistant programs, who had rated the importance of these recommendations. Their results provided insight into whether there is a willingness in the educational community to base its educational efforts on these recommendations. Their findings showed that the respondents rated the importance of offering patient-centered education rather highly. Given this finding, the next question is how dental/dental hygiene educators can translate this objective into their classroom and clinic activities. Inglehart et al. (2002) argued that OHRQoL could serve as a portal to patient-centered education by shaping the content and thus the focus of educational efforts in classrooms, clinics, and community settings. Explicitly encouraging students to reflect on how health and disease affect patients' quality of life, and which role quality of life concerns can play for their patient's utilization versus avoidance of health care services may be a valuable way to educate patient-centered future providers.

Oral-Health-Related Quality of Life and Behavioral Scientists—Concluding Remarks

Ten years ago, a chapter on OHRQoL would not have been included in a volume on behavioral science contributions to dentistry. The concept would have been too new and unexplored to justify an inclusion. Today, this situation is quite different. Over the past few years, an increasing number of publications showed that OHRQoL is a powerful concept that can help researchers in the oral health sciences, clinicians, and educators alike to reflect on the ultimate objectives they have for their work (Inglehart & Bagramian, 2002b). For behavioral scientists working in dentistry, this concept can open doors by helping them to communicate the important role that the patient and the patient's behavior has for oral health and disease and for oral health care interactions. This chapter showed the way OHRQoL can be of importance in a wide range of settings. It was written with the goal of raising interest in this concept, and challenging researchers in the oral health sciences, clinicians, and dental educators to consider this concept provided by the behavioral sciences in their professional activities.

References

Andrews, F. M., & McKennell, A. C. (1980). Measures of self-reported well-being: their affective, cognitive and other components. *Social Indicators Research, 8,* 127–55.

Atchison, K. A. (2002). Understanding the "quality" of quality care and quality of life. In Inglehart, M. R., & Bagramian, R. A. (eds.), *Oral Health-Related Quality of Life.* Chicago, IL: Quintessence Publishing, Inc., 13–28.

Atchison, K. A., & Dolan, T. A. (1990). Development of the Geriatric Oral Health Assessment Index. *Journal of Dental Education, 54,* 680–687.

Bryant, P. S., & Kleinman, D. V. (2002). Research on oral health-related quality of life: current status and future directions. In Inglehart, M. R., & Bagramian, R. A. (eds.), *Oral Health-Related Quality of Life.* Chicago, IL: Quintessence Publishing, Inc., 2002.

Campbell, A. (1976). Subjective measures of well-being. *American Psychologist, 31,* 117–24.

Chen, M., Andersen, R. M., Barmes, D. E., Leclercq, M. H., & Lyttle, C. S. (1997). *Comparing Oral Health Care Systems: A Second International Collaborative Study.* Geneva: World Health Organization.

Cimprich, B., & Paterson, A. G. (2002). Health-related quality of life: conceptual issues and research applications. In Inglehart, M. R., & Bagramian, R. A. (eds.), *Oral Health-Related Quality of Life*. Chicago, IL: Quintessence Publishing, Inc., 2002.

Cohen, L. K., & Jago, J. D. (1976). Toward the formulation of sociodental indicators. *International Journal of Health Services, 6*, 681–698.

Eklund, S. A., & Burt, B. A. (2002). Tooth loss, dental caries, and the quality of life: a public health perspective. In Inglehart, M. R., & Bagramian, R. A. (eds.), *Oral Health-Related Quality of Life*. Chicago, IL: Quintessence Publishing, Inc..

Engel, G. L. (1977). The need for a new medical model: a challenge for biomedicine. *Science, 196*, 129–136.

Filstrup, S. L., Briskie, D., da Fonseca, M., Lawrence, L., Wandera, A., & Inglehart, M. R. (2003). Early childhood caries and quality of life—child and parent perspectives. *Journal of Pediatric Dentistry, 25(5)*, 431–440.

Flamenbaum, M. H., Inglehart, M. R., Eboda, N., Feigal, R., & Peters, T. (2003). Chemomechanical vs. Traditional Caries Removal in Children—Operator and Child Perspective. Paper presented at the Meeting of the American Association of Dental Research, San Antonio, March 2003. (Abstract in *Journal of Dental Research*, 2003).

General Accounting Office. (2000). *Dental Disease Is a Chronic Problem Among Low Income Populations*. General Accounting Office Publication GAO/HEHS 00-72. Washington, DC: Government Printing Office.

Giddon, D. B. (1978). The mouth and the quality of life. *The New York Journal of Dentistry, 48(1)*, 3–10.

———. (1987). Oral health and the quality of life. *Journal of the American College of Dentists, 54(2)*, 10–15.

Gift, H. D. (1992). Research directions in oral health promotion for older adults. *Journal of Dental Education, 56*, 626–631.

Gift, H. D., & Atchison, K. A. (1995). Oral health, health, and health-related quality of life. *Medical Care, 33* (Supplement), NS 57–77.

Gift, H. D., & Redford, M. (1992). Oral health and the quality of life. *Clinics in Geriatric Medicine, 8*, 673–683.

Gift, H. D., Atchison, K. A., & Drury, P. F. (1998). Perceptions of the natural dentition in the context of multiple variables. *Journal of Dental Research, 77*, 1529–1538.

Gray, S. A., Inglehart, M. R., & Sarment, D. (2002). Dentures and Quality of Life—A Cross-Sectional Analysis. Paper presented at the Meeting of the American Association of Dental Research, March 2002.

Henson, B., Inglehart, M. R., Eisbruch, A., & Ship, J. (2001). Preserved salivary output and xerostomia-related quality of life in head and neck cancer patients receiving parotid-sparing radiotherapy. *Oral Oncology, 37*, 84–93.

Heydecke, G., Tedesco, L. A., Kowalski, C., & Inglehart, M. R. (2004). Complete dentures and oral health-related quality of life—do coping styles matter? *Community Dentistry & Oral Epidemiology, 32(4)*, 297–306.

Inglehart, M. R., & Bagramian, R. A. (2002a). Oral health-related quality of life: an introduction. In Inglehart, M. R., & Bagramian, R. A. (eds.). *Oral Health-Related Quality of Life*. Chicago, IL: Quintessence Publishing, Inc., 2002.

Inglehart, M. R., & Bagramian, R. A., eds. (2002b). *Oral Health-Related Quality of Life*. Chicago, IL: Quintessence Publishing, Inc..

Inglehart, M. R., Tedesco, L. A., & Valachovic, R. W. (2002). Using oral health-related quality of life to refocus dental education. In Inglehart, M. R., & Bagramian, R. A. (eds.). *Oral Health-Related Quality of Life*. Chicago, IL: Quintessence Publishing, Inc..

Institute of Medicine. Committee on the Future of Dental Education. (1995). *Dental Education at the Crossroads: Challenges and Changes*. Washington, DC: National Academy Press, 1995.

Jokovic, A., Locker, D., Stephens, M., Kenny, D., Tompson, B., & Guyatt, G. (2002). Validity and reliability of a questionnaire for measuring child oral-health-related quality of life. *Journal of Dental Research, 81(7)*, 459–63.

Khan, F. A., Sayed, S., Johnson, R., & Inglehart, M. R. (2004). Treatment Cooperation with Orthodontic Treatment—The Role of Psychosocial Factors. Paper presented at the Meeting of the American Association of Dental Research in Baltimore, MD, March 2005.

Kressin, N. R. (1996). Associations among different assessments of oral health outcomes. *Journal of Dental Education, 60*, 502–506.

Locker, D. (1988). Measuring oral health: a conceptual framework. *Community Dental Health, 5*, 3–18.

Peterson, C. (2002). Quality of life as a psychologist views it. In Inglehart, M. R., & Bagramian, R. A. (eds.). *Oral Health-Related Quality of Life*. Chicago, IL: Quintessence Publishing, Inc., 2002.

Reisine, S. (1988). The effects of pain and oral health on quality of life. *Community Dental Health, 5*, 63–68.

Reisine, S. T. (1985). Dental health and public health: the social impact of dental disease. *American Journal of Public Health, 75*, 27–30.

Sheiham, A., Maizels, J., & Maizels, A. (1987). New composite indicators of dental health. *Community Dental Health, 4*, 407–414.

Slade, G. D. (1997a). Derivation and validation of a short form oral health impact profile. *Community Dentistry and Oral Epidemiology, 25*, 284–90.

———. (2002). Assessment of oral health-related quality of life. In Inglehart, M. R., & Bagramian, R. A. (eds.). *Oral Health-Related Quality of Life*. Chicago, IL: Quintessence Publishing Inc., 2002.

Slade, G. D., ed. (1997b). *Measuring Oral Health and Quality of Life*. Chapel Hill, NC: Department of Dental Ecology, School of Dentistry, University of North Carolina.

Slade, G. D., and Spencer, A. J. (1994). Development and evaluation of the oral health impact profile. *Community Dental Health, 11*, 3–11.

Somerman, M. J. (2002). Quality of life and basic research in the oral health sciences. In Inglehart, M. R., & Bagramian, R. A. (eds.). *Oral Health-Related Quality of Life*. Chicago, IL: Quintessence Publishing, Inc., 2002.

Strauss, R. P., & Hunt, R. J. (1993). Understanding the value of teeth to older adults: influences on the quality of life. *Journal of the American Dental Association, 124* (January), 105–10.

U.S. Department of Health and Human Services. (2000). *Oral Health in America: A Report of the Surgeon General*. NIH—publication 00-4713. Rockville, MD: U.S. Department of Health and Human Services, National Institute of Dental and Craniofacial Research, National Institutes of Health.

World Health Organization. (1948). *Constitution of the World Health Organization*. Geneva: World Health Organization.

Stress and Inflammation: A Bidirectional Relationship

Salomon Amar

Introduction

The molecular and biochemical bases for interactions between the immune and central nervous systems are the focus of intense research due to the deleterious effects of immune dysregulation. Immune cytokines not only activate immune function but also recruit central stress-responsive neurotransmitter systems in the modulation of the immune response and in the activation of behaviors that may be adaptive during injury or inflammation. Peripherally generated cytokines, such as interleukin-1, signal hypothalamic corticotropin-releasing hormone (CRH) neurons to activate pituitary-adrenal counterregulation of inflammation through the potent anti-inflammatory effect of glucocorticoids.

Corticotropin-releasing hormone not only activates the pituitary-adrenal axis but also sets in motion a coordinated series of behavioral and physiologic responses, suggesting that the central nervous system may coordinate both behavioral and immunologic adaptation during stressful situations. The pathophysiologic perturbation of this feedback loop, through various mechanisms, results in the development of inflammatory syndromes, such as rheumatoid arthritis, and behavioral syndromes, such as depression.

Thus, diseases characterized by both inflammatory and emotional disturbances may derive from common alterations in specific central nervous system pathways (for example, the CRH system). In addition, disruptions of this communication by genetic, infectious, toxic, or pharmacologic means can influence the susceptibility to disorders associated with both behavioral and inflammatory components and potentially alter their natural history. These concepts suggest that neuropharmacologic agents that stimulate hypothalamic CRH might potentially be adjunctive therapy for illnesses traditionally viewed as inflammatory or autoimmune.

It is the molecular and biochemical mechanisms by which the peripheral immunologic apparatus signals the brain to participate in maintaining immunologic and behavioral homeostasis. Although many neurohormonal systems play a role in this interaction, we focus primarily on the interaction between peripherally generated cytokines and the hypothalamic-pituitary-adrenal (HPA) axis. In this interaction, immune signals to corticotropin-releasing hormone (CRH) neurons in the hypothalamus promote the release of CRH into the hypophyseal portal system and thus activate pituitary-adrenal counterregulation of inflammation through the potent anti-inflammatory effects of the glucocorticoids (Woloski et al., 1985; Bernton et al., 1987; Sapolsky et al., 1987; Berkenbosch et al., 1987; Breder, Dinarello, & Saper, 1988; Fontana, Weber, & Dayer, 1984; Bernardini et al., 1988; Sternberg, 1988; Sternberg, Hill, et al., 1989; Sternberg, Young, et al., 1989; Wick et al., 1987; Mason, MacPhee, & Antoni, 1990; Sundar et al., 1990; Sternberg and Wilder, 1989). Recent data show that centrally directed CRH promotes various other physiologic and behavioral changes that are adaptive during stressful situations, which suggests that immune signals to CRH neurons could have consequences beyond modulation of immune function.

Perturbations in the communication between the immune system and the brain could theoretically produce disease states that include not only inflammatory diseases, such as rheumatoid arthritis, but also affective disorders, such as major depression. This concept suggests that disease states characterized by both inflammatory and emotional disturbances may derive from coherent alterations in specific central nervous system pathways and may also respond to the same therapeutic agents.

Living organisms survive by maintaining a complex dynamic equilibrium that is often threatened by intrinsic or extrinsic disturbing forces. The steady state required for successful adaptation is maintained by counteracting and reestablishing forces that consist of a complex repertoire of molecular, cellular, physiologic, and behavioral responses. These adaptive responses provide a selective advantage for survival, and a substantial portion of our cellular machinery is dedicated to the goal of maintaining a steady state.

We refer to this steady state as homeostasis. Stressors are the disturbing forces or threats to homeostasis, and adaptive responses include physical or mental reactions that attempt to counteract the effects of the stressors or disturbing forces in order to reestablish homeostasis. Thus, we define stress as a state of disharmony or threatened homeostasis. The adaptive responses can be specific to the stressor, or they can be generalized and nonspecific. Responses of the latter type generally occur only if the magnitude of the threat to homeostasis exceeds a certain threshold. The stereotypic activation of general adaptation mechanisms during periods of stress is referred to as the "general adaptation or stress syndrome" (Selye, 1950); however, a person's adaptive response to disturbing forces may itself serve as a stressor capable of producing pathologic changes.

Neurobiology of Stress

Psychological and emotional stress commence with impulses arising from high cortical centers of the brain that are relayed through the limbic system to the hypothalamus. Chemical mediators, including norepinephrine (NE), serotonin, and acetylcholine, are released and activate cells of the paraventricular nucleus of the hypothalamus to produce corticotropin-releasing factor (CRF), the coordinator of the stress response (Selye, 1950; Gold et al., 1988). CRF enters the portal venous system of the hypothalamus, travels to, and activates the corticotropes of the anterior pituitary gland to produce proopiomelanocortin (POMC), a polyprotein that is subsequently cleaved to form adrenocorticotropic hormone (ACTH), β-endorphin, and alpha melanocyte-stimulating hormone (α-MSH). CRF also stimulates the locus coeruleus, a dense collection of autonomic cells in the brainstem, to secrete NE at sympathetic nerve endings.

Activation of the sympathetic nervous system (SNS) centrally is also transmitted to the adrenal medulla, where chromaffin cells are stimulated by sympathetic fibers in the splanchnic nerve to produce epinephrine (E). Virtually all the E and approximately 10% of circulating NE are elaborated by the adrenal medulla. ACTH stimulates the adrenal cortex to produce corticosteroids, which, together with the catecholamines E and NE produced by the SNS, are the major stress hormones. Glucagon and growth hormone, also released with acute stress, are considered to be stress hormones. The renin–angiotensin system also participates in the stress response. SNS innervation of the kidney may result in the production of renin, which initiates a series of reactions whereby renin and angiotensin-converting enzyme (ACE) produce angiotensin II, a powerful vasoconstrictor that elevates the blood pressure and heart rate. Although CRF is the major coordinator of the stress response, other neuropeptides such as substance P (SP), which is present in the brain as well as primary sensory neurons, may participate in the stress response by activating the HPA axis and the SNS.

Inflammation and the Stress Response

Neuroendocrine hormones triggered during stress may lead to immune dysregulation or altered or amplified cytokine production, resulting in atopic, autoimmune diseases or decreased host defense. The stress response and induction of a dysregulation of cytokine balance can trigger the hypothalamic-pituitary-adrenal axis and sympathetic nervous system.

Inflammatory stimuli may also lead to activation of aspects of the stress response. The inflammatory response is the most primitive of protective mechanisms; rudiments of it existed before the development of the nervous system. In response to psychological stress or certain physical stressors, an inflammatory process may occur by release of various types of transmitter substances of the neuroendocrine-immune (NEI) network including epinephrine, norepinephrine, acetylcholine, substance P (SP), vasoactive intestinal peptide, glucagon, insulin, cytokines, growth factors, and other inflammatory mediators from sensory nerves and the activation of mast cells or other inflammatory cells. Central neuropeptides, particularly corticosteroid releasing factor (CRF), and perhaps SP as well, initiate a systemic stress response by activation of neuroendocrinological pathways such as the sympathetic nervous system, hypothalamic pituitary axis, and the renin-angiotensin system, with the release of the stress hormones (i.e., catecholamines, corticosteroids, growth hormone, glucagons, and renin). These, together with cytokines induced by stress, initiate the acute-phase response (APR) and the induction of acute-phase proteins, essential mediators of inflammation. Central nervous system norepinephrine may also induce the APR perhaps by macrophage activation and cytokine release.

The increase in lipids with stress may also be a factor in macrophage activation, as may lipopolysaccharide, which might induce cytokines from hepatic Kupffer cells, subsequent to an enhanced absorption from the gastrointestinal tract during psychologic stress. The brain may initiate or inhibit the inflammatory process. The inflammatory response is contained within the psychological stress response, which evolved later. Moreover, the same neuropeptides (i.e., CRF and possibly SP as well) mediate both stress and inflammation. Cytokines evoked by either a stress or inflammatory response may utilize similar somatosensory pathways to signal the brain. Other instances whereby stress may induce inflammatory changes are reviewed. It is postulated that repeated episodes of acute or chronic psychogenic stress may produce chronic inflammatory changes that may result in atherosclerosis in the arteries or chronic inflammatory changes in other organs as well.

Although the "stress" response is activated by these stimuli, the resultant physiological changes also equip an organism to deal with infection. Thus, corticosteroids and catecholamines, the major stress hormones, actually initiate a response characterized by production of cytokines and acute-phase reactants as in an inflammatory state. The inflammatory response, therefore, is contained within the "stress response" that is evoked by psychogenic stimuli. The coupling has obvious survival advantage for an animal engaged in, or recuperating from, combat. The immune system evolved from the inflammatory system and, like the latter, is intimately involved in the protection of the host. It, too, is coupled with the stress response, that is, the brain and immune systems interact in a negative feedback loop (Selye, 1950; Gold et al., 1988; Black, 2002).

Repeated episodes of acute or chronic psychological stress could also induce an acute-phase response (APR) and subsequently a chronic inflammatory process such as atherosclerosis. Such stress can induce an APR and inflammation, and has been extended to include a chronic inflammatory process(s), characterized by the presence of certain cytokines and acute-phase reactants (APR), which is associated with certain metabolic diseases. The loci of origin of these cytokines, particularly interleukin 6 (IL-6), and their induction, has been considered. Evidence is presented that the liver, the endothelium, and fat cell depots are the primary sources of cytokines, particularly IL-6, and that IL-6 and the acute-phase protein (APP), C-reactive protein (CRP), are strongly associated with, and likely play a dominant role in, the development of this inflammatory process, which leads to insulin resistance, non-insulin-dependent diabetes mellitus type II, and metabolic syndrome X. The fact that stress can activate an APR, which is part of the innate immune inflammatory response, is evidence that the inflammatory response is contained within the stress response or that stress can induce an inflammatory response. The evidence that the stress, inflammatory, and immune systems all evolved from a single cell, the phagocyte, is further evidence for their intimate relationship. It appears that the inflammatory response is contained within the stress response and is adaptive in that an animal may be better able to react to an organism introduced during combat. The argument is made that humans reacting to stressors that are not life-threatening but are "perceived" as such, mount similar stress/inflammatory responses in the arteries, and that if repetitive or chronic may culminate in atherosclerosis (Black, 2003; Black & Garbutt, 2002).

Surgical Stress

General anesthesia accompanied by surgical stress may influence the inflammatory responses that are essential for maintaining the homeostatic state during the postoperative course. Severe dysregulation of the inflammatory process may provoke or aggravate postoperative complications, for example, increased susceptibility to infections, inadequate stress reactions, and hypercatabolism. Anesthetics have been suspected of impairing various functions of the immune system either directly, by disturbing the functions of immune-competent cells, or indirectly by modulating the stress response. In the past, conflicting data on the possible immunological side effects of anesthetics have been published. Potential reasons for these controversial findings include heterogeneous patient study groups with diverse preexisting diseases, lack of standardization of surgical procedures, major differences in the length and severity of surgical tissue injury, and a small number of randomized studies. Although the immunological effects are of minor consequence in subjects with normal immune functions, the suppression of cellular and humoral immunity following surgery and general anesthesia may be relevant in patients with preexisting immune disorders (Schneemilch, Schilling, & Bank, 2004).

Molecular Implications

A wide range of environmental stress and human disorders involves inappropriate regulation of NF-κB, including cancers and numerous inflammatory conditions. Transgenic mice that express luciferase under the control of NF-κB, enabling real-time noninvasive imaging of NF-κB activity in intact animals have been developed. It was shown that, in the absence of stimulation, strong, intrinsic luminescence is evident in lymph nodes in the neck region, thymus, and Peyer's patches. Treating mice with stressors, such as TNF-α, IL-1α, or lipopolysaccharide (LPS), increases the luminescence in a tissue-specific manner, with the strongest activity observable in the skin, lungs, spleen, Peyer's patches, and wall of the small intestine. Liver, kidney, heart, muscle, and adipose tissue exhibit less-intense activities. Exposure of the skin to a low dose of UV-B radiation increases luminescence in the exposed areas. In ocular experiments, LPS- and TNF-α-injected NF-κB-luciferase transgenic mice exhibit a 20–40-fold increase in lens NF-κB activity, similar to other LPS- and TNF-α–responsive organs. Peak NF-κB activity occurs 6 h after injection of TNF-α and 12 h after injection of LPS. Peak activities occur, respectively, 3 and 6 h later than that in other tissues. Mice exposed to 360 J/m^2 of UV-B exhibit a 16-fold increase in NF-κB activity 6 h after exposure, characteristically similar to TNF-α–exposed mice. Thus, in NF-κB-luciferase transgenic mice, NF-κB activity also occurs in lens epithelial tissue and is activated when the intact mouse is exposed to classical stressors. Furthermore, as revealed by real-time noninvasive imaging, induction of chronic inflammation resembling rheumatoid arthritis produces strong NF-κB activity in the affected joints. Models for monitoring NF-κB activation both in tissue homogenates and in intact animals after the use of classical stress activators are now available to further our knowledge of the relationship between stress and inflammation (Carlsen et al., 2004).

Conclusions

Disorders in which abnormalities in immune function are mediated by the NEI network include allergic diseases: allergic rhinitis, atopic dermatitis, and gastrointestinal allergies and asthma through overproduction of neuropeptides and cytokines. The multiple roles of Th2 cells in maintaining allergic inflammation and altering the balance between Th1 and Th2 responses are important mechanisms for allergic inflammation and tissue damage. In addition, several autoimmune diseases mediated by the NEI network such as rheumatoid arthritis, systemic lupus erythematosus, and diabetes mellitus can be attributable to immune dysregulation.

Understanding the NEI network will contribute to novel treatments for immediate and late allergic reactions. Chronic stress or depression could lead to decreased host defenses, decreased response to vaccines, viral susceptibility, or malignancy. Treatment of allergic, autoimmune diseases and asthma should include stress management and behavioral intervention to prevent stress-related immune imbalances.

Acknowledgments

This work was supported by grants from the National Institutes of Health: RO1 DE14079; PO1 DE 13191; RO1 DE 15989 RO1 DE 15345; RO1 HL 76801.

References

Berkenbosch, F., van Oers, J., del Rey, A., Tilders, F., & Besedovsky, H. (1987). Corticotropin- releasing factor-producing neurons in the rat activated by interleukin-1. *Science, 238*, 524–36.

Bernardini, R., Luger, A., Gold, P. W., Chiarenza, A., Legakis, J., & Chrousos, G. P., Petraglia, F., ed. (1988). Cytokines stimulate pituitary-adrenal function via activation of the CRH neuron. *New Trends in Brain and Female Reproductive Function.* Rome: CIG Edizioni Internazionali..

Bernton, E. W., Beach, J. E., Holaday, J. W., Smallridge, R. C., & Fein, H. G. (1987). Release of multiple hormones by a direct action of interleukin-1 on pituitary cells. *Science, 238,* 519–21.

Black, P. H. (1994a). Central nervous system–immune system interactions: pyschoneuroendocrinology of stress and its immune consequences. *Antimicrobial Agents and Chemotherapy, 38,* 1–6.

——. (1994b). Immune system-central nervous system interactions: immunomodulatory consequences of immune system mediators on the brain. *Antimicrobial Agents and Chemotherapy, 38,* 7–12.

——. (2002). Stress and the inflammatory response: a review of neurogenic inflammation. *Brain, Behavior and Immunity, 16,* 622–53.

——. (2003). The inflammatory response is an integral part of the stress response: implications for atherosclerosis, insulin resistance, type II diabetes and metabolic syndrome X. *Brain, Behavior, and Immunity, 17*(5), 350–64.

Black, P. H., & Garbutt, L. D. (2002). Stress, inflammation and cardiovascular disease. *Journal of Psychosomatic Research, 52* (1), 1–23.

Breder, C. D., Dinarello, C. A., & Saper, C. B. (1988). Interleukin-1 immunoreactive innervation of the human hypothalamus. *Science, 240,* 321–24.

Carlsen, H., Alexander, G., Austenaa, L. M., Ebihara, K., & Blomhoff, R. (2004). Molecular imaging of the transcription factor NF-kappaB, a primary regulator of stress response. *Mutation Research, 551*(1–2), 199–211.

Fontana, A., Weber, E., & Dayer, J. M. (1984). Synthesis of interleukin 1/endogenous pyrogen in the brain of endotoxin-treated mice: a step in fever induction? *Journal of Immunology, 133,* 1696–98.

Gold, P. W. (1988). Stress-responsive neuromodulators. *Biological Psychiatry, 24*(4), 371–74.

Mason, D., MacPhee, I., & Antoni, F. (1990). The role of the neuroendocrine system in determining genetic susceptibility to experimental allergic encephalomyelitis in the rat. *Immunology, 70,* 1–5.

Sapolsky, R., River, C., Yamamoto, G., Plotsky, P., & Vale, W. (1987). Interleukin-1 stimulates the secretion of hypothalamic corticotropin releasing factor. *Science, 238,* 522 24.

Schneemilch, C. E., Schilling T., & Bank, U. (2004). Effects of general anesthesia on inflammation. *Best Practice and Research: Clinical Anaesthesiology,* 18, 493–507.

Selye, H. (1950). Stress. Montreal: Acta.

Sternberg, E. M. (1988). Monokines, lymphokines and the brain. In Cruse, J. M., Lewis, R. E., Jr. (eds.), *The Year in Immunology,* vol. 5. Basel: Karger.

Sternberg, E. M., & Wilder, R. L. (1989). The role of the hypothalamic-pituitary-adrenal axis in an experimental model of arthritis. *Progress in Neuro Endocrin Immunology, 2,* 102–8.

Sternberg, E. M., Hill, J. M., Chrousos, G. P., Kamilaris, T., Listwak, S. J., & Gold P. W., et al. (1989). Inflammatory mediator-induced hypothalamic-pituitary-adrenal axis activation is defective in streptococcal cell wall arthritis-susceptible Lewis rats. *Proceedings of the National Academy of Sciences of the United States of America*, vol. 86, 2374–78.

Sternberg, E. M., Young, W., III, Bernardini, R., Calogero, A. E., Chrousos, G. P., & Gold, P. W., et al. (1989). A central nervous system defect in biosynthesis of corticotropin- releasing hormone is associated with susceptibility to streptococcal cell wall arthritis in Lewis rats. *Proceedings of the National Academy of Sciences of the United States of America*, 86, 4771–75.

Sundar, S. K., Cierpial, M. A., Kilts, C., Ritchie, J. C., & Weiss, J. M. (1990). Brain IL-1-induced immunocupression occurs through activation of both pituitary-adrenal axis and sympathetic nervous system by corticotropin-releasing factor. *Journal of Neuroscience, 10*, 3701–6.

Wick, G., Kromer, G., Neu, N., Fassler, R., Ziemiecki, A., & Muller, R. G., et al. (1987). The multi-factorial pathogenesis of autoimmune disease. *Immunology Letters, 16*, 249–57.

Woloski, B. M., Smith, E. M., Meyer, W. J., III, Fuller, G. M., & Blalock, J. E. (1985). Corticotropin-releasing activity of monokines. *Science, 230*, 1035–37.

Saliva in Health and Disease

Mahvash Navazesh

Introduction

The public and health professionals' image of saliva is changing drastically and rapidly because of abundant information about the role of saliva in health and disease that is made available for public consumption via the internet and the media. In the view of most people, saliva was created for licking envelopes and stamps.

People rarely paid attention to saliva unless they were nervous, developed dry mouth, and had to deliver a public speech. Indeed, dry mouth caused by anxiety was used as a diagnostic aid by ancient societies in a lie detector test known as the *Rice Test* (Mandel, 1993). An accused was given a mouthful of dry rice to chew and swallow. If the accused was anxious because of guilt, the emotional inhibition of salivation resulting from increasing activity of the sympathetic nervous system would have interfered with adequate bolus formation and swallowing. That was interpreted as proof of wrongdoing and resulted in beheading of the accused.

What used to be described as 99% water, today is viewed as a fountain of information that reflects an individual's state of health and disease. Hundreds of publications in recent years have focused on the etiology of and associated complications with salivary gland hypofunction. The quality and quantity of saliva, like urine and blood, are affected by a variety of medical conditions and medications, as well as the psychological status of the patient. The public and professionals are used to blood and urine tests, but not a saliva test, as a routine practice for risk assessment and disease prevention. Although a saliva test is less invasive than a blood test, and needs less privacy than a urine test, it has not been part of the everyday practice of medicine and dentistry in the past. However, saliva diagnostic tests are becoming more commonly utilized by physicians, some dentists, and law enforcement agents (Tu, Kapur, & Israel, 1992).

This chapter is written in an attempt to enhance awareness among oral health care providers of the significant role that saliva plays in health and disease and the significant role that they could play in the early detection and recognition of salivary gland hypofunction, systemic disease, psychological states, as well as the prevention of associated complications.

Formation

Saliva is produced by three pairs of major glands and numerous minor salivary glands within the oral cavity. The parotid, submandibular, and sublingual salivary glands contribute to 90% of total saliva secretions. Minor salivary glands contribute to the remaining 10%. The saliva secreted by the major and minor glands collectively is referred to as whole saliva. In the resting (unstimulated) state, approximately two-thirds of the volume of whole saliva is produced by submandibular glands. Upon stimulation, the parotid glands account for at least 50% of whole saliva volume in the mouth. Sublingual glands contribute to a small percentage of unstimulated and stimulated whole saliva. Minor salivary glands contribute significantly to the lubrication of the oral mucosa because they contain a large amount of proteins. Unlike some minor salivary glands that are pure mucous in nature, parotid glands are purely serous and produce waterlike secretions. Submandibular and sublingual glands are mixed.

In general, the acinar (secretory) cells are responsible for production of the primary saliva. The ductal cells are responsible for further modifications of saliva until it is secreted in the mouth. Saliva is 99% water and 1% proteins and salts. The normal daily production of saliva ranges from 0.5 to 1.5 liters. The average whole unstimulated saliva flow rate is approximately 0.3–0.4 ml/min. This rate decreases to 0.1 ml/min during sleeping hours and increases to approximately 4.0 to 5.0 ml/min during eating, chewing, and other stimulating conditions. Saliva is always hypotonic to plasma. The higher the saliva flow rate the greater the tonicity of saliva will be. Salivary gland secretion is mainly controlled by the autonomic nervous system. Parasympathetic stimulation produces copious (watery) saliva, whereas sympathetic stimulation produces more viscous saliva (Bardow, Pedersen, & Nauntofte, 2004).

Function

Saliva plays a significant role in the protection of the intraoral structures against insults introduced by different microbial pathogens and chemical and mechanical irritants. The functions of saliva are listed in table 4.1.

Saliva contains three buffer systems (bicarbonate, phosphate, and protein) and helps to maintain an acceptable pH in the range of 6.0–7.5 within the

Table 4.1   Functions of Saliva

- Buffering capacity
- Remineralization of teeth
- Lubrication capacity
- Repair of soft tissues
- Digestion
- Antimicrobial capacity

oral cavity. When a substance is placed in the oral cavity, the saliva flow will increase based on its taste, consistency, and concentration. When the volume of saliva is about 1.1 ml, the urge for swallowing will occur. The salivary stimulation, dilution of tastant, and swallowing will go on until the concentration of the tastants reaches a point where it no longer stimulates the flow rate. The oral clearance of different substances will be prolonged in the absence of saliva, leading to potential harm to intraoral hard and soft tissues. Saliva is supersaturated with respect to calcium hydroxyapatite under normal physiologic conditions, which prevents demineralization of the dentition. The salivary protein pellicle further protects teeth against irritants.

Human saliva contains α amylase and lipase, which may play a role in starch digestion and triglyceride breakdown in neonates with pancreatic dysfunction. Salivary mucins play a significant role in lubricating the intraoral structures and serve as a barrier against microbial invasion. Lysozyme and lactoferrin are examples of other proteins with antimicrobial properties. Lactoferrin is believed to have antibacterial, antifungal, and antiviral properties. Salivary peroxidase has antibacterial properties, whereas histatins have been associated with antibacterial and antifungal properties. Salivary epidermal growth factor enhances the oral mucosal healing process and protects the esophageal mucosa. In addition to these proteins with specific functions, other enzymes may serve as diagnostic markers, such as pseudocholinesterase for mental disease (Giddon & Lisanti, 1962). Saliva contains other organic components, such as glucose, urea, cortisol, sex hormones, and blood group substances, which have also been utilized in saliva as screening/diagnostic tools.

Dysfunction

Multiple medical conditions and medications can affect the quality and quantity of saliva (Antilla, Knuuttila, & Sakki, 1998; Bergdahl & Bergdahl, 2000; Bergdahl, Bergdahl, & Johansson, 1997; Sreebny & Schwartz, 1997). This chapter will focus only on the common factors associated with chronic salivary gland hypofunction in adults (table 4.2). Less-frequent, uncommon, and/or acute conditions such as dehydration, salivary gland neoplasm, sialosis, sialadenosis, sialorrhea, sialolithiasis and sialadenitis will not be covered here. Salivary cortisol level is increased as a response of the adrenal cortex to stressors such as chronic dental anxiety, stressful computer task requirements, viewing anxiety-provoking videos, and masticatory muscle ac-

Table 4.2   Chronic Conditions Associated with Salivary Gland Hypofunction in Adults

Medications
- Antidepressants (lithium, tricyclics)
- Antipsychotics
- Antihistamines
- Antiemetics
- Antiretroviral therapy (protease inhibitors)
- Decongestants
- Appetite suppressants
- Diuretics

Irradiation

Chemotherapy

Medical conditions
- Sjögren's syndrome
- Viral infections (HIV, HCV)
- Uncontrolled diabetes
- Alzheimer's disease
- Hypertension
- Depression

tivity caused by clenching teeth. Relaxation modalities such as viewing soothing videos, listening to music, and acupuncture treatment could lower the saliva cortisol and amylase levels (Bakke et al., 2004; Benjamins, Asscheman, & Schuurs, 1992; Blom & Lundeberg, 2000; Bosch et al., 1996; Brennan et al., 2002; Hasegawa, Uozumi, & Ono, 2004; Hill & Walker, 2001; Miluk-Kolasa et al., 1994; Neudeck, Jacoby, & Florin, 2001; Piollet et al., 1984; Stones et al., 1999; Takai et al., 2004). As noted earlier, subjective dry mouth may have a psychological origin. Psychological processes are often accompanied by disturbed oral sensations, and, in fact, most individuals have experienced a dry mouth during a period of acute stress. Together with depression, mental stress has been reported to be associated with a dry mouth condition, either as a result of the illness itself or as an adverse effect of drugs used in management of the psychological state (Bergdahl et al., 1997; Bolwig & Rafaelsen, 1972; Davies & Gurland, 1961). Stress may play a role, and the more anxiety there is the lower the whole unstimulated saliva content of IgA. However, it has proved difficult to separate the effects of anxiety on salivary flow and immunoglobulin levels independently. These findings are in keeping with studies of saliva during daily relaxation. The secretory IgA rate increased significantly after relaxation (Green, Green, & Santoro, 1988).

Studies of cortisol in depressed patients have given interesting results, provided technical aspects of steroid assays are controlled. In depression, there seem to be differences in salivary cortisol between patients with endogenous and nonendogenous depression. Generally, there is a correlation between plasma ACTH levels and salivary cortisol, but this relationship is not present in patients with endogenous depression, suggesting either a drug effect or a disturbance of regulation of cortisol secretion (Galard et al., 1991). Self-induced vomiting and binge eating are features of bulimia nervosa. Saliva function has been studied in this group and it is known that approximately 25% have sialadenosis (Riad, Barton, & Wilson, 1991; Roberts et al., 1989). Some studies have shown that parotid function is reduced in bulimics; that is, resting and stimulated flow rates are reduced in those with sialadenosis, and total protein and amylase levels are increased. Other studies of parotid and submandibular gland function have shown no difference in function in relation to controls, and amylase levels were equivalent.

Xerostomia is a common oral complaint associated with more than five hundred medications (Sreebny & Schwartz, 1988). Polypharmacy is the most common cause of xerostomia (subjective complaint of dry mouth) and salivary gland hypofunction (objective evidence of reduced saliva flow rate) in the elderly. The most frequent types of medications with xerogenic potential are those with anticholinergic or sympathomimetic actions. Salivary gland hypofunction is a greatly overlooked condition, and many patients who take xerogenic medications may not know that they are at risk for oral complications such as dental caries and fungal infections. Therefore, the absence of a subjective complaint of oral dryness does not indicate adequate saliva production. Accordingly, the diagnosis of drug-induced hyposalivation requires measurements of saliva output or flow rate. In addition to the xerogenic medications taken by mouth, other chemotherapeutic modalities like chemotherapy and radiation therapy lead to qualitative and quantitative salivary changes. There is an association between the severity of salivary gland hypofunction and the degree of exposure to radiation. The management of oropharyngeal cancer often involves administration of 60-GY to 70-GY radiation, which can lead to a 95% reduction in the amount of salivary secretions in the involved areas (Davies et al., 2001). The severity of xerostomia and salivary gland hypofunction has also been associated with the total number of chemotherapeutic drugs used for the management of various malignancies.

Xerostomia is one of the most common complaints among patients who have undergone radiation therapy and/or chemotherapy (Hainsworth et al., 2002; Nagler, 1998; Pow et al., 2003; Singh, Scully, & Joyston-Bechal, 1996). Unlike inflammatory changes associated with over-the-counter and prescription drugs that are temporary in nature, and could resolve on their own if the drugs were discontinued, the salivary changes associated with radiation and chemotherapy could be permanent.

Chronic medical conditions could also affect the salivary flow rate and composition via different mechanisms. For example, in Sjögrens syndrome, an autoimmune disorder, the salivary gland tissue is replaced by inflammatory (CD4 T cell) lymphocytes leading to a dry mouth sensation caused by saliva hyposecretion (Fox, Stern, & Michelson, 2000; Fox & Stern, 2002). In HIV-infected patients, the salivary glands may be affected because of tissue replacement by CD8 T cell infiltration as part of a diffuse infiltrated lymphocytosis syndrome or due to persistent enlargement of the parotid glands leading to dry mouth caused by HIV infection per se. In addition to the disease process, antiretroviral medications, such as protease inhibitors, independently increase the risk for xerostomia and salivary gland hypofunction in this patient population. Hepatitis C virus (HCV) may also lead to salivary gland disorders caused by lymphocytic infiltration (CD20 cells) (Ferreiro et al., 2002; Henderson et al., 2001; Loustaud-Ratti et al., 2001; Mariette, Loiseau, & Morinet, 1995; Scott et al., 1997).

Patients with uncontrolled diabetes, depression, or Alzheimer's disease are also reported to experience salivary gland hypofunction and xerostomia (Lin et al., 2002; Ship et al., 1990; Sreebny et al., 1992). However, the mechanism behind the salivary gland dysfunction in these patients may be more hormonal and neurogenic in nature than inflammatory. Xerostomia and salivary gland hypofunction, as stated before, are common in elderly adults. It is currently believed that the impact of aging on the function of the major salivary glands is of no clinical significance. In general, salivary gland function is age stable across the human life span in healthy adults. The frequent signs and symptoms associated with salivary gland hypofunction that are commonly seen in geriatric patients are caused by the medical conditions commonly seen in, and xerogenic medications often utilized by, this age group.

Complications

The most common signs and symptoms associated with chronic salivary gland hypofunction and xerostomia are listed in table 4.3. Infection and inflammation are the most common associated signs (fig. 4.1). The quality of life has been reported to be reduced in patients with chronic salivary gland hypofunction (Ackerstaff et al., 2002). Since the patients may not present with any complaints, despite reduced saliva output, practitioners are often faced with irreversible complications in late stages of the disease. Chronic salivary gland hypofunction increases susceptibility to coronal and root den-

Table 4.3 Common Signs and Symptoms Associated with Chronic Salivary Gland Hypofunction

SIGNS
- Dry, chapped lips; desiccated, dry and fissured tongue
- Angular cheilitis/pseudomembranous and erythematous candidiasis
- Dental caries (cervical and root caries in particular)
- Gingivitis

SYMPTOMS
- None (often may be asymptomatic)
- Difficulty swallowing, chewing, speaking, licking stamps
- Bad taste, breath
- Sore mouth, lips, tongue
- Burning mouth, lips, tongue
- Difficulty wearing removable intra-oral prostheses
- Frequent need to sip water with food
- Frequent awakening at night with dry mouth
- Dry mouth, nose, throat

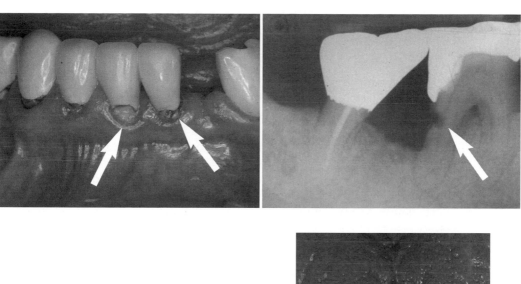

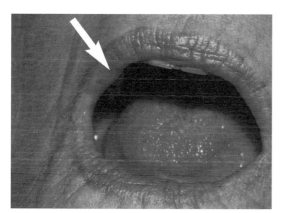

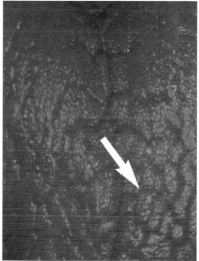

Fig. 4.1. Clinical and radiographic evidence of recurrent dental caries and dry lips and tongue in a patient with chronic salivary gland hypofunction.

tal caries. A low saliva flow rate leads to a prolonged oral sugar clearance time and could lead to root surface caries. It also could increase the risk for the development of periodontal disease by promoting plaque and calculus formation. Fungal infection caused by *Candida albicans* is another example of a common infection in the presence of chronic salivary gland hypofunction (Pedersen et al., 1999). Figure 4.1 represents the clinical oral findings in a patient with severe salivary gland hypofunction.

Clinical Significance

Because saliva plays such an important role in the maintenance of oral and systemic health, it is imperative to identify those individuals who are at risk for salivary gland hypofunction and prevent them from experiencing the

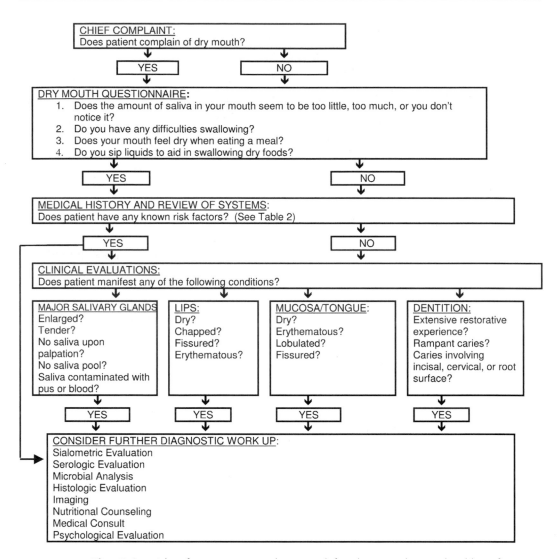

Fig. 4.2. Identifying patients with or at risk for chronic salivary gland hypofunction. (Adapted with permission of the publisher by Navazesh et al., 2002.)

possible associated complications. It is also critical to properly manage those who are affected by salivary gland hypofunction and attempt to eliminate the causative factors. The necessary steps to facilitate these processes are summarized in figure 4.2.

Evaluation of salivary gland function should be included in the first visit for every new patient examination as well as ongoing observations during subsequent visits for care delivery. Regardless of presenting complaints, there are standard questions that could identify at-risk patients. The four questions listed in figure 4.2 are some examples. The severity of any *yes* response to any of these questions could be further evaluated utilizing a 100 mm visual analog scale. During the medical history taking and review of systems, the presence, duration, and severity of any medical conditions and

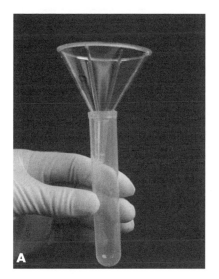
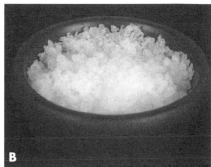
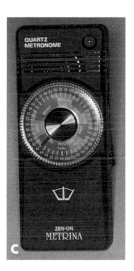
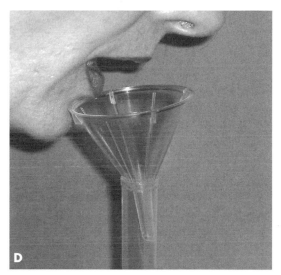

Fig. 4.3.   Salivary collection setting including (a) graduated test tube and funnel, (b) crushed ice (only if further laboratory analysis is indicated), (c) a metronome (to control chewing frequency), and (d) patient demonstrating saliva collection.

potential xerogenic medications should be documented. During clinical evaluation, the size, consistency, and response to palpation of salivary glands should be documented as well as changes involving other soft and hard tissue structures such as dry lips, fissured tongue, carious teeth, or inflamed gingiva. Based on the subjective reports and objective findings, one may choose to perform further diagnostic tests such as sialometric, serologic, microbiologic, or histologic evaluations and imaging. Most of these diagnostic tests are known to health care providers. The least known test is sialometric evaluation, and therefore, it is discussed in detail below. The setting for saliva collection is shown in figure 4.3.

Unstimulated saliva. Collecting whole saliva is easier and more cost-effective than collecting saliva from an individual gland (parotids, submandibular/sublingual) in a private practice setting. It is possible, of course, to collect from individual salivary glands by cannulation or more conveniently by using a Lashley or Curby cup (Lashley, 1999). Whole saliva can be collected under unstimulated (resting) and stimulated conditions. Patients are instructed not to drink, eat, smoke, perform oral hygiene, or put anything into their mouths for 90 minutes before the collection time. The dentist or designated staff member collects the saliva in a quiet environment, with the patient sitting in an upright position, head tilted forward and eyes open, with minimal body and orofacial movements. The patient is asked to swallow saliva first, then stay motionless and allow the saliva to drain passively for five minutes over the lower lip into a preweighed test tube fitted with a funnel. After the five-minute collection period, the patient is asked to void the mouth of saliva by spitting into a funnel.

Stimulated saliva. The clinician then collects stimulated saliva by asking the patient to chew on a piece of unflavored gum base at approximately 70 chews per minute. The patient will void the mouth of saliva by spitting into the collection tube every minute for a total of five minutes. The clinician then calculates the salivary flow rate by dividing the amount (weight or volume) of collected saliva by the duration of the collected period (five minutes). There is no general agreement about what constitutes a normal salivary flow rate. However, researchers generally consider an unstimulated flow rate of 0.1 to 0.2 ml per minute (or grams per minute) and a chewing stimulated flow rate of 0.7 ml/minute (or g/minute) for men and 0.5 ml/minute for women to be abnormally low. Currently, scientists use a 0.1 ml/minute unstimulated whole saliva flow rate as a criterion for the diagnosis of Sjögren's syndrome.

The management of patients with salivary gland hypofunction may include enhancement of daily oral hygiene, regular oral professional evaluations and care, hydration, lubrication, stimulation of salivary glands, nutritional counseling, and avoidance of irritants such as alcohol, tobacco, and sugar-containing salivary stimulants. Medications available by prescription, such as pilocarpine hydrochloride (Salagen) and cevimeline hydrochloride (Evoxac), have been the areas of focus for stimulation of salivary glands in multiple patient populations and clinical trials in recent years.

Gene therapy in animal models has also been investigated in recent years for the management of salivary gland dysfunction caused by irradiation to the head and neck areas. The ductal cells of the salivary glands are genetically reengineered and transformed to fluid-producing cells via gene therapy. More recently, gene therapy has been utilized for the management of Sjögren's syndrome in an animal model (Kok et al., 2003). An immunomodulatory gene delivered locally to the salivary glands is shown to be effective in lowering the inflammatory response and limiting the functional damage induced by the inflammatory process. The clinical application of gene therapy for the management of salivary gland dysfunction in humans will be invaluable and a reality in the future.

Current Diagnostic Values and Future Directions

Qualitative and quantitative changes of saliva may be utilized for the detection of and exposure to chemicals and pathogens or quantification of the severity of or susceptibility to different conditions (Kaufman & Lamster, 2002; Tabak, 2001). For example, the salivary levels of alcohol (ethanol), tobacco (nicotine, cotinine), cocaine, marijuana, opiate, and methadone correspond well with their concentrations in serum and are utilized as screening tools by insurance companies and law enforcement agencies to evaluate possible exposure to these chemicals. The presence in saliva of antigens or antibodies of the pathogens, such as HIV-1; HIV-2; hepatitis A, B, C; measles; mumps; or rubella, may be used to evaluate possible exposure to these pathogens. Salivary levels of microorganisms *(Streptococcus mutants* and *Lactobacillus acidophilus)* and *Candida albicans* are routinely used to assess susceptibility to dental caries and oral candidiasis, respectively (Fox, 2004; Kaufman & Lamster, 2000). Saliva could also be used to monitor disease progression and response to pharmacotherapeutic agents. Insulin, cortisol, aldosterone, estrogens, progesterone, lithium, theophilline, and caffeine are some examples. Potential salivary biomarkers for diabetes, ovarian cancer, breast cancer, oral cancer, preterm labor and exposure to the coronovirus in severe acute respiratory syndrome (SARS) have been the focus of scholarly activities by multiple scientists in recent years. With the remarkable advances in the areas of gene therapy (Voutetakis et al., 2004), microarray chip technology, and gene mapping, saliva will continue to serve as a fountain of opportunity for the advancement of science, and for risk assessment, disease prevention, and therapeutic modalities. When one licks an envelope or a stamp, a much more detailed message is transmitted than meets the eye.

For further information, the readers are encouraged to visit the following websites:

http://www.ada.org
http://www.cdc.gov
http://www.iadr.com
http://www.nidcr.nih.gov
http://www.sjogrens.org
http://www.nidcr.nih.gov

References

Ackerstaff, A. H., Tan, I. B., Rasch, C. R., Balm, A. J., Keus, R. B., Schornagel, J. H., et al. (2002). Quality-of-life assessment after supradose selective intra-arterial cisplatin and concomitant radiation (RAD-PLAT) for inoperable stage IV head and neck squamous cell carcinoma. *Archives of Otolaryngology—Head & Neck Surgery, 128,* 1185–90.

Antilla, S. S., Knuuttila, M. L., & Sakki, T. K. (1998). Depressive symptoms as an underlying factor of the sensation of dry mouth. *Psychosomatic Medicine, 60,* 215–18.

Bakke, M., Tuxen, A., Thomsen, C. E., Bardow, A., Alkjaer, T., & Jensen, B. R. (2004). Salivary cortisol level, salivary flow rate, and masticatory muscle activity in response to acute mental stress: a comparison between aged and young women. *Gerontology, 50*(6), 383–92.

Bardow, A., Pedersen, A. M. L., & Nauntofte, B. (2004). Saliva. In T. S. Miles, B. Nauntofte, & P. Svenson (eds.), *Clinical Oral Physiology*. Copenhagen: Quintessence.

Benjamins, C., Asscheman, H., & Schuurs, A. H. (1992). Increased salivary cortisol in severe dental anxiety. *Psychophysiology, 29*(3); 302–5.

Bergdahl, M. & Bergdahl, J. (2000). Low unstimulated salivary flow and subjective oral dryness: association with mediation, anxiety, depression, and stress. *Journal of Dental Research, 79*, 1652–58.

Bergdahl, M., Bergdahl, J., & Johansson, I. (1997). Depressive symptoms in individuals with idiopathic subjective dry mouth. *Journal of Oral Pathology & Medicine, 26*, 448–50.

Blom, M., & Lundeberg, T. (2000). Long-term follow-up of patients treated with acupuncture for xerostomia and the influence of additional treatment. *Oral Diseases, 6*(1), 15–24.

Bolwig, T., & Rafaelsen, O. (1972). Salivation in affective disorders. *Psychological Medicine, 2*, 232–38.

Bosch, J. A., Brand, H. S., Ligtenberg, T. J., Bermond, B., Hoogstraten J., & Amerongen, A. V. N. (1996). Psychological stress as a determinant of protein levels and saliva induced aggregation of *Streptococcus gordonii* in human whole saliva. *Psychosomatic Medicine, 58*(4), 374–82.

Brennan, M. T., Shariff, G., Lockhart, P. B., & Fox, P. C. (2002). Treatment of xerostomia: a systematic review of therapeutic trials. *Dental Clinics of North America, 46*(4), 847–56.

Davies, A. N., Broadley, K., & Beighton, D. (2001). Xerostomia in patients with advanced cancer. *Journal of Pain and Symptom Management, 22*, 820–50.

Davies, B. M., & Gurland, J. B. (1961). Salivary secretion in depressive illness. *Journal of Psychosomatic Research, 5*, 269–71.

Ferreiro, M. C., Prieto, M. H., Rodriguez, S. B., Vasquez, R. I., Iglesias, A. C., & Dios, P. D. (2002). Whole stimulated salivary flow in patients with chronic hepatitis C virus infection. *Journal of Oral Pathology & Medicine, 31*, 117–20.

Fox, P. C. (2004). Salivary enhancement therapies. *Caries Research, 38*, 241–46.

Fox, R. I., & Stern, M. (2002). Sjögren's syndrome: mechanisms of pathogenesis involved interaction of immune and neurosecretory systems. *Scandinavian Journal of Rheumatology Supplement, 116*, 3–13.

Fox, R. I., Stern, M., & Michelson, P. (2000). Update in Sjögren's syndrome. *Current Opinion in Rheumatology, 12*, 391–98.

Galard, R., Gallart, J. M., Catalyn, R., Schwartz, S., Arguello, J. M., & Castellanos, J. M. (1991). Salivary cortisol levels and their correlation with plasma ACTH levels in depressed patients before and after the DST. *American Journal of Psychiatry, 148*, 505–8.

Giddon, D. B., & Lisanti, V. F. (1962). Cholinesterase-like substance in the parotid saliva of normal and psychiatric patients. *Lancet, 1*, 725–26.

Green, M. L., Green, R. G., & Santoro, W. (1988). Daily relaxation modifies serum and salivary immunoglobulins and psychophysiologic symptom severity. *Biofeedback & Self Regulation, 13*, 187–99.

Hainsworth, J. D., Meluch, A. A., McClurkan, S., Gray, J. R., Stroup, S. L., Burris, H. A., III, et al. (2002). Introduction paclitaxel, carboplatin, and infusional 5-FU followed by concurrent radiation therapy and weekly paclitaxel/carboplatin in the treatment of locally advanced head and neck cancer: a phase II trial of the Minnie Pearl Cancer Research Network. *Cancer, 8*, 311–21.

Hasegawa, H., Uozumi, T., & Ono, K. (2004). Psychological and physiological evaluations of music listening for mental stress. *Hokkaido Igaku Zasshi, 79*(3), 225–35.

Henderson, L., Muir, M., Mills, P. R., Spence, E., Fox, R., McCruden, E. A., et al. (2001). Oral health of patients with hepatitis C virus infection: a pilot study. *Oral Diseases, 7*, 271–75.

Hill, C. M., & Walker, R. V. (2001). Salivary cortisol determinations and self-rating scales in the assessment of stress in patients undergoing the extraction of wisdom teeth. *British Dental Journal, 191*(9), 513–15.

Kaufman, K., & Lamster, I. B. (2000). Analysis of saliva for periodontal diagnosis: a review. *Journal of Clinical Periodontology, 27*, 453–65.

———. (2002). The diagnostic applications of saliva—a review. *Critical Reviews in Oral Biology and Medicine, 13*(2), 197–212.

Kok, M. R., Yamano, S., Lodde, B. M., Wang, J., Couwenhoven, R. I., Yakar, S., et al. (2003). Local adeno-associated virus-mediated interleukin 10 gene transfer has disease-modifying effects in a murine model of Sjögren's syndrome. *Human Gene Therapy, 14*(17), 1605–18.

Lashley, K. S. (1999). The human salivary reflex and its use in psychology. *Psychological Review, 23*, 446.

Lin, C. C., Sun, S. S., Kao, A., & Lee, C. C. (2002). Impaired salivary function in patients with noninsulin-dependent diabetes mellitus with xerostomia. *Journal of Diabetes and its Complications, 16*, 176–79.

Loustaud-Ratti, V., Rishe, A., Liozon, E., Labrousse, F., Soria, P., Rogez, S., et al. (2001). Prevalence and characteristics of Sjögren's syndrome or Sicca syndrome in chronic hepatitis C virus infection: a prospective study. *Journal of Rheumatology, 28*, 2245–51.

Mandel, I. D. (1993). Salivary diagnosis: promises, promises. In D. Malamud & L. Tabak (eds.), *Annals of the New York Academy of Sciences: Vol. 694. Saliva As a Diagnostic Fluid* (pp. 1–10). New York: The New York Academy of Sciences.

Mariette, X., Loiseau, P., & Morinet, F. (1995). Hepatitis C virus in saliva. *Annals of Internal Medicine, 122*, 556.

Miluk-Kolasa, B., Obminski, Z., Stupnicki, R., & Golec, L. (1994). Effects of music treatment on salivary cortisol in patients exposed to presurgical stress. *Experimental & Clinical Endocrinology, 102*(2), 118–20.

Nagler, R. M. (1998). Effects of radiotherapy and chemotherapeutic cytokines on a human salivary cell line. *Anticancer Research, 18*, 309–14.

Neudeck, P., Jacoby, G. E., & Florin, I. (2001). Dexamethasone suppression test using saliva cortisol measurement in bulimia nervosa. *Physiology & Behavior, 72*(1–2), 93–98.

Pedersen, A. M., Reibel, J., Nordgarden, H., Bergem, H. O., Jensen, J. L., & Nauntofte, B. (1999). Primary Sjögren's syndrome: salivary gland function and clinical oral findings. *Oral Diseases, 5*, 128–38.

Piollet, I., Lepine, J. P., Guechot, J., Philip, E., Rouillon, F., Fiet, J., et al. (1984). Plasma and saliva DST (dexamethasone suppression test) in depression. Clinical applications and kinetic approach. *Encephale, 10*(6), 279–80.

Pow, E. H., McMillan, A. S., Leung, W. K., Wong, M. C., & Kwong, D. L. (2003). Salivary gland function and xerostomia in southern Chinese following radiotherapy for nasopharyngeal carcinoma. *Clinical Oral Investigations, 74*, 230–34.

Riad, M., Barton, J. R., & Wilson, J. A. (1991). Parotid salivary secretory pattern in bulimia nervosa. *Acta Oto-Laryngologica, 111*, 392–95.

Roberts, M. W., Tylenda, C. A., Sonies, B. C., & Elin, R. J.(1989). Dyspaghia in bulimia nervosa. *Dysphagia, 4*, 106–11.

Scott, C. A., Avellini, C., Desinan, L., Pirisi, M., Ferraccioli, G. F., Bardus, P., et al. (1997). Chronic lymphocytic sialadenitis in HCV-related chronic liver disease: comparison of Sjögren's syndrome. *Histopathology, 30*, 41–48.

Ship, J. A., DeCarli, C., Friedland, R. P., & Baum, B. J. (1990). Diminished submandibular salivary flow in dementia of the Alzheimer type. *Gerontology, 46*, 61–66.

Singh, N., Scully, C., & Joyston-Bechal, S. (1996). Oral complications of cancer therapies: prevention and management. *Clinical Oncology (Royal College of Radiologists), 8*, 15–24.

Sreebny, L. M., & Schwartz, S. S. (1988). A reference guide to drugs and dry mouth. *Gerodontology, 4,* 66–70.

——. (1997). A reference guide to drugs and dry mouth—2nd edition. *Gerodontology, 14,* 33–47.

Sreebny, L. M., Yu, A., Green, A., & Valdini, A. (1992). Xerostomia in diabetes mellitus. *Diabetes Care, 15,* 900–904.

Stones, A., Groome, D., Perry, D., Hucklebridge, F., & Evans, P. (1999). The effect of stress on salivary cortisol in panic disorder patients. *Journal of Affective Disorders, 52*(1–3), 197–201.

Tabak, L. A. (2001). A revolution in biomedical assessment: the development of salivary diagnostics. *Journal of Dental Education, 65*(12), 1335–39.

Takai, N., Yamaguchi, M., Aragaki, T., Eto, K., Uchihashi, K., & Nishikawa, Y. (2004). Effect of psychological stress on the salivary cortisol and amylase levels in healthy young adults. *Archives of Oral Biology, 49*(12), 963–68.

Tu, G., Kapur, B., & Isreal, Y. (1992). Characteristics of a new urine, serum, and saliva alcohol reagent strip. *Alcohol Clinical & Experimental Research, 16,* 222–27.

Voutetakis, A., Kok, M. R., Zheng, C., Bossis, I., Wang, J., Cotrim, A. P., et al. (2004). Reengineered salivary glands are stable endogenous bioreactors for systemic gene therapeutics. *Proceedings of the National Academy of Sciences, 101,* 3053–58.

Biofeedback in the Treatment of Myofascial Pain Disorder and Temporomandibular Joint Pain

A. G. Forgione and Bruce L. Mehler

This chapter is an introduction to biofeedback for the dental student and dental professional pursuing postgraduate studies. Following a review of the literature on biofeedback treatment in dentistry, technical and practical aspects of surface electromyography (sEMG) are presented in some depth because of both its utility as a training modality and its growing use in the study of the muscular components of the cranio-cervical-mandibular system and occlusion.

Introduction

Elevated muscle activity, muscle imbalance, muscle irritability, weakness, poor control, or muscle-substitution patterns frequently appear either as causes or as functional symptoms in cases of temporomandibular and my-ofascial pain disorders. Consequently, the ability to objectively monitor muscle activity appears to offer promise both as an important assessment tool and as a modality for treatment using biofeedback training techniques.

Biofeedback is a therapeutic method that involves (fig. 5.1) the amplification of a human biological signal, which is then usually presented visually or audibly to sense receptors (the eyes and ears) designed by nature for detection of stimuli in the external world (exteroceptive stimuli). The body's capacity for fine discrimination of interoceptive signals is crude when compared with the normal operation of these exteroceptive sense receptors. The biofeedback method allows the patient or therapist or both to observe subtle

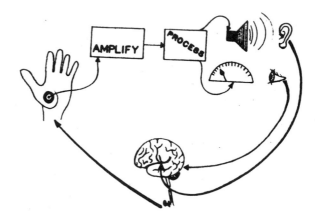

Fig. 5.1. Schematic of a biofeedback loop.

changes in internal activity and provides information (feedback) that can be utilized to modify these physiological events in a desired direction while they are in process. In the treatment of pain conditions, biofeedback training is typically directed at decreasing inappropriate psychophysiological arousal, although the role for rehabilitative training focused on learning adaptive patterns of muscle activation in cases of inappropriate muscle inhibition and substitution during dynamic motion should not be overlooked.

Figure 5.2 shows that there are three avenues of entry to the nervous system to obtain low arousal states:

1. The *central nervous system,* which requires broad methods to evoke patterns of response (i.e., hypnosis, yoga, cognitive behavior therapy, and meditation)
2. The *autonomic nervous system*, which is quieted by diaphragmatic breathing (pranayama)
3. The *somatic-motor system,* which may be addressed through surface electromyography (sEMG) as well as other techniques such as Jacobsonian progressive muscle relaxation and massage.

Figure 5.3 shows various types of biofeedback devices and the avenue of entry commonly employed. Monitoring the central nervous system, as through EEG (electroencephalography), is an area of active investigation but has not been demonstrated to have a direct application at this time in dentistry. The autonomic system has been monitored by the GSR (galvanic skin response), GSP (galvanic skin potential), heart rate, blood volume, and hand temperature. Even though temperature feedback devices are currently fairly inexpensive, the use of thermal feedback to induce general quiescence has not become popular in dental practice. The same can be said of every other feedback method except surface electromyographic biofeedback (sEMG). The interested reader is referred to Basmajian (1989) and Schwartz and Andrasik (2003) for a broader description of biofeedback devices.

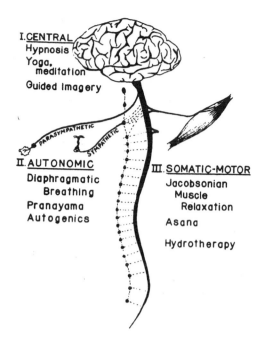

Fig. 5.2. Methods of "relaxation."

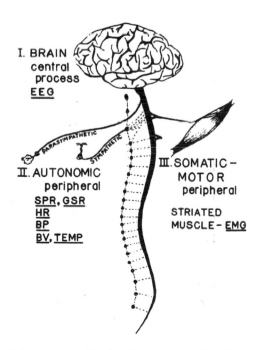

Fig. 5.3. Types of biofeedback devices for the avenues of entry.

Historical Development

Self-regulation, the practice of voluntary modification of one's own physiological activity, motor behavior, or conscious processes, has been a human endeavor for ages. It is impossible to date the origin of Zen and yoga meditation. Stoyva (1978) reported that in 1901, Bair taught subjects to wiggle their ears if they received feedback information. His biofeedback device was a system of levers and a kymograph. In 1888, Charles Fere (Fowles, 1986) reported that the surface resistance of the skin varied as a function of cognitive activity and sensory stimulation. A direct approach to the autonomic nervous system was opened.

Budyznski and Stoyva published in 1969 on a new method to produce deep muscle relaxation by "analog information feedback." Frontalis muscle tension was reduced to a greater degree with biofeedback than with no feedback. In 1973, they applied their method, which provided immediate auditory and visual feedback to the masseter muscle of forty subjects and no feedback to a control group of forty. In this paper, they outlined a shaping technique to provide gradual relaxation by successive approximations to the deeply relaxed state. Graduated steps reduce the chance of error, which would have occurred had the steps been too large. Eighty males were assigned to groups of twenty. Two experimental groups received the shaping method with the biofeedback of either an auditory signal or a visual signal. There was no difference between the auditory signal or the visual biofeedback signal. Both control groups, one a steady tone, the other, no tone, received no feedback. Their tension levels were significantly higher than the biofeedback groups. It was in this paper that Budyznski and Stoyva proposed a method for treatment of nocturnal bruxism and myofascial pain dysfunction syndrome.

Budyznski and Stoyva's work was followed in 1975 by clinical reports by Carlsson, Gale, and Ohman and by Gessel on the use of EMG biofeedback in temporomandibular disorders (TMD) and Cannistraci (1976) on biofeedback and bruxism. Most major texts on biofeedback now include discussions on applications with dental patients (Cannistraci & Fritz, 1989; Glaros & Lausten, 2003).

Meta-analysis

Crider and Glaros (1999) examined outcome evaluations of treatments performed with sEMG to determine the efficacy of these studies and to estimate treatment effect size. Thirteen studies of sEMG biofeedback treatment for TMD were analyzed, consisting of six controlled, four comparative treatment, and three uncontrolled trials. Three types of outcome were used: pain reports, clinical exam findings, and ratings of global improvement.

Five of the six controlled trials found EMG biofeedback treatments to be superior to no treatment or psychological placebo controls for at least one of the three types of outcome. Data from twelve studies contributed to a meta-analysis that compared pretreatment- to posttreatment-effect sizes for EMG biofeedback treatments to effect sizes for control conditions. Mean effect sizes for both reported pain and clinical exam outcomes were substantially larger for biofeedback treatments than for control conditions. In addition, 69% of patients who received EMG biofeedback treatments were rated as symptom-free or significantly improved, compared with 35% of patients treated with a variety of placebo interventions. Follow-up outcomes for EMG biofeedback treatments showed no deterioration from posttreatment levels. The authors concluded that the outcomes of these studies support the efficacy of EMG of biofeedback treatments for TMD.

Another meta-analysis (fifty-one studies) was performed by Fernandez and Turk (1989). The results supported their view that there are long-term advantages when using cognitive behavioral skills training (CBST) over dental and pharmacological techniques in managing TMD-related pain. Flor and Birbaumer (1993) compared CBST, biofeedback, and conservative medical treatment in chronic back and TMD. Treatment with biofeedback produced the most change. At six and twenty-four months, only the biofeedback group maintained the significant decrease in pain severity.

Gardea, Gatchel, and Mishra (2001) ran a study that eliminated many shortcomings in earlier research. Chronic patients were assigned to one of three biobehavioral treatment groups—biofeedback, CBST, a combination of biofeedback and CBST, or a no-treatment comparison group with each group performing a one-year follow-up. The major finding was that for pain scores, the biofeedback and combined groups showed the greatest improvement. The combined group showed the greatest improvement on pain-related disability. The one year follow-up showed that the biofeedback group was most effective in reducing TMD pain.

Dahlstrom (1989), in an exhaustive review, examined twelve studies that used sEMG. In one study, Carlsson and Gale (1977) treated eleven TMD patients in six to eight sessions finding that eight were significantly improved. Dohrman and Laskin (1978) treated sixteen myofascial pain disorder (MPD) patients with masseter muscle biofeedback training and eight patients with "placebo feedback." Mean levels of masseter activity were significantly reduced in patients in the experimental group. Only one biofeedback patient required further treatment while five of the eight controls required additional intervention. In another study (Stenn, Mothersill, & Brooke, 1979), masseter activity was measured in eleven longstanding subjects. Six of the patients were given masseter feedback with relaxation training for eight sessions. The remaining five were given relaxation training and masseter activity recorded with no feedback. All patients also received cognitive behavior modification. A significant reduction of masseter activity in all subjects occurred with no difference between groups. There was a significant reduction in number of symptoms and signs of MPD in all subjects. This study shows that multiple modes of therapy increase the probability of successful treatment, but, given a choice, biofeedback alone appears to be most effective.

Of all types of biofeedback, only sEMG is close to meeting the needs of dentistry. Biofeedback of surface EMG provides the dentist with a method of treating TMDs and a method of performing assessments of muscle status and function should the need arise. In spite of its emergence in the 1960s, however, one is hard put to find sEMG biofeedback in the curriculum of many dental schools.

In the near future, however, the potential of biofeedback is that it will play a more significant a role in assessment and treatment. Physical therapy has made rapid advances in muscle assessment in many body areas but not in mandibular function. The door is open to make muscular assessments part of the patient record in the years to come.

Biofeedback in Clinical Practice

Surface EMG biofeedback employs instrumentation to monitor subtle changes in muscular physiological activity and to deliver that information to a patient to assist in learning to modify the activity in a desired direction. In this learning environment, the dentist or an assistant frequently assumes the role of a coach, helping the patient understand (discriminate) the feedback information, suggesting strategies to employ to move in the desired direction, providing encouragement (reinforcement) for targeted behavior, and adjusting training goals (shaping) as needed. In a way, biofeedback becomes the setting of a social interaction that is inexorably bound with the instrument. Even though this can be said of almost any treatment, the interaction with the instrument maintains some distance between clinician and patient. This can be useful in situations where the patient has difficulty learning the task; the clinician does not have to take on the role of "judging" the patient, telling them they have to relax, but instead the clinician can become an ally who assists the patient in trying to learn from the machine. The use of a device maintains constancy, which reduces variability.

A feedback device can be as simple as a mirror that is used to visually demonstrate to a patient when one shoulder is being held higher than another and when they are in balance. But typically, biofeedback devices are electronic instruments that can detect extremely small physiological changes and provide direct feedback (information) about activity in the form of visual or auditory signals. Biofeedback devices may be relatively basic units that indicate physiological changes by means of a moving light bar or a simple tone that changes in pitch as a physiological variable changes. Alternatively, computer-based systems are available that monitor a range of physiological parameters at the same time and that provide detailed visual and auditory display options, as well as offering extensive data reduction and report-generation capabilities.

In some instances, the feedback may be indirect, where the clinician observes the instrument and provides the patient with cues indicating whether activity is moving in a desired or nondesired direction. More commonly in dental practice, the meaning of the feedback signal is simply explained ("down means lower muscle tension") and suggestions are provided to start the feedback process ("focus on slowing your breathing and allow your jaw to gradually drop"). Biofeedback displays can be quite engaging, and some patients will respond to a visual display of unbalanced bilateral masseter or trapezius activity by immediately trying to bring the two signals into balance. Other patients will require more active guidance. For an extended consideration of biofeedback principles and clinical technique, the edited volumes by Basmajian (1989) and Schwartz and Andrasik (2003) are standard references.

There are many approaches to relaxation training for pain and stress management ranging from progressive muscle relaxation to techniques involving varying emphasis on the use of imagery, breathing, autogenic phrasing, or hypnotic suggestion (Lehrer & Woolfolk, 1993; Turk, Meichenbaum, & Genest, 1983). The question is sometimes posed as to whether a particular relaxation training technique or biofeedback is more effective as a treatment modality. It can be argued that in many situations, it is the combination of relaxation training and biofeedback that is effective. For many patients, biofeedback monitoring during (or before and after) a relaxation training session helps to demonstrate that the relaxation training procedure is producing a measurable change in their bodies. This may be the crucial step in helping a patient "buy into" the prescription that they practice the relaxation procedure outside of the clinic. In a similar fashion, knowing that their progress is going to be visible on the biofeedback device influences the motivation of some patients to practice at home between clinic sessions since their progress can be measured objectively with a screen.

While this chapter focuses on muscle-related biofeedback, it is important to note that some patients may present with anxiety or stress-related symptoms. These problems are not in the realm of dentistry unless fear of dental treatment is the focus. This area is covered in other parts of this book (see part II, Anxiety, Fear, and Pain). It is suggested that the novice devote himself or herself to one method. The view that patients can use sEMG as a method of relaxation training is sound and supported by research.

Electromyography as a Measure of Muscle Activity

Electromyography (EMG) measures muscle activity by detecting changes in electrical potential that are associated with muscle action potentials. Muscle action potentials are similar to the action potentials that are generated in nerve cells, involving rapid changes in the relative concentrations of ionic charges across the cell membrane. When a motor neuron stimulates a muscle fiber, a wave of depolarization propagates bidirectionally along the length of the fiber resulting in a cascade of molecular interactions that cause the fiber to contract. Muscle activity, such as the contraction of the masseter muscle to close the jaw, is the result of the summed activity of many muscle fibers. The overall strength of a muscle contraction is a function of both the number of fibers recruited and the frequency of firing of individual fibers.

Surface electromyography (sEMG) is a noninvasive technique that places relatively large recording electrodes on the surface of the skin over a muscle or muscles of interest. Like fine-wire EMG, sEMG provides a measure of the summed electrical activity of groups of muscle fibers, but does so for a much larger area of muscle and without the discomfort and complications of inserting a lead through the skin. With proper instrumentation and recording technique, sEMG is a highly reliable measure of muscle activity across repetitions and testing days, obtaining reliability coefficients superior to that of invasive-wire EMG recordings (Giroux & Lamontagne, 1990; Komi & Buskirk, 1970) and providing more information about functional activity level (Sihvonen et al., 1991). It should be noted that EMG does have some limitations in that it can not detect activity in deep muscle groups except when contractions from these groups are relatively strong (Wolf et al., 1991).

Detecting the EMG Signal

The magnitude of the EMG signal that appears at the surface of the skin is extremely low when compared to the forms of electrical energy with which we are familiar. A fully charged standard flashlight battery has a rated electrical potential of 1.5 volts. In comparison, a surface EMG reading from the forearm of a relaxed individual might be measured at 1.5 microvolts, one millionth the voltage of the battery. Besides this low-level electrical activity from muscle at the skin surface, external sources of electrical activity may also be present. These other sources are referred to as "noise" and include radio frequency waves (from radio and television stations, cell phones, microwaves) and interference from power-line sources (fluorescent lights, dimmer switches, heating units, air-conditioner motors, X-ray machine power supplies). These additional sources of electrical signal may be present at the level of several hundred microvolts, easily masking muscle activity. As late as the 1960s and 1970s, quality sEMG recordings were typically carried out in special wire-mesh enclosures to shield the subject from these external noise sources. Advances in electronics and instrumentation design have allowed sEMG recording to move out of the laboratory and made it into a practical measure that can be carried out in most office settings. A basic understanding of some of these features is important in determining the suitability of an sEMG unit for various dental applications. Proper clinical technique can also affect the quality of sEMG recordings. Both issues are addressed in the following sections.

Surface EMG Sensors and Recording Techniques

Sensor Placement

Modern surface EMG systems are based on a differential amplifier design that involves the placement of two active (sensing) contacts on the surface of skin over the muscle of interest. Ideally, the two active contacts should be positioned so that an imaginary line drawn between them runs in parallel with the orientation of the muscle fibers. Since the muscle action potentials propagate along the length of the muscle fiber, the instantaneous electrical potential will differ at two points along the length of the muscle at a given moment in time while the signal from external electrical noise sources will tend to be at the same level at both points. The EMG instrument cancels out (subtracts) the signal that is common at the two points (the noise component) and amplifies the remaining (differential) signal that represents muscle activity. If the active contacts are placed perpendicular (across the muscle fibers), the temporal characteristics of the EMG signal at the two points will be similar and more of the muscle signal will be canceled along with the external noise sources.

A third contact, known as the reference, is generally placed an equal distance from the two active contacts, either over the muscle of interest or on a more distant, electrically neutral location such as the ear lobe. (Alternate terms for the third contact are "ground," which dates back to the time when electrical recording devices were literally grounded to the earth, and "common" since the electrical activity from both active contact points are referenced to this common location.) Multichannel instruments (units that are designed to measure activity from more than one muscle at a time) may use a single reference contact for the entire system or may utilize a reference sensor for each pair of active contacts.

Preamplified Sensors

Classic EMG systems have long cables connecting the sensing contacts to the instrument. These cables can act as antennas, picking up electrical noise along their length and, because of the very low voltage of the EMG signal, can be susceptible to artifact from cable sway when subjects move during dynamic activity. Some EMG systems offer preamplified sensors, often called active electrodes, that place noise rejection circuitry and an amplification stage at or near the skin site. These amplified sensor assemblies tend to be larger than nonamplified, but offer advantages in noise and artifact rejection, particularly when assessments are conducted that involve movement.

Types of Electrodes

Most current surface EMG sensor systems are designed to use disposable electrodes that combine a conductive metal contact surrounded by adhesive foam or tape to affix the sensor to the skin. The metallic contact may be flat (for use with or without a thin film of conductive electrode gel) or may be cup shaped (to be filled with electrode gel). When using cup-style electrodes, it is important to make sure the cup is filled completely; air pockets or gaps between the gel and the skin reduce the effective contact area and degrade signal quality. Overfilling the electrode cup can result in the gel being forced under the adhesive when the electrode is pressed onto the skin. This can result in the sensor coming loose from the skin. If the gel spreads across the skin and makes contact between closely spaced sensors (bridging), this will decrease the quality of the recording. Pregelled electrodes are available, however, they tend to be more expensive and have limited shelf life (as the gel tends to dry out). If the signal quality of pregelled electrodes is suspect, applying a thin film of electrode gel to the pregelled surface will generally "revive" the electrode. Electrodes that have dark gray or black surface are silver/silver chloride and should always be used with electrode gel.

Skin Preparation

Oils, dirt, and dry skin cells all impact significantly on the conductivity of the pathway between the skin and the sensor. Cleaning the skin with isopropyl alcohol is strongly recommended regardless of how "clean" the skin surface may appear. The introduction of preamplified sensors with "dry" recording capability has greatly increased the ability of high-end instruments to detect EMG activity under poor recording conditions, however, signal quality can invariably be improved by wiping the skin with alcohol and applying electrode gel. Hair tends to push the electrode away from the skin surface. Where hair is thick, it may be necessary to shave the site to obtain a reliable recording.

Quantifying EMG Activity

When reading about or discussing EMG readings with colleagues, it is important to be aware that various methods may be used for quantifying the EMG signal. The details of the different approaches are not as important as recognizing that a given level of muscle activity can be assigned a different numerical value depending on whether peak-to-peak, peak, root mean square (RMS), or integrated average methodology is used. A sign wave varying in amplitude by +/- one volt is quantified as 2.0 volts peak-to-peak, 1.0 volt peak, 0.707 volts RMS, and 0.637 integrated average. To put this in more familiar terms, the electrical power from a standard wall outlet would be rated as 310, 155, 110, or 99 volts, respectively. A research study of averaged resting values for the masseter muscle in asymptomatic patients using peak-to-peak quantification would be likely to report values more than twice as large as the values that would be expected using RMS quantification.

It is also important to take into account the frequency characteristics of a particular model of EMG instrument when comparing data from different settings. Instruments employing wideband filters (see discussion on frequency below) will detect more of the underlying EMG signal than instruments using a more restrictive frequency range. For a more in-depth consideration of surface EMG, the classic work in the field is Basmajian and DeLuca (1989). More easily accessible references are the companion works of Cram and Kasman (1998) and Kasman, Cram, and Wolf (1998).

Considerations in Selecting an sEMG Instrument

Surface EMG instruments intended for biofeedback applications are available in stand-alone and computer-based configurations. A typical stand-alone instrument is battery powered and easily portable. Early designs often quantified EMG activity by means of a scaled meter with a moving needle to represent instantaneous readings. Current units are more likely to use a series of LEDs that light up sequentially (a light bar) to represent changing levels of activity. A digital display may also be included to provide more precise quantification. High-end units may provide options to display peak values or averaged values on the digital display. The term "channel" is generally used to describe the number of sites that can be monitored at the same time. Most stand-alone EMG units are single-channel designs, although some dual-channel units exist. In the hands of a competent therapist, a stand-alone sEMG device with simple auditory or visual feedback capacity can be very useful for carrying out basic biofeedback-assisted relaxation training. Dual-channel capability is a distinct plus for evaluating and training patients with muscle-imbalance problems. (It is appropriate to note that two single-channel units can fill the same role as a dual-channel instrument.)

Multichannel computer-based systems that can automatically record and display patterned muscle activity over time provide a valuable tool in assessing muscular-skeletal-dentition dynamics as a function of posture and bite, and in response to bite guards, splints, and other dental appliances. The capacity to measure more than one pair of muscles at a time enhances the practitioner's ability to develop a full picture of potentially complex muscle interactions. In these situations, computer-based systems providing two, four, or even eight channels of sEMG are worth considering.

Computer-based systems generally consist of an instrumentation unit that is connected to a standard PC-style computer using a dedicated interface card, serial port, or USB connection. Computer requirements (operating system, processor speed, memory, etc.) vary greatly and should be checked with the manufacturer before acquiring a system. Most systems are designed to allow the computer to run other applications when not being used for EMG monitoring. Software for the instrument may be designed specifically for biofeedback, may support both assessment and biofeedback training protocols, or may be intended primarily for research. The ease of use of software packages varies significantly and should be evaluated carefully when selecting an instrument.

Laptops and Electrical Interference

Computers must be properly grounded or their connection to the electrical system and/or their power supplies can be significant sources of electrical interference that can overwhelm the noise-rejection capabilities of the EMG unit. This is not generally an issue for desktop computers since grounded power supplies are standard. If you are acquiring a laptop computer for EMG use, select a model with a grounded transformer (a power supply with a three-prong power cord). If this is not an option, it may be necessary to run the laptop on battery power. (Make sure that the power cord is disconnected from the wall, not just at the back of the computer, as the built-in transformer that is part of the power-cord assembly continues to radiate significant electrical interference.)

Frequency Range

As mentioned previously, the electrical potential measured by the sEMG represents the grouped activity of many muscle fibers firing in varying sequence and at different rates. At the surface of the skin, this activity spans a frequency range from several cycles per second through approximately 500 Hz, with the dominant energy falling in the range of 50 to 150 Hz (Basmajian & De Luca, 1985; De Luca, 1994). Activity above 500 Hz is most likely external electrical artifact, and appropriately designed sEMG instruments use hardware circuits and/or sophisticated mathematical transformations in software processing to reduce these higher frequency signals. The lower range of the EMG signal can be contaminated with external noise from wall power and from biological sources such as EKG and EEG activity. Early biofeedback instrument designs frequently limited (filtered out) signals below 100 Hz. to minimize these sources of artifact. Subsequent research has demonstrated that the spectral characteristics of the EMG signal sift dramatically into the lower frequency range as muscles become fatigued (Basmajian & De Luca, 1985; Cram & Kasman, 1998). This may result in a situation where significant muscle activity (tension) is present, but is ignored by the filter design of some instruments.

Removing higher frequency signals is known as low-pass filtering; removing signals at the lower end of the frequency spectrum is known as high-pass filtering. The resulting range of signals that are "passed" by the combined filters is known as the bandpass. All things being equal, it is suggested that the ideal low-end settings for a sEMG biofeedback system should be in the range of 10 to 35 Hz. and the upper boundary in the 300 to 500 Hz range. As an example, the instruments in use at the Craniofacial Pain Center employ a 25-to-450-Hz bandpass. The addition of a notch filter set specifically to suppress wall-power interference at 60 Hz (50 Hz in some countries) is often a useful feature in units intended primarily for use in a dental office surrounded by a variety of motorized devices.

Selecting Muscles for Training

It is important to consider the training goal and individual characteristics of a particular patient when selecting a muscle site or muscles for biofeedback training. Perhaps the most common image of biofeedback-assisted relaxation training is of a patient sitting in a reclining chair with EMG sensors aligned horizontally across the patient's forehead (which will pick up undifferentiated activity from each frontalis, the corrugator, the temporalis, and contributions from the masseters if they are sufficiently activated). This generalized frontal placement does not allow for any specificity of muscle training but is often useful when the patients carry elevated tension levels broadly through their facial musculature and the training goal aims at general relaxation. (Cram and Kasman [1998] provide a detailed atlas of both generalized and muscle-specific placements.) However, it is important to recognize that while some patients may present with generalized patterns of muscle tension, muscular problems can be quite site specific in others (Mehta & Forgione, 1994). For a patient who presents with elevated resting activity in the right masseter and modest or low levels of activity in the left, training to bring the two muscles more into balance may be more significant than lowering overall levels of muscle activity. Clinicians should also be aware of the phenomena of referred muscle pain (Simons et al., 1999). Unremarkable temporalis or frontalis EMG levels may be recorded in a patient complaining of pain in the temporal-frontal region while additional investigation may reveal hyperactivity in the sternocleidomastoid or upper trapezius muscles, which can refer pain to these areas. Multisite assessment of a particular patient's pattern of muscle activity at rest and during functional activation of the musculature of mastication is strongly recommended.

Summary

The advances of technology have allowed miniaturization of very sensitive recording devices that make real-time monitoring of the muscles of cranio-cervical-mandibular system a straightforward office procedure. The biobehavioral treatment TMDs, including surface EMG biofeedback training, is a conservative approach that is less expensive than more traditional treatment and is a reversible procedure. There is at this time an adequate number of studies to suggest the value of including biofeedback in dental practice.

References

Basmajian, J. V., & De Luca, C. J. (1985). *Muscles Alive.* 5th ed. Baltimore: Williams and Wilkins.

Basmajian, J. V., ed. (1989). *Biofeedback: Principles and Practice for Clinicians.* 3d ed. Baltimore: Williams & Wilkins.

Budyznski, T. H., & Stoyva, J. M. (1969). An instrument for producing deep muscle relaxation by means of analog information feedback. *Journal of Applied Behavior Analysis, 2,* 231–37.

——. (1973). An electromyographic feedback technique for teaching voluntary relaxation of masseter muscle. *Journal Dental Research, 52,* 116.

Cannistraci, A. J. (1976). A method to control bruxism: biofeedback-assisted relaxation therapy. *Journal of the American Society for Preventative Dentistry, 6,* 12–15.

Cannistraci, A. J., & Fritz, G. (1989). Dental applications of biofeedback. In J. V. Basmajian (ed.), *Biofeedback: Principles and Practices for Clinicians.* 3d ed. Baltimore: Williams & Wilkins.

Carlsson, S. G., & Gale, E. N. (1977). Biofeedback in the treatment of long-term temporomandibular joint pain. *Biofeedback and Self-Regulation, 2,* 161–71.

Carlsson, S. G., Gale, E. N., & Ohman, A. (1975). Treatment of temporomadibular joint syndrome with biofeedback training. *Journal of the American Dental Association, 91,* 602–05.

Cram, J. R., & Kasman, G. S. (1998). *Introduction to Surface Electromyography.* Gaithersburg, MD: Aspen Publishers, Inc.

Crider, A. B., & Glaros, A. G. (1999). A meta-analysis of EMG biofeedback treatment of temporomandibular disorders. *Journal of Orofacial Pain, 13,* 29–37.

Dahlstrom, L. (1989). Electromyographic studies of craniomandibular disorders: a review of the literature. *Journal of Oral Rehabilitation, 16(1),* 1–20.

De Luca, C. J. (1994). *Surface Electromyography: Detection and Recording.* Monograph. Boston: NeuroMuscular Research Center, Boston University.

Dohrman, R. S., & Laskin, D. M. (1978). An evaluation of electromyographic biofeedback in the treatment of myofacial pain-dysfunction syndrome. *Journal of the American Dental Association, 96,* 656–62.

Fernandez, E., & Turk, D. C. (1989). The utility of cognitive coping strategies for altering pain perception: a meta-analysis. *Pain, 38,* 123–35.

Flor, H., & Birbaumer, N. (1993). Comparison of efficacy of electromyographic biofeedback, cognitive-behavioral therapy, and conservative medical interventions in the treatment of chronic musculo-skeletal pain. *Journal of Consulting and Clinical Psychology, 61,* 653–58.

Fowles, D. C. (1986). The eccrine system and electrodermal activity. In M. G. H. Coles, E. Donchin, & S. W. Porges (eds.), *Psychophysiology: Systems, Processes, and Applications.* New York: The Guilford Press.

Gardea, M. A., Gatchel, R. J., & Mishra, K. D. (2001). Long-term efficacy of behavioral treatment of temporomandibular disorders. *Journal of Behavioral Medicine, 24(4)*, 341–89.

Gessel, A. H. (1975). Electromyographic biofeedback and tricyclic antidepressants in myofascial pain-dysfunction syndrome: psychological predictors of outcome. *Journal of the American Dental Association, 91*, 1048–52.

Giroux, B., & Lamontagne, M. (1990). Comparisons between surface electrodes and intermuscular wire electrodes in isometric and dynamic conditions. *Electromyography and Clinical Neurophysiology, 30*, 397–405.

Glaros, A. G., & Lausten, L. (2003). Temporomandibular disorders. In M. S. Schwartz & F. Andrasik (eds.), *Biofeedback: A Practitioner's Guide*. 3d ed. New York: Guilford Press.

Kasman, G. S., Cram, J. R., & Wolf, S. L. (1998). *Clinical Applications in Surface Electromyography*. Gaithersburg, MD: Aspen Publishers, Inc.

Komi, P. V., & Buskirk, E. R. (1970). Reproducibility of electromyographic measurements with inserted wire electrodes and surface electrodes. *Electromyography, 4*, 357–67.

Lehrer, P. M., & Woolfolk, R. L. (1993). *Principles and Practice of Stress Management*. 2d ed. New York: Guilford Press.

Mehta, N., & Forgione, A. G. (1994). The effect of macroposture and body mechanics on dental occlusion. In H. Gelb (ed.), *New Concepts in Craniomandibular and Chronic Pain Management*. Japan: Ishikawa.

Schwartz, M. S., & Andrasik, F. (eds.). (2003). *Biofeedback: A Practitioner's Guide*. 3d ed. New York: Guilford Press.

Sihvonen, T., Partanen, J., Hanninen, O., & Soimakallio, S. (1991). Electric behavior of low back muscles during lumbar pelvic rhythm in low back pain patients and healthy controls. *Archives of Physical Medicine and Rehabilitation, 72*, 1080–87.

Simons, D. G., Travell, J. G., Simons, L. S., & Travell, J. G. (1999). *Travell & Simons' Myofascial Pain and Dysfunction: The Trigger Point Manual*. 2d ed. Baltimore: Williams & Wilkins.

Stenn, P. G., Mothersill, K. J., & Brooke, R. I. (1979). Biofeedback and a cognitive behavioral approach to treatment of myofascial pain dysfunction syndrome. *Behavior Therapy, 10*, 29–36.

Stoyva, J. (1978). Editorial. *Biofeedback and Self-Regulation, 3*, 329.

Turk, D. C., Meichenbaum, D., & Genest, M. (1983). *Pain and Behavioral Medicine: A Cognitive-Behavioral Perspective*. New York: Guilford Press.

Wolf, L. B., Segal, R. L., Wolf, S. L., & Nyberg, R. (1991). Quantitative analysis of surface and percutaneous electromyographic activity in lumbar erector spinae of normal young women. *Spine, 16(2)*, 155–61.

Hypnosis in Dentistry

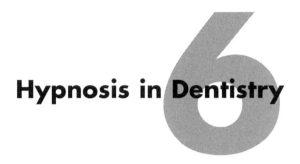

Bruce Peltier

If M. Mesmer had no other secret than how to put the imagination into motion effectively, for health purposes, would not that still be a marvelous blessing? If the medicine of imagination is best, should we not practice the medicine of imagination?

— B. Franklin and others, 1784

Hypnosis has been available to dentistry for centuries, yet it is underutilized and widely misunderstood. This chapter describes the essential nature of hypnosis and recommends applications that should be learned and used by every competent modern dentist. The subject is too vast and complex to be covered here, consequently, the goal of this chapter is to introduce hypnosis, dispel inhibiting myths, and provide a map along with encouragement for exploration. A proper understanding of hypnosis can enhance the experience of both dentist and patient, and dentists who fail to apply basic hypnotic principles are letting their patients down.

A Brief History of Clinical Hypnosis

Hypnosis has a storied past, filled with mystery and misunderstanding. Hypnotic practice has suffered by being caught between implausibly exaggerated claims and overwrought skepticism. The literature on hypnosis is littered with reports such as Ewin's 1992 study titled "Hypnotherapy for warts (verruca vulgaris): 41 consecutive cases with 33 cures" and Willard's (1977) purportedly successful research on "breast enlargement through visual imagery and hypnosis." Nonetheless, it has survived over the centuries while other nonphysical forms of healing have not. The American Medical Association officially endorsed hypnosis as a treatment modality in 1958, recommending its inclusion in mainstream medical training (Wester, 1987).

While trance was exploited by ancient healers, the modern history of clinical hypnosis begins with the Viennese physician Anton Mesmer. Mesmer studied gypsy and religious healing practices and became intrigued with the "laying on of hands," which seemed to produce medical results. His work in "animal magnetism" was eventually discredited when a distinguished panel of investigators, including Benjamin Franklin, Antoine Lavoisier, and Dr. Joseph Guillotin acknowledged that Mesmer had achieved physical outcomes. They found, however, that his "cures" (including "crises" and convulsions) were not the result of animal magnetism, as Mesmer claimed, but "that this new agent may be only the imagination itself, the power of which is so great that it is little understood" (Franklin et al., 1784).

The "father" of clinical hypnosis was a Scottish physician named James Braid (Kroger, 1977). He replaced the concept of animal magnetism with his term "hypnosis," derived from the Greek word for sleep, *hypnos*. This turned out to be an unfortunate naming, as comparisons of hypnosis to sleep are inaccurate and misleading. Interest in medical applications of hypnosis was great in nineteenth-century Europe, where Bernheim, Charcot, Janet, and Freud all conducted extensive explorations into its usefulness. Unfortunately, Freud discarded hypnosis, partly because it bypassed the very resistance and defenses that his approach was designed to explore. Hypnosis did not fit his theoretical view, and Freud's powerful influence diminished collegial interest. Janet was prophetic at the time, however, when he said, "if my work is not accepted today, it will be tomorrow when there will be a new turn in fashion's wheel which will bring back hypnotism as surely as our grandmother's styles" (Kroger, 1977, p. 4).

The physical and psychological trauma of two world wars accelerated interest in hypnosis. Military doctors returned home from battlefields to continue their study of trance and healing.

The next wave of interest in hypnosis was generated in the second half of the twentieth century by the charismatic and somewhat eccentric psychiatrist, Milton Erickson. His innovations and publications excited a generation of physicians, psychologists, and dentists, and his views shaped the way that modern clinical hypnosis is understood. Erickson understood hypnosis in a broader way than his predecessors, and he eventually focused on the ways that humans influence each other subconsciously, both in and out of formal trance states. Zeig (1987) observed, "To Erickson, hypnosis was not merely a trance state within a person; it was a special context for communication" (p. 394). Erickson actually caused a paradigm shift in the ways that hypnosis is understood and practiced, and those changes are described later in this chapter.

The Nature of Hypnosis

Hypnotic interventions can add to clinical practice in the following ways (Holroyd, 1987):

- Enhanced rapport
- Increased suggestibility
- Positive use of attention and awareness
- Utilization of dissociation
- Access to the mind-body relationship
- Use of imagery
- Responsiveness to the doctor's messages

Since patients and doctors typically fail to avail themselves of the benefits of hypnosis due to misconceptions, it is wise to begin with those. A multitude of myths and misunderstandings blur our ability to take advantage of something that is inexpensive (or free), generally harmless, relatively easy to do, and filled with potential benefit. Here are four important problematic myths.

Myth #1: Hypnosis is a trance state. This is the most pervasive misconception. While hypnosis has historical roots in formal trance induction, trance is only one aspect of the hypnotic continuum. This myth is problematic for dentistry because deep trances can be time-consuming, because only small numbers of people are capable of the kind of trance states that yield reliable dental anesthesia or analgesia, because most people are frightened by the prospect of entering a deep trance at the suggestion of a hypnotist, and because stage hypnotists have made fools of volunteers in public. Most of the value of dental hypnosis lies in qualities of hypnosis that do *not* involve deep trance states or lengthy inductions.

Myth #2: Hypnosis involves loss of control. Most people do not cherish the idea of losing control, especially in a dental office. Much of the difficulty that patients have with visits to the dentist involve a real or perceived loss of control, and the thought of giving over more control to a dentist is not attractive to most patients. If anything, properly conducted hypnotic interventions help people gain control and manage themselves more autonomously and effectively.

Myth #3: Hypnosis is dangerous. People (doctors and patients) are concerned that odd or bizarre things might happen when a dentist hypnotizes a patient, especially if the dentist is inexperienced in hypnosis. The procedures and skills described in this chapter have little or no chance of harming patients, especially if the dentist does not attempt to coerce patients.

Myth #4: The doctor must possess an elaborate set of skills and must exercise them charismatically. There are hypnotic skills that are complex, and the learning curve for a hypnotic practitioner can be long (and interesting, even thrilling), but the basic skills required to hypnotically enhance a dental practice can be taught to doctors, hygienists, assistants, and front office staff in a relatively short period of time. They do require diligence and focus, but they are worth it, both in terms of patient experience and worker satisfaction.

Defining Hypnosis and Using It

Novices think exclusively about trance when they think of hypnosis, but there are other ways to define hypnosis that open the door to widespread

Table 6.1   Clinical Hypnosis Map

Forms
    Trance
- light
- heavy

    Nontrance
- language
- indirect suggestion
- stories
- modeling

Styles
- authoritarian-direct
- permissive-indirect

Uses
- suggestion
- uncovering
- developing imagery resources
- relaxation

and efficient application in dental care. There exists no single, well-accepted definition of hypnosis. Carol Erickson reports (personal communication) that her father, Milton, once said, "I've been doing hypnosis for fifty years, thinking about it for fifty years, and I still don't really know what it is." In fact, as Lynn and Rhue (1991) observe in their book on theories of hypnosis, "There is no question that hypnosis has eluded a single, simple definition."

What follows is a description of a "map" of hypnosis. An outline of this map can be found at table 6.1. This description is quite basic in nature, and the map is not the territory.

Forms

It is useful to divide hypnosis into two forms: *trance* and *nontrance.*

Trance

Trance is a "state" of consciousness that allows special focus. It does not only happen in hypnosis or meditation, and there are countless variations of natural trance states in everyday life. In fact, it is best to think of consciousness as variegated. When people think of hypnosis, they usually have heavy trance states in mind. Deep trances represent a stereotype of hypnosis. Heavy trance states can be interesting, to be sure, and they can even be useful in the hands of a skilled hypnotherapist or dentist. But only a small number of people are capable of easily or conveniently entering very deep trance states. The majority are not (Moss, 1977, p. 323; American Society of Clinical

Hypnosis, 1973, p. 6). Most people can learn to enter a moderately deep state given time, practice, and concentration, but this can prove inefficient or impractical in a real-life dental practice. When Milton Erickson used deep trance, he often spent hours preparing his patient for the experience (Hammond, 1990, p. 21), and he spent a lifetime preparing himself.

There are many varieties of consciousness that we all experience every hour of every day. These variations can harm us (the flashback of the person with post-traumatic stress disorder, for example) and help us (when we imagine that we can accomplish something difficult). We drift in and out of various trancelike states all the time. We stare out a window. We gaze at an attractive person who happens to walk by (and lose our previous train of thought!). We absorb ourselves in a good novel. These are common examples of natural trances.

It is useful to (somewhat artificially) divide trance states into "heavy" states and "light" trance states. It is the variety of trance that interests the modern clinical hypnotist, along with the way that focus-of-attention works in trance states. For example, most people have experienced the inconvenience of a cracked car windshield. It's an annoyance at first, but we rather quickly learn to stare right through the crack to focus on the highway. It isn't long before we don't even notice the crack at all. Many people talk on cell phones while they drive cars. In spite of what seems to be a dangerously compromised capacity, there apparently have not been a significant number of highway disasters as a result. This is a function of how we can focus our attention in variable ways, and this is one key to the use of trance hypnosis in dental practice. Patients who have trouble in the dental chair are not managing their focus optimally for the experience. You could not drive a stick-shift automobile if you focused exclusively and obsessively on how the shift stick felt in your hand or on the possibility that a shifting error might cause your demise.

Many patients enter the dental office already in a trance state. Such a "state" can impair practice or enhance it, depending upon the ability of the dental team to recognize and utilize it. "Focused attention can lead to comfort as well as discomfort" (Zeig, 1987, p. 396).

Nontrance Hypnosis

Nontrance hypnosis can be defined as "a way of communicating and influencing which bypasses critical-analytical thought." This definition opens the door to the numerous ways that we influence each other on a moment-to-moment basis. We are not even aware that most of the influencing happens. When you motion to someone with your hand, they walk through a doorway ahead of you. When you lower your voice, you send a message that something is important or private. When you raise your eyebrows, you might send a message that something is strange or unexpected. These ways of influencing are powerful because they are unexamined. They tend to bypass the resistance of one's critical thinking or belief system. We are always sending messages and influencing each other, and the nonverbal messages are usually more powerful than the verbal ones. You can tell a patient that there is nothing to fear, but the sound of the high-speed drill can send a more compelling and ominous message. More to the point, you can welcome a patient to your operatory and tell them how glad you are to see them, but the speed of your speech and your rushed physical movement send a different message. The nonverbal message bypasses reason and powerfully influences the brain and mind. Verbal messages are overwhelmed and lost.

Language

Language can be hypnotic in a similar way, when the use of words and sentence structure influence by bypassing critical-analytical thought processes. The essential factor is *implication*. What we imply is often more powerful than what we say. Even if it is not, it cannot be ignored, for it changes the meaning of the verbal message. For example, the word "try" is hypnotic. It is often meant to communicate "please do this," but its deeper, more powerful implication can be "make some efforts in that direction, but fail to actually accomplish it." There are some words in dentistry that are so toxic that they should be used cautiously, if at all. Examples include, "pain," "painful," "shot," "hurt," "needle," "drill," and many others that serve only to alarm people or call to mind images or feelings that threaten. They communicate danger to many people.

Pediatric dentists tend to be quite aware of the power of specific words, and dental students are given lists of translations to learn to use with kids. Hurt or pain are called "bother" or "discomfort." The explorer is referred to as the "tooth counter" and the perio probe is called the "ruler." Xylocaine is called "sleepy juice." The word "discomfort" is, itself, an interesting example of hypnotic communication. There is a principle in hypnosis that asserts that one cannot *not* think of something. (Even the grammar-checker on my computer balks at this sentence!). You cannot not think of an elephant. In order to "not" think of an elephant, you have to (positively) think of it and then "try" to not think of it (that elephant). It really cannot be done. "Not think of an elephant" is a self-canceling phrase, similar to the sentence "Everything I say is a lie." (That phrase has trance inducing qualities, as well. Try to make logical sense out of it and see what happens.) The word "pain" simply implies or reminds one of hurtful, dangerous scenarios. "Discomfort" contains the word "comfort" inside of it for many people at some irrational, unspoken level.

Indirect Suggestion

Indirect suggestion is another form of hypnotic influence, and it does not involve formal trance states. You can communicate something without explicitly saying it or even saying it at all. In fact, you can even communicate an injunction by asking for its opposite, and sometimes this proves to be a more powerful way. For example, you can add the word "yet" to the end of a sentence and change its meaning. "You haven't experienced the new ways that dentists can get people numb yet" implies that the individual will have that experience. "You haven't figured out how to breathe in a way that allows you to be comfortable while we do impressions yet" implies that you will teach yourself how to get through the impression process soon (or at least some time in the future) without gagging. If you look closely at the sentence, you can see that it also implies that there will be more impressions taken in the future.

You can imply that patients will do something in the future by asking them not to do it now. "Please don't get too relaxed just yet. I have to ask you a few medical history questions before we get started." This sentence sends the message, by implication, that you will relax when the "real" dentistry happens.

You can preempt resistance or criticism with a sentence like this: "This might sound a little odd, but many people tell me that they actually enjoy coming here for their dentistry." or "This is going to sound silly, but. . ." or "I know you're not going to believe this, but many people don't even feel it when I give them anesthetic." Such a sentence opens the door for people to say to themselves, "Let me be the judge of that" or "I'll see about that," rather than, "I know I can't stand injections" or "I hate the dentist's office."

Stories

Stories are hypnotic, and powerful influencers use them. A story has a way of capturing one's imagination and, once again, influencing in a way that bypasses critical-analytic reasoning. We process information from stories differently than we process a direct injunction (in the form of "You should do X."), and we generally offer less resistance. A good story causes a person to focus in a special way on what is being said and to listen for implication, meanings, and "lessons." It's often better to tell a hopeful or cautionary tale rather than to give a directive ("Don't do that, because you might get hurt"). You have a greater chance of influencing a child by telling a story about another child who is now blind than you do if you simply tell that child that he or she shouldn't point a BB gun at other people.

A smart dentist collects stories about patients and dentistry and life so that he or she can use those stories to make points with patients. "I once had a patient" stories are important tools in a hypnotic dentist's kit. These stories can be used to communicate expected behavior: a story about a patient who did not follow specific postoperative instructions can be very powerful! A story about a phobic patient who had a wonderful experience in your dental practice is quite useful, especially if it includes hints about how the specific behaviors (theirs and the dentist's) that created the positive experience.

Modeling

Modeling is a fourth form of nontrance hypnotic influence. People respond more powerfully to authentic models than they do to advice from others. All members of the dental practice, including dentists, hygienists, assistants, and front-office staff, must model a positive, friendly, safe, comfortable, can-do attitude. These attitudes are contagious, and they send important messages about safety and competence. How could patients feel comfortable if the dental office is dingy or if staff members seem sad or angry or hurried? Imagine how a nervous patient assesses the situation when the doctor seems disorganized or frustrated or bored. There is nothing that can be said to cancel the powerful physical, visual, sensual, and behavioral messages modeled by the dental team. The physical behavior of the dentist creates an atmosphere of safety or danger, of caring or impersonality, of warmth or coldness. A disorganized dentist sends a terrible message, and a gentle and confident hand on the shoulder or jaw, or a reassuring smile can send an overwhelmingly positive message that bypasses critical-analytic reasoning or resistance. The hypnotic dentist develops a set of gestures that are trance enhancing. The way that a dentist moves and uses his or her hands can promote a feeling of safety, comfort, and confidence.

"Spa dentistry" seems to be on the right track, in this regard, with headphones for music and DVDs, comfortable chairs, warm blankets, "lifescape" glasses that create the sensation of babbling brooks or a day at the ocean, and even the smell of fresh-baked cookies!

Styles

There are two different styles of hypnotic communication, a direct-authoritarian style and an indirect-permissive style. Both can be effective when applied appropriately.

Authoritarian

The traditional way to use hypnosis is *authoritarian*. The "hypnotist" is thought to be in charge of the trance and situation. Forceful suggestions are used to direct a patient into a deep trance state and to cause linear behavior change. "Your eyes are feeling sleepy and your eyelids are feeling heavy," is an example of an authoritarian way of trance induction. A direct induction might include phrases like, "at the count of three your eyes will close and you will go into a deep trance." The most authoritarian approach of all is exemplified by the televised "healer" who smacks a subject on the forehead and shouts, "Sleep!" Such an approach can be useful in a dental office when used by a well-trained, confident hypnotist and a cooperative patient, but, like deep-trance states, such an approach is not typically practical or even appropriate.

Permissive

Modern clinical hypnotists favor more *permissive* tactics, which take advantage of the opportunities for trance and suggestion that naturally present themselves in dental practice. Most patients enter the dental office with a special kind of focus, and the hypnotic dentist might need only say, "Just go ahead and let yourself relax for a few moments before we get started." The dentist offers choices and follows up on those taken by the patient. "You can go ahead and close your eyes while we examine your teeth or you can keep them open and pay close attention to what we do." The dentist observes the patient's choice and reinforces it. "That's right. Stay focused on the handle of the lamp while I begin to work. Continue to breathe comfortably and relax more and more as your mouth remains open and relaxed." Indirect suggestions for comfort and cooperation can then be used. "Many people are pleasantly surprised at how comfortable they can become in a dental chair."

Uses

Hypnotic phenomena can be used to enhance dentistry in several ways. First of all, *relaxation* usually (but not necessarily) accompanies light trance or hypnotic rapport, and relaxation is fundamentally incompatible with anxiety. This is the simplest benefit of trance and, often, out-of-trance hypnosis, and it is helpful and important to patients and dentists. If this were the only benefit of hypnosis, the endeavor would be worthwhile.

The second benefit is from the enhanced power the *suggestions* have as a result of hypnosis. It is widely assumed that suggestions given to someone in a trance state have a good chance of being accepted uncritically and remembered powerfully or subconsciously. Even if they are not completely accepted, they are likely to be heard very clearly by someone in a moderate or deep trance, and the whole point of nontrance hypnosis is to influence through direct or indirect suggestion. Dentists and their team can make all kinds of useful suggestions; suggestions for relaxation, for a comfortable impression-taking or radiographic session, for comfort during injections, for comfort during appointments, for minimal swelling and bleeding after an extraction, for accurate cooperation with postoperative home treatment, for flossing and brushing, and for clenching and bruxing, to give a few examples.

A third application of hypnosis, the development of *imagery resources,* is very important to dentistry. Images tend to communicate more powerfully than words. Imagine "the taste of butterscotch" and compare it with a description of its recipe. Light trance states ("close your eyes") can be used to help patients find an internal source of strength, comfort, or self-efficacy that can enable them to survive or thrive in a dental appointment. For example, a dentist or assistant can simply ask the patient to sit back, relax comfortably, notice their breathing, and let their breathing become relaxed. They can then make the following suggestion:

> You can close your eyes now or later, or you can keep them open. It really doesn't matter. Most people enjoy having them closed to do this. Go inside of yourself for a few moments and find something that will help you right now. Maybe you will find an image that feels good. Perhaps you have a favorite place where you love to go to feel relaxed and comfortable, and safe. Perhaps you can imagine a person who has a way of making you feel good in some way. It could even be a visual image or a favorite color or sound. I don't exactly know what you will come up with. Let me know by raising your hand slightly as a signal that you've found something that works for you.

Patients can then keep that imagery resource in mind while the dental appointment proceeds. As an example, I once treated a patient with a significant dental phobia. In my psychology office, he took several sessions to establish a solid mental relationship with a purple kaleidoscopic image and used it to get through an oral surgery appointment that involved the extraction of several broken teeth and root tips. He was genuinely thrilled with his successful passage through a long-avoided procedure. All that the oral surgeon had to do was to allow this patient a few moments to gather his imagery resource and get it locked into focus.

The fourth use of hypnosis may not be directly useful to dentists, but is extremely useful to psychologists and could certainly be useful in a coordinated treatment effort between practitioners of those two specialties. It is called "uncovering." Light to moderate trance states are used to help patients reveal things to themselves that might be related or responsible for problems such as dental fears, phobias, or even bruxism. This is an occasion to note that hypnotic skills do not somehow allow a dentist to practice psychology nor would it help a psychologist to practice dentistry. Hypnosis is extremely unlikely to cause any harm as long as dentists use it to practice dentistry and not psychotherapy. If a dentist suspects that a patient is restricted by a deeper psychological malady, the dentist should coordinate care with a psychologist trained in hypnosis and familiar with dentistry. Effective hypnotic practice might require a dentist to find a hypnotic psychologist and involve him or her in the dental practice, so that appropriate and regular exchange of referrals is possible. Many patients will benefit from such a collaborative arrangement. The psychologist can spend three to ten sessions with a patient to get the patient ready for comfortable and efficient dental care, and can accompany such patients to the dental office for the first few transitional dental appointments.

Recommendations for Dentists

1. *There is much more to learn about natural and clinical hypnosis, including trance, hypnotic communication, direct and indirect suggestion, imagery, and physical relaxation.*

   This chapter scratches the surface. A list of recommended readings is at the end of this chapter. Hypnosis cannot be learned from books, of course. Hands-on, supervised training is available, but since interest in hypnosis is presently in a period of quiescence, you may have to assert effort to find good training. You will be able to find a few expert psychologists or dentists in any urban center who would be willing to provide training.

   Hypnosis attracts quacks. Be careful about collaborating with practitioners who do not possess a legitimate license to practice psychology or psychotherapy. That said, some of the "quacks" who make themselves available through the internet or neighborhood newspaper ads are actually quite skilled at trance induction. The problem is that they do not have training in safe, scientifically based psychotherapy.

   The American Society of Clinical Hypnosis provides regular training for beginning, intermediate, and advanced uses of hypnosis, along with a journal and list of teachers and practitioners. Information can be found on its website. The organization welcomes dentist members.

2. *Do not fall for or promote the prevailing myths associated with hypnosis. Do not focus on deep trance states and dramatic outcomes.*

   A healthy use of hypnotic communication can promote a focus on the positive, enhance acceptance, increase emphasis on choice and personal autonomy, decrease resistance to suggestion, and promote an attitude of wonder about possibilities. The shift from an anxious grip on frightening or threatening images to an open attitude that wonders about lovely possibilities can be nearly effortless sometimes. A lovely experience is just around the corner.

3. *Teach yourself how to communicate in ways that bypass conscious resistance.*

   Watch others and learn how these things work. Study your own interactions with staff, patients, and your own children, grandchildren, nephews, and nieces. Be flexible and experimental in your own communications. Teach yourself gestures to communicate what you would like patients to do. Offer choice in your practice and do not attempt to coerce others.

4. *Examine your practice environment to understand the implicit messages that it sends to patients (and perhaps to your team).*

   Obviously, it is best to create a practice that welcomes people into a safe, calm, and competent place. Observe verbal, nonverbal, visual, auditory, olfactory, and kinesic cues. A high-paced, impersonal, production-oriented practice probably will not send optimal, implicit, hypnotic messages to wary patients.

   Good luck with your hypnotic adventures. A wonderful world of possibility awaits you.

References

American Society of Clinical Hypnosis. (1973). A syllabus on hypnosis and a handbook of therapeutic suggestions.

Ewin, D. (1992). Hypnotherapy for warts (verruca vulgaris): 41 consecutive cases with 33 cures. *The American Journal of Clinical Hypnosis, 35 (1),* 1–6.

Franklin, B., Majault, M. J., Le Roy, J. B., Sallin, C. L., Bailly, J. S., D'Arcet, J., de Bory, G., Guillotin, J. I., & Lavoisier, A. L. (1784). *Rapport des commissaires charges par le Roi, de l'examen du magnetisme animal.* (Reprinted in *Skeptic,* 1996, 4 [3], 66–83.)

Hammond, C. (1990). *Handbook of hypnotic suggestions and metaphors.* New York: W. W. Norton.

Holroyd, J. (1987). How hypnosis may potentiate psychotherapy. *American Journal of Clinical Hypnosis, 29(3),* 194–200.

Kroger, W. (1977). *Clinical and experimental hypnosis in medicine, dentistry, and psychology.* 2d ed. Philadelphia: J. B. Lippincott.

Lynn, S., & Rhue, J. (1991). *Theories of Hypnosis: Current Models and Perspectives.* New York: Guilford Press.

Moss, A. (1977). Hypnodontics: hypnosis in dentistry. In W. S. Kroger, *Clinical and Experimental Hypnosis in Medicine, Dentistry, and Psychology.* 2d ed. Philadelphia: J. B. Lippincott.

Wester, W. (1987). *Clinical Hypnosis: A Case Management Approach.* Cincinnati: Behavioral Science Center, Inc., Publications.

Willard, R. (1977). Breast enlargement through visual imagery and hypnosis. *The American Journal of Clinical Hypnosis, 19(4),* 195–99.

Zeig, J. (1987). *The Evolution of Psychotherapy.* New York: Brunner/Mazel.

Recommended Readings

These readings are presented in order of complexity. Beginners are urged to start at the top of the list and work their way down.

1. Zilbergeld, B., Edelstien, M. G., & Araoz, D. (eds.) (1986). *Hypnosis: Questions & Answers.* New York: W. W. Norton. This book has long been out of print but can be found on used-book-dealer websites. It is very accessible to the novice and is a good source to start with.

2. Yapko, M. (1995). *Essentials of Hypnosis.* New York: Brunner/Mazel. This is a good, linear, beginning book for those who want to learn about the basics of applied clinical hypnosis.

3. Lynn, S., & Rhue, J. (1991). *Theories of Hypnosis: Current Models and Perspectives.* New York: Guilford Press. This is a "theories" book that describes various views of hypnosis. It is excellent for the person interested in trying to figure out what hypnosis is. It reports on several very different descriptions of the basic elements of hypnosis.

4. Hammond, C. (1990). *Handbook of Hypnotic Suggestions and Metaphors.* New York: W. W. Norton. This is a large book, filled with specifically worded suggestions and metaphors for an extremely wide range of medical and dental issues, including phobias and fears, TMJ, bruxism, gag reflex, extractions, tongue thrusting, and flossing.

5. Sheikh, A. (1984). *Imagination and Healing.* Farmingdale, NY: Baywood Publishing. This book is a comprehensive introduction to the use of imagery in clinical practice.

6. Rosen, S. (ed) (1982). *My Voice Will Go with You.* New York: W. W. Norton. This book is an accessible introduction to a difficult subject matter: the work of Milton Erickson. It includes stories that Erickson used along with examples of reframing, indirect suggestion, and observations by Erickson and others about his work.

7. O'Hanlon, W. *Taproots: Underlying Principles of Milton Erickson's Therapy and Hypnosis.* New York: W. W. Norton. This book attempts to distill and catalogue some of the more complex aspects of Erickson's work.

8. Watzlawick, P., Weakland, J., & Fisch, R. (1974). *Change: Principles of Problem Formation and Problem Resolution.* New York: W. W. Norton. This is the most complex of the books listed and perhaps the most intriguing. It is certainly the most charming. It describes the role of paradox in human behavior and is a book to read and reread, especially if you think you understand what's going on in the world.

Anxiety, Fear, and Pain

Emotional and Environmental Determinants of Dental Pain

7

Daniel W. McNeil, John T. Sorrell, and Kevin E. Vowles

Narrative

Pain associated with the oral cavity, and surrounding regions of the body, is both universal and commonplace in the human experience. Consistent with a biopsychosocial model, the experience and expression of dental pain are subject to individual biological parameters, general principles of learning as well as each person's individual difference psychological factors, and social (including cultural) influences. These factors are, of course, interactive in their effect on behavior, such as when an individual experiences nociception during the drilling of a tooth restoration. That person's experience of the sensations (cognitive interpretation and emotional response) certainly is driven by his or her basic biological predispositions (e.g., tendency toward hypertension in response to stressors in general, including dental procedures), social factors (e.g., the dentist's "chairside" manner in interacting with the patient), and psychological factors such as prior history (e.g., a past dental appointment that is remembered as "traumatic"), learned psychological responses to such situations (e.g., coping by using self-distraction), among a myriad of other possible influences.

This chapter focuses on psychological factors, specifically certain *emotional* ones (such as anxiety and fear), that affect pain in humans in the orofacial region, but specifically focusing on dental (intraoral) pain. It also is focused on certain social considerations, specifically those that are involved in the immediate *environment* of the dental operatory (such as issues of predictability and control). In the dental office or clinic, these environmental determinants also take the form of such stimuli as the dentist him/herself, dental hygienists, dental assistants, and other personnel, as well as other aspects of the setting (e.g., clinic setting with multiple dental chairs in close proximity versus an individual office with a single chair).

Dental pain typically is related to inflammatory diseases involving the dental pulp or periodontal tissues (Holland, 2001). Such pain, however, can spread to other sites from the teeth or be referred to the teeth from other regions; somatoform disorders, including pain syndromes, also can be manifested in toothache (Holland). Pain in the hard and soft tissues of the oral cavity must be understood in the context of pain in the orofacial region more generally. The definition of "orofacial pain" from the American Academy of Orofacial Pain suggests that it is "pain conditions that are associated with the hard and soft tissues of the head, face, neck, and all of the intraoral structures" (Okeson, 1996, p. 1), which includes acute dental and procedural pain. To the layperson, dental pain may be most associated with toothache or procedural pain related to restoration, extraction, endodontic therapy, orthodontics, or periodontal surgery.

Holland (2001) suggests that dental pain can be of pulpal origin (e.g., hypersensitive dentin, reversible pulpitis, irreversible pulpitis) or periodontal origin (e.g., associated with periodontal disease, pericoronitis, periadicular periodontitis, postendodontic pain, cracked-tooth syndrome, postextraction pain). Additionally, Holland indicates that the pain can be referred from the teeth to another site (e.g., masticatory muscles), or from other bodily regions to the teeth. Neuralgias can present as tooth pain; there is tooth pain with no known organic etiology (e.g., "phantom tooth pain" or *atypical odontalgia)* (Holland). In the literature, there presently is a dearth of high-quality epidemiological data on dental pain (Pau, Croucher, & Marcenes, 2003). Even less is known about pain associated with the soft tissues in the intraoral region (LeResche, 2001).

There is a body of empirical evidence concerning toothache, such as the finding that toothache pain is associated with certain verbal descriptors that can distinguish it from other types of general bodily pain. Research with the *McGill Pain Questionnaire* (Melzack, 1975) has found that toothache is associated with the sensory words "throbbing, boring, and sharp"; an affective word, "sickening"; evaluative words, "annoying"; and temporal words, "constant and rhythmic" (Dubuisson & Melzack, 1976). These verbal descriptors have even been found to discriminate between tooth pain that suggests irreversible disease versus a potentially treatable condition (Grushka & Sessle, 1984).

Contemporary definitions of pain in general, and orofacial pain in particular, specifically promote the idea that there are numerous environmental and emotional factors that are involved in the manifestation of such states, in addition to neurobiological ones. As a general state, "pain" is defined by the International Association for the Study of Pain as "an unpleasant sensory and emotional experience associated with actual or potential tissue damage, or described in terms of such damage" (Merskey & Bogduk, 1994, p. 210). Suggestions that pain is controlled in some large part by environmental, social, or cultural forces, however, may be scoffed at or even met with complete rejection and anger by the person expressing such pain, particularly when it is of high intensity. Undoubtedly, intensity of pain, as well as other qualities of the sensory experience such as duration, affect how it is perceived and expressed, but these responses, too, are modulated by environmental and emotional factors. Sometimes, as in the case of very high intensity, acute pain, it captures much of a person's attention and controls much of the person's behavior, although there still are ramifications in that person's environment (e.g., social mobilization of others to encourage seeking treatment to resolve toothache pain) and emotional state (e.g., fear about receiving dental care, which may or may not be overwhelmed by the pain).

Conceptual Issues in Understanding Dental Pain

Pain has numerous meanings socioculturally. It fundamentally is a construct (Cleeland, 1986) rather than being a disease entity in itself. While it may be a manifestation of an advancing or receding pathological state, it largely is symptomatic. In some cases of chronic pain syndrome in which organic pathology is low or apparently wholly absent, the expression of pain and associated disability is the principal pathological focus. To the person experiencing dental (and/or other) pain, however, particularly when it is intense, it is entirely real and may capture most or all of the person's attention and behavior, and may seem entirely sensory. (It is recognized, however, that there are those cases, albeit very small in number relative to all cases of dental pain, in which patients purposely malinger oral pain, such as when they are seeking drugs.) Pain can be a strong motivating force that drives behavior, such as when pain overwhelms fear in a dentally phobic person who finally presents himself for treatment of an abscess. In fact, stimulus intensity often is overlooked but may typically be the primary factor in determining whether a highly fearful person responds to pain or to fear (Vowles et al., in press). It is not whether a patient is experiencing fearful or painful sensations, but how much of each affect that person. Like pain, fear exists along a continuum of intensity, and is not an all-or-nothing response.

Dental pain can provoke the same response in very different groups of patients, such as those who seek preventive oral health care, versus those who seek dental care only symptomatically (e.g., when there is a problem such as pain). The intensity of the pain, likely in part, determines the rapidity with which a person seeks such care. In other instances, individuals may regard lower intensity pain as a state to be endured, hoping that it "goes away."

Pain fundamentally is a warning signal, with adaptive, evolutionary-based qualities, and strong motivational functions (McNeill & Dubner, 2001). It is a protective state, one that allows humans to survive in an environment that can be dangerous, and in which diseases can become life-threatening. Dental pain, for example, is highly functional (if troublesome) in that it signals the possibility of an ongoing disease state that must be interrupted if remaining tooth structure is to be saved and restored, and to prevent systemic disease. In persistent pain, the responsivity extends beyond an expected recuperative period; it can become chronic and nonfunctional, such as in some cases of temporomandibular disorder.

The meaning of pain, and whether it is expected and of known etiology, also is important in terms of an individual's responsivity. Lang (1985) highlights the importance of meaning, in addition to stimulus and response properties, in emotional responding. Postoperative dental pain, for example, may be expected and regarded as normal if the sensations are predicted by the dentist and if experienced in the context of the dentist's supportive chair-side manner. The response to postoperative pain of similar sensory qualities, after treatment in which the patient feels ignored or poorly treated, however, may be much more negative. There may be requests for pharmacological interventions, particularly if the pain is unexpected and regarded as a sign of continuing, unresolved problems, rather than an indication of the natural recovery process.

In some instances, states that dental patients refer to as "pain" might be classified differently by external observers. This difference in perspective may make little difference to the person experiencing that state as painful, however.

Describing one's current state as painful can be powerful, engendering sometimes rapid and highly responsive action on the part of those in the immediate environment, particularly in those who may have caused the pain. When the patient in a dental chair, for example, says to the dentist, "That hurts!", the function likely is to get the dentist to stop what she or he is doing, and to modify the present course of action (e.g., by inquiring about the patient's feelings, administering additional anesthetic). Interestingly, external observers (and the dentist him/herself) may believe that a more accurate statement by the patient might have been, "I'm afraid." Nevertheless, as presented so clearly by Bochner (1988), "All pain, whatever its origin is real to the sufferer" (p. 41). The words we use to describe internal states in health care settings have functions, not only to communicate meaning (Davis et al., 2005), but perhaps to attempt to elicit certain outcomes (e.g., to take a break from a lengthy dental procedure).

Emotional Determinants

A variety of states, including anxiety, fear, stress, panic, and depression, among others, are potentially important in the experience and expression of pain (Keefe et al., 2001). These states may predispose individuals to experiencing nociception as painful, might be concomitants of pain, or may be secondary to pain. In some instances, such as in some cases of fear, the emotional response actually may attenuate pain (Vowles et al., in press). In the case of dental pain, anxiety and fear are important foci, as they are very frequently associated. Fear about pain is the most important determinant of overall dental fear (McNeil & Berryman, 1989).

Anxiety and Fear of Pain Models in Dentistry

A predominant perspective of anxiety and fear is based on a diathesis-stress model in which persons have a biological predisposition to develop problematic levels of anxiety and/or fear. It is not until an environmental stressor is encountered that the disorder manifests (Barlow, 2002), although the disorder may develop in the absence of a genetic vulnerability or environmental trigger. Fear of pain models in dentistry are adopted from broader theoretical conceptualization of fear, anxiety, and fear of pain. Sorrell and McNeil (2005) reviewed four primary fear of pain models and applied them in the dental context. The models reviewed include Mowrer's two-factor theory, Davey's model of the conditioning process in learned fears, fear-avoidance model, and the expectancy model of fear. Each will be outlined here and accompanied by examples to illustrate the applicability and process of emotions in the dental environment.

Mowrer's Two-Factor Theory

Mowrer's (1939) two-factor theory was among early theoretical conceptualizations that attempted to bring meaning and understanding to fear and avoidance behavior. Indeed, it is a theory that makes up part of Davey's model as well as the fear-avoidance model. Using a classical conditioning framework, Mowrer postulated that a neutral stimulus acquired aversive properties in the presence, and temporal contiguity of, a fear-evoking event. It is the reduction in fear that consequences avoidance of the aversive stimuli that maintains such behavior. When aversive stimuli are avoided, fear is reduced and avoidance behavior is maintained (i.e., negative reinforcement). The process begins with arbitrary stimuli, such as the sights, sounds, and odors of a dental operatory, such as the dental chair, drilling sounds, and characteristic smells of a dental office (conditioned stimuli—CS), which are present in the patient's environment just prior to a pain stimulus in the patient's mouth, such as an upper palate injection (unconditioned stimulus—UCS). The patient then responds with fear (unconditioned response—UCR). In the future when dental operatory stimuli (e.g., chair, drilling, and/or smell) elicit a fear response, they have become conditioned stimuli, and fear in their presence is a conditioned response (conditioned response—CR). When the patient who has developed the conditioned response to dental stimuli then avoids the dental office by canceling or not showing for an appointment, the associated reduction of fear is a relief and continues the vicious cycle of avoidance behavior (i.e., no visits to the dental office). Although this model was accepted for many years as critical in understanding behavior, newer models of fear and avoidance were developed to account for shortcomings in two-factor theory (e.g., the role of cognitive factors in fear learning) (see Craske, 1999, for a review). Among the revised conditioning conceptualizations was Davey's model of the conditioning process.

Davey's Model

Considering a more diverse approach to learned fears, Davey (1989a) developed a model for dental phobias and anxieties that suggests two explanations in which painful dental-related events may not lead to future fears of dental pain. Latent inhibition, he asserts, may moderate the conditioning process because a patient may have had several years of treatment in the absence of an aversive dental experience. With many positive experiences between a CS (e.g., dental chair) and the absence of an UCS (e.g., pain), a CR (e.g., fear) is much more difficult to establish when the UCS eventually occurs in the presence of the CS. Thus, the association that has developed over many years of painless treatment between attending the dentist and good oral health is too strong for a UCS-CR association to be established effectively. Moreover, if a painful experience establishes a CS-UCS (UCR) association, the strength of the CR depends on the patient's evaluation of the UCS (Davey, 1989a, 1989b; Davey & Craigie, 1997). Pain may be experienced prior to root canal therapy when an injection of anesthesia is administered. However, the knowledge that having a root canal procedure should help to reestablish good oral health will moderate a significant fear response (Davey, 1989a). The addition of this cognitive component to a dental fear model was novel relative to Mowrer's theory and helped pave the way for more recent models related to fear of pain.

Fear-Avoidance Model

The fear-avoidance model (Lethem et al., 1983) is a conceptualization that predominantly has been applied with chronic musculoskeletal pain-related problems (Vlaeyen & Linton, 2000). However, it is a model that as well can be applied to patient behavior in the dental environment (Sorrell & McNeil, 2005). The fear-avoidance model asserts that physical strain or injury is followed by the experience of pain, which leads to either of two methods of responding. A patient can develop little or no fear to interrupt with her ability to approach pain-related contexts or stimuli and return to a level of functioning prior to injury, or she can begin to catastrophize about the pain and the environment in which it occurred, which leads to increased fear of pain, avoidance, and disability. In the context of the dental environment, disability is equated to long-term avoidance of oral health care, and potential exacerbation of oral diseases. The fear-avoidance model is well supported primarily throughout the general fear of musculoskeletal pain literature (e.g., Vlaeyen et al., 2001), however, the utility of this model in dentistry is profound.

Consider the following example to illustrate how the fear-avoidance model is applicable to the dental environment. Two middle-aged patients arrive for root canal therapy with their endodontist. The endodontist has the same difficulty completely numbing both patients prior to drilling. As a result, the experience of pain is great for both patients at the outset of treatment, which is followed by the administration of more anesthesia to adequately anesthetize the affected area. Both patients endure the remainder of treatment without incident. Richard leaves the endodontist's office complaining about how terrible the pain was during the procedure. Richard focuses on all the terrible outcomes that potentially could have occurred. His catastrophizing begins to increase his overall fear of dental pain. Sally, however, leaves the clinic in some discomfort in the area of her mouth where there was pain but feels satisfied with the medication she is given for swelling and pain. Her experience and thoughts do not contribute to the development of fear of dental pain. When it is time for these patients to return for follow-up treatment to remove the temporary filling and permanently seal the root canal, Richard experiences considerable fear and pain while Sally has neither. Sally receives treatment and returns to her everyday activities. Richard cancels his appointment, fearing that going to the endodontist will result in more pain and discomfort. The longer Richard avoids having his root canal treatment completed, the more likely it is to become infected, potentiating pain exacerbation and discomfort. Although his pain continues,

Richard believes that staying away from the endodontist is better for him than subjecting himself to additional pain that may be experienced in the dental environment.

Expectancy Model of Fear

The *expectancy model of fear* (Reiss & McNally, 1985) is another fear of pain conceptualization that is quite relevant in dentistry. The expectancy model is based on two components to fear: expectations that certain events and/or experiences (heart palpitation, embarrassment, or losing control of emotions) will occur in particular situations, and anxiety sensitivity, which refers to the belief that those expected experiences are dangerous or threatening. Taken together, these factors influence behavioral responses in the context of (potential) threat, and in particular avoidance and escape behavior.

It is believed that anxiety sensitivity is a predisposing variable linked to responding with fear to anxiety-related events (Reiss, 1991) and operates as a vulnerability to the development of an anxiety disorder (Craske, 1999). The vast majority of empirical support for the expectancy model is taken from research on anxiety disorders (e.g., Taylor et al., 1992) and chronic pain (e.g., Greenberg & Burns, 2003; Zvolensky et al., 2001). Gross (1992a) applied the expectancy model of fear to dental avoidance with the development of the Pain Sensitivity Index (PSI). Using the PSI, Gross found that pain sensitivity among dental patients predicted pain intensity, and pain intensity predicted dental avoidance. Although Gross asserts that anxiety sensitivity and pain sensitivity are distinct constructs, they both are founded on the same model of fear learning and are closely related (Gross, 1992a; 1992b).

Norton and Asmundson (2003) integrated anxiety sensitivity, as it relates to physiological responding, into the fear-avoidance model of chronic pain. The authors indicated that although the fear-avoidance model focuses on cognitive and behavioral aspects of pain responding, it does not highlight the contributions of physiological arousal toward pain avoidance. The amended fear-avoidance model suggests that anxiety sensitivity will impact avoidance behavior at the level of pain catastrophizing; physiological activity (e.g., muscle tension), along with anxiety sensitivity, will contribute to fear of pain (see Norton & Asmundson for a review). Thus, it is a patient's experience of physiological arousal during dental treatment, and the belief that treatment may lead to pain or lasting harm (e.g., a catastrophe in the dental chair, such as myocardial infarction) that initiates dental fear. The maintenance of avoidance behavior occurs through negative reinforcement. Fear is reduced when the dental office is avoided, and the reduction of fear increases the likelihood of the response (i.e., avoidance) in the future.

Individual Differences and Pain Sensitivity

Earlier investigations into individual differences related to dental pain focused broadly on dental fear. Results from these studies suggest that patients with higher levels of dental fear responded with more sensitivity to pain (i.e., less pain tolerance) during treatment (e.g., Kleinknecht & Bernstein, 1978), are more likely to report dental pain (Vassend, 1993), are more likely to have irregular dental attendance (Milgrom et al., 1985) and to poorly re-call the actual intensity of dental pain (Klepac et al., 1980) compared to pa-tients with a low level of dental fear.

Catastrophizing

A cognitive tendency to focus and ruminate on negative outcomes in threat-ening events, catastrophizing is an individual difference variable that has implications in dentistry. When catastrophizing was examined among pa-tients during dental hygiene treatment, results revealed that even when gen-der and oral hygiene status were controlled statistically, catastrophizing sig-nificantly predicted pain (Sullivan & Neish, 1998). Therefore, it appears that excessive focus on pain sensations during dental treatment could be a way in which catastrophizing increases pain (Sullivan & Neish). In addition to dental treatment, evidence shows that catastrophizing serves an important role in the maintenance of other oral-health-related problems such as tem-poromandibular disorder (Turner et al., 2001).

Emotions are powerful determinants of pain responding in dentistry. The link among anxiety, fear, and pain in oral health care is particularly strong. Nevertheless, a variety of social and other environmental factors, such as communication between patient and provider, as well as the ability to pre-dict, and the ability to control, aspects of dental procedures, also are critically important in affecting dental pain.

Environmental Determinants

The social aspects of the dental situation are extremely important in the overall environment for the dental patient. Dental treatment typically can be accomplished only with the presence of a provider. The behavior of the provider(s), in some large part, helps to determine the patient's conceptual-ization of, and response to, nociception. Additionally, other experienced as-pects of the environment, such as predictability and control, impact pain responding.

Communication and Relationship with Dental Providers

There is a conceptual basis for the assertion that the effectiveness of continu-ing treatment that maintains oral health status is at least partially predicated on the social aspects of the relationship between patient and provider (Grembowski, Anderson, & Chen, 1989; Kent & Blinkhorn, 1991). Patients' views of the quality of this relationship predict a number of outcomes, includ-ing treatment adherence, appointment attendance, and satisfaction (Sandell, Camner, & Sarhed, 1994; Sinha, Nanda, & McNeil, 1996). The data available from studies of chronic pain also suggest that pain responding is affected by social variables (Flor et al., 1995; Payne & Norfleet, 1986; Skevington, 1995). Taken together, these two areas of findings suggest that the specific characteristics of oral health care providers, and the office or clinic in which they work, have the potential to lessen or exacerbate pain responding.

In the oral health literature, communication between patients and providers is perhaps the most well established determinant of pain responding. Riley, Gilbert, and Heft (2004) indicated that patient attitudes about past appointment quality differentiated between individuals who had discussed an orofacial pain problem with a health care provider or only with a layperson, such as a spouse, relative, or friend. Patient perceptions of appointment quality were assessed via a series of standardized questions broadly assessing the nature of interaction and communication within the clinic, as understood by the patient. It is noteworthy that those individuals who perceived poorer quality relations with health care providers, and were less likely to have talked with a provider about a pain problem, would be at greater risk for the development of health problems associated with not receiving appropriate dental care. In addition, encouraging patient communication regarding worries or pain intensity may serve to increase perceptions of prediction and control, as discussed subsequently (Maggirias & Locker, 2002).

In addition to perception of communication quality on the part of the patient, the actual content of communications appears to have an effect on pain responding. In Gryll and Katahn's (1978) classic study on this topic, two facets of communication content were found to have an effect on pain responding. First, when the provider communicated confidence in the effectiveness of a particular intervention, the patients reported that it was more effective at relieving pain than when the provider noted ambivalence regarding the intervention's efficacy. Second, providers who were instructed to be "warm and friendly" and to actively elicit discussion and questions from their patients also were associated with lesser pain reports relative to more neutral and less-talkative providers. Although the findings of this study are relatively dated, and it has yet to be replicated or followed up, they are significant in that they illustrate the importance of what is said to patients, and the way in which it is said.

Distraction

Distraction serves to shift the patient's attention away from the environmental procedural cues, and away from the sensory aspects of a painful situation, to another, typically more pleasant stimulus (Kent & Blinkhorn, 1991). Distraction is particularly well suited to most dental settings, as well as other situations that involve acute, transient pain (e.g., child immunizations). It appears that the more sensory systems that are involved in the distraction, the more effective it becomes, as watching a television program or playing a video game have been found to be more effective at reducing patient discomfort relative to listening to an audiotape (Seyrek, Corah, & Pace, 1984). More recently, researchers have made use of more technologically advanced methods of distraction (i.e., virtual reality), which also appear to be effective at decreasing reports of discomfort in dental settings (Frere et al., 2001), while not interfering with the clinical aspects of procedures. Children reported less discomfort when allowed to begin with an easier, or less painful, procedure and to "work up" to the more difficult procedures (Kaakko et al., 2003).

Predictability and Controllability

Predictability and controllability in regard to dental experiences are broadly defined as whether or not persons are informed about what will occur during dental treatment, and whether or not they are able to influence what happens during the treatment situation, respectively. Predictability, more specifically, is defined as the degree to which the presence or absence of a given signal indicates the onset, offset, duration, or intensity of a noxious stimulus or threatening event. Controllability is defined as having the ability to alter the onset, offset, duration, or intensity of an aversive dental experience (Arntz & Schmidt, 1989; Foa, Zinbarg, & Rothbaum, 1992; Zvolensky, Lejuez, & Eifert, 2000). Although having control over the influence of an aversive stimulus implies a degree of predictability, this relation is unidirectional in that predictability does not suggest having control (Zvolensky et al.). Indeed, predictability and controllability are multifaceted concepts that affect patients in many aspects of the dental environment (Walker, 2001), including in the experience of dental pain. Given the overwhelming impact that predictability and controllability have on pain and distress in general medical settings (Ludwick-Rosenthal & Neufeld, 1988), considerable research and clinical utility of these concepts have accumulated in dental arenas.

Predictability of aversive events (such as dental pain) has been closely linked to the development and maintenance of problematic levels of fear and anxiety (Zvolensky, Eifert, et al., 2000). Many aspects of the dental experience can be unpredictable, and the effects of unpredictability on dental pain can be pronounced. Knowing when or if an endodontist will probe a tooth that is not adequately anaesthetized during root canal therapy, or how long an injection will take when anesthesia is administered, are examples of the potentially vague, unpredictable nature of the dental environment, which can lead to greater pain responding. Patients lacking predictability about a tooth extraction procedure, for example, displayed greater pain behavior compared to patients who were informed and able to predict what would occur in treatment (Auerbach et al., 1976).

In a similar study, Auerbach and colleagues (1983) found that when tooth extraction patients had a preference for procedure- and sensory-related information and actually then received predictability about treatment, pain and distress responding was significantly reduced compared to patients who received predictability but had no such preference for information. Moreover, dental patients given detailed predictability about procedural and sensory aspects of treatment experienced reductions in both pain *and* anxiety (Corah, Gale, & Illing, 1979). The positive impact of predictability on pain, anxiety, and fear is particularly important given the overwhelming negative impact of anxiety and fear on dental pain responding (Jerremalm, Jansson, & Ost, 1986; Kent, 1984; Klepac, 1975; Klepac et al., 1980). Evidence consistently suggests that fear and anxiety negatively impact patients' ability to accurately predict dental pain experiences (e.g., Van Buren & Klein-knecht, 1979) and that fearful individuals may overpredict aversive events to protect themselves from the negative impact of underpredictions (e.g., potentially increased pain) (Arntz & Hopmans, 1998). Therefore, if enhancing predictability about dental procedures decreases anxiety about treatment and increases the accuracy of patient's predictions about pain, the detrimental impact of anxiety on dental pain likely would be reduced as well.

The vast majority of attempts to ameliorate dental anxiety, fear, and pain, and increase predictability during dental treatments has been with the use of information. Providing information as a method to enhance predictability about treatment was among the first interventions implemented in medical procedures (Ludwick-Rosenthal & Neufeld, 1988). The rationale for this methodology is based on research that suggests predictability to reduce the impact of aversive stimuli on pain and distress responding (Staub, Tursky, & Schwartz, 1971). High levels of information about nitrous oxide sedation, relative to low levels, leads to higher pain threshold and tolerance ratings for tooth pulp stimulation (Dworkin et al., 1984). A broad array of information can be provided to patients, including information about the dental procedure and sensory aspects of treatment (Reading, 1979). It appears that patients benefit best from a combination of both procedural and sensory information (Miller, Combs, & Stoddard, 1989). When information about treatment is used in this way, patients are better able to accurately predict what events will occur, when they will occur, and how long they will last, which likely influences the cognitive appraisal of threat (Corah & Boffa, 1970) and allows for use of individual coping strategies (Staub et al., 1971).

Although enhancing predictability about dental treatment is beneficial for some patients, individual differences exist. Miller (1995) reviewed individual difference factors and highlighted two behavioral coping styles that influence the effects of predictability. Patients who are characterized as "monitors" are more concerned and distressed with their medical condition, experience greater side effects, are more knowledgeable about their situation, and are less satisfied and more demanding about the psychosocial aspects of their care compared to patients who are characterized as "blunters." Miller concludes that patients respond better during treatment when the information they receive matches their coping style. More detailed information seems best for those with a monitoring style and less treatment-relevant information for those with a blunting style. Too much information for blunters may disrupt their avoidance coping and too little information for monitors may limit their procedural focus.

Similar to the influences of predictability, the importance of controllability for individual health and coping is pronounced and the implications of control on health are broad (Shapiro, Schwartz, & Astin, 1996). Although controllability is a multifaceted concept, it often is discussed in terms of control and perceived control. Walker (2001) describes the former to involve human responding, which leads to a change in an event and the latter to refer to the belief that an event is under control. Both forms of control have implications with regard to general pain and specifically to dental pain responding. For example, perceived control over anxiety-related events has been shown to predict pain tolerance and endurance (Feldner & Hekmat,

2001), and perceived control can decrease autonomic arousal during painful stimulation (Geer, Davison, & Gatchel, 1970). Taken together, these data suggest that perceived control influences how persons respond behaviorally and physiologically to pain while other factors such as pain-related anxiety and fear may affect the reported experience of pain intensity (Carter et al., 2002; McCracken, Zayfert, & Gross, 1992). Furthermore, giving accessibility to actual control mechanisms during pain stimulation can increase tolerance (Kanfer & Goldfoot, 1966; Kanfer & Seidner, 1973).

In dental settings, perceived control has had similar pain-reducing effects as in experimental contexts. Studies demonstrate strong evidence for the decreasing effects of perceived control on pain responding during treatment (e.g., Corah, Gale, & Illing, 1979; Thrash Marr, & Boone, 1982). Literature examining actual control during dental treatment, however, has been plagued with somewhat mixed results. It was found, for example, that control was beneficial for patients who used a signaling device that communicated to the dentist that treatment was uncomfortable and the procedure needed to stop until the patient felt ready to proceed (Corah, 1973). A similar study using a different sample of dental patients demonstrated somewhat different effects. Greater physiological responsivity was found among patients who had control during treatment relative to patients without control (Corah, Bissell, & Illig, 1978). When results were examined with the consideration of the patient's locus of control, which generally refers to one's beliefs about accountability for what happens to one, it was determined, however, that patients with an external locus of control had greater physiological responding during treatment compared to those with an internal locus of control. In other words, patients who generally believe that the outcome of life events is largely determined by factors outside of their control (i.e., external locus of control) benefit very little from acquiring control in the dental environment, and dental patients who believe that they have a meaningful influence on the outcome of life events (i.e., internal locus of control) derive more benefit from control during treatment. Based on these data, it appears that locus of control may be closely linked to the patient's desired and felt control in dental settings.

Desire for control is the degree to which patients want to influence what occurs in an aversive dental situation; felt control indicates the level of control experienced (Law, Logan, & Baron, 1994). When desired control and felt control mismatch (specifically for high desire/low felt control patients), dental fear is the highest (Baron, Logan, & Hoppe, 1993; Logan et al., 1991), and pain-related distress is the greatest (Baron & Logan, 1993; Logan et al., 1991). Interventions designed to increase felt control among high desire/low felt control patients have reversed high distress ratings during dental treatment (see Baron & Logan for a review). Furthermore, there is discussion about the benefits of relinquishing control to others who perhaps are more suited to control a given situation and minimize danger in that potentially noxious setting (Walker, 2001). Indeed, regardless of how much control a patient has during a dental procedure, treatment ultimately must be completed despite fear, anxiety, or pain experienced.

In allowing a dentist to use his or her expertise to perform a procedure, a patient can resign attempts to control the situation and use energies elsewhere to cope during treatment. Moreover, the act of giving up control (e.g., eliminating the struggle to reduce fear or pain in dental environments) in and of itself can be considered a form of gaining control when all other attempts to control have failed (e.g., acceptance-based coping; Hayes, 2004). Although relinquishing control to others and using acceptance-based approaches in the dental environment may differ conceptually, the functions of reducing fear, anxiety, and pain may be similar and await empirical investigation.

Dental Personnel as Threatening Stimuli

For highly fearful patients, dentists and other dental personnel can be "fear stimuli" that occasion negative reactivity (e.g., verbal reports of distress, psychophysiological responding, and even, in extreme cases, escape in the form of the patient leaving the operatory). Like the "white coat effect" (Pickering & Friedman, 1991) that can be manifested in a rise of blood pressure in patients when they are being assessed or treated by physicians or other health care providers, even the sight of the dentist can be fear evoking. A telling cartoon (*Francie*) in this area is that in which a dentist is just entering one end of a long operatory, and a patient is seated alone in a dental chair at the other end. As the dentist enters, the patient, with no other external provocation whatsoever, says "OW!" (Shepherd, 1991). This example portrays both the stimulus value of the dentist as being associated with pain, and the overlapping mixture of words that can be used to describe fearful and/or painful states (Davis et al., 2004).

Dental Personnel as Relief Stimuli

While most often associated with being a fearful stimulus, dentists and allied personnel also can be viewed as offering relief to those suffering with dental pain. In this case, dentists help relieve an ongoing aversive state (e.g., pain) in patients, so the conditioning process that takes place is negative reinforcement. The encounter with the dentist as a stimulus may be reinforcing because an aversive (i.e., painful) situation (e.g., toothache) is removed. Some patients in certain situations, therefore, are extremely grateful to their dentists. There are, however, many other aspects to such situations (e.g., discomfort that is associated with the procedures involved in addressing oral disease causing toothache pain). Consequently, single, or even a few, positive conditioning events with a dentist frequently may not override highly fearful patients' prior fearful learning history.

Gender, Culture, and Lifespan Issues

The social environment, interacting with one's gender and cultural background, determine in part, one's reactions to pain, and how one constructs ideas about its meaning. Root canal therapy in dentistry, for example, is a frequent symbol for pain that has been co-opted by advertisers in the United States in the service of marketing (and the likely dis-service of public health issues in dentistry) (Sorrell, 2003). Certain less economically advantaged cultural groups in less-developed nations, for example, may expect dental care to be painful, and therefore do not complain about nociception, but rather regard dental care as a privilege. In some North American cultural groups, on the other hand, there may be the expectation that there should be very little, or no, discomfort or pain associated with visits to the dentist.

There has been some attention to ethnic and racial differences in orofacial pain. Lipton and Marback (1984) suggest that while the factors that affect the reporting of pain differ among cultural groups, the reporting of pain may be more similar, except in the arena of emotions associated with pain. Weisenberg et al. (1975) found that black, white, and Puerto Rican emergency dental patients were similar in terms of specific reports about dental pain, as well as electrodermal activity, but differed in their tendency to adopt avoidance strategies. Finally, Riley, Gilbert, and Heft (2003) investigated orofacial pain symptoms, and found sex-differentiated socioeconomic (SES) differences, with persons of lower SES reporting greater pain and having greater behavioral impact from the pain, relative to those with higher SES.

The gender and cultural status of the dentist, hygienist, and other dental personnel in the office or clinic contribute to determining a patient's response to nociception, and whether they even label it as pain. Responses may be different, for example depending on gender matching or discontinuity between provider and patient, or between experimenter and subject (Carter et al., 2002; Rollman, Lautenbacher, & Jones; Vowles et al., in press). Consistent with a literature on sex difference in verbal reports of fear in many (but not all) areas, women indicated more fear, and men less fear, in response to dental pain (Liddell & Locker, 1997). In this same study, relative to men, women indicated greater avoidance of pain, less acceptance of pain, and greater desire for control.

A recent review of dental pain articles suggests that younger individuals, and those of lower socioeconomic status, are more likely to report pain, and that older adults and persons of higher socioeconomic status are less prone to do so (Pau et al., 2003). The prevalence of certain types of dental pain (e.g., toothache) decrease with age, while others (e.g., burning mouth syndrome) may be much more common in those over thirty years of age or in the very elderly (LaResche, 2001).

Summary and Conclusions

Emotional and environmental factors, individually and in combination, clearly affect dental pain at all levels of processing and response, interacting with neurobiological influences. Dental pain is affected by emotions, particularly fear, anxiety, and depression (Eli, 1992), emotional processes such as catastrophizing, as well as individual difference factors such as pain sensitivity, and memory of pain. Moreover, aspects of the environment are powerful determinants of dental pain, such as issues of communication between patient and provider, distraction, predictability, and control. Finally, sociocultural factors, including socioeconomic status, gender, race and ethnicity, and age all affect the experience and expression of dental pain.

References

Arntz, A., & Hopmans, M. (1998). Underpredicted pain disrupts more than correctly predicted pain, but does not hurt more. *Behavior Research and Therapy, 36*, 1121–29.

Arntz, A., & Schmidt, A. J. M. (1989). Perceived control and the experience of pain. In A. Steptoe & A. Appels (eds.), *Stress, Personal Control and Health* (pp. 131–62). London: John Wiley & Sons.

Auerbach, S. M., Kendal, P. C., Cuttler, H. F., & Levitt, N. R. (1976). Anxiety, locus of control, type of preparatory information, and adjustment to dental surgery. *Journal of Consulting and Clinical Psychology, 4*, 809–18.

Auerbach, S. M., Martelli, M. F., & Mercuri, L. G. (1983). Anxiety, information, interpersonal impacts, and adjustment to a stressful health care situation. *Journal of Personality and Social Psychology, 44*, 1284–96.

Barlow, D. H. (2002). *Anxiety and Its Disorders: The Nature and Treatment of Anxiety and Panic.* 2d ed. New York: Guilford Press.

Baron, R. S., & Logan, H. (1993). Desired control, felt control, and dental pain: recent findings and remaining issues. *Motivation and Emotion, 17*, 181–204.

Baron, R. S., Logan, H., & Hoppe, S. (1993). Emotional and sensory focus as mediators of dental pain among patients differing in desired and felt dental control. *Health Psychology, 12*, 381–89.

Bochner, S. (1988). *The Psychology of the Dentist-Patient Relationship.* New York: Springer-Verlag.

Carter, L. E., McNeil, D. W., Vowles, K. E., Sorrell, J. T., Turk, C. L., Ries, B. J., & Hopko, D. R. (2002). Effects of emotion on pain reports, tolerance, and physiology. *Pain Research and Management, 7*, 21–30.

Cleeland, C. S. (1986). How to treat a "construct." *Journal of Pain and Symptom Management, 1*, 161–62.

Corah, N. L. (1973). Effect of perceived control on stress reduction in pedodontic patients. *Journal of Dental Research, 52*, 1261–64.

Corah, N. L., & Boffa, J. (1970). Perceived control, self-observation, and response to aversive stimulation. *Journal of Personality and Social Psychology, 16*, 1–4.

Corah, N. L., Bissell, G. D., & Illing, S. J. (1978). Effect of perceived control on stress reduction in adult dental patients. *Journal of Dental Research, 57*, 74–76.

Corah, N. L., Gale, E. N., & Illing, S. J. (1979). Psychological stress reduction during dental procedures. *Journal of Dental Research, 58*, 1347–51.

Craske, M. G. (1999). *Anxiety Disorders: Psychological Approaches to Theory and Treatment.* Boulder, CO: Westview Press.

Davey, G. (1989a). Dental phobias and anxieties: evidence for conditioning processes in the acquisition and modulation of a learned fear. *Behavior Research and Therapy, 27*, 51–58.

———. (1989b). UCS revaluation and conditioning models of acquired fears. *Behavior Research and Therapy, 27*, 521–28.

Davey, G., & Craigie, P. (1997). Manipulation of dangerousness judgments to fear-relevant stimuli: effects on a priori UCS expectancy and a posteriori covariation assessment. *Behavior Research and Therapy, 35*, 607–17.

Davis, A. M., McNeil, D. W., Fluharty, K. K., Perry, J. E., & Bowers, E. J. (2004, November). *Understanding fear and pain using multidimensional scaling techniques.* Poster presented at the meeting of the Association for Advancement of Behavior Therapy, New Orleans, LA.

Dubuisson, D., & Melzack, R. (1976). Classification of clinical pain descriptors by multiple group discriminant analysis. *Experimental Neurology, 51,* 480–87.

Dworkin, S. F., Chen, A. C. N., Schubert, M. M., & Clark, D. W. (1984). Cognitive modification of pain: information in combination with N_2O. *Pain, 19,* 339–51.

Eli, I. (1992). *Oral Psychophysiology: Stress, Pain, and Behavior in Dental Care.* Boca Raton, FL: CRC Press.

Feldner, M. T., & Hekmat, H. (2001). Perceived control over anxiety-related events as a predictor of pain behaviors in a cold pressor task. *Journal of Behavior Therapy & Experimental Psychiatry, 32,* 191–202.

Flor, H., Breitenstein, C., Birbaumer, N., & Furst, M. (1995). A psychophysiological analysis of spouse solicitousness towards pain behaviors, spouse interaction, and pain perception. *Behavior Therapy, 26,* 255–72.

Foa, E. B., Zinbarg, R., & Rothbaum, B. O. (1992). Uncontrollability and unpredictability in post-traumatic stress disorder: an animal model. *Psychological Bulletin, 112,* 218–38.

Frere, C. L., Crout, R., Yorty, J., & McNeil, D. W. (2001). Effects of audiovisual distraction during dental prophylaxis. *Journal of the American Dental Association, 132,* 1031–38.

Geer, J. H., Davison, G. C., & Gatchel, R. I. (1970). Reduction of stress in humans through nonveridical perceived control of aversive stimulation. *Journal of Personality and Social Psychology, 16,* 731–38.

Greenberg, J., & Burns, J. W. (2003). Pain anxiety among chronic pain patients: specific phobia or manifestation of anxiety sensitivity. *Behavior Research and Therapy, 41,* 223–40.

Grembowski, D., Anderson, R. M., & Chen, M. (1989). A public health model of the dental care process. *Medical Care Review, 46,* 439–96.

Gross, P. R. (1992a). Is pain sensitivity associated with dental avoidance? *Behavior Research and Therapy, 30,* 7–13.

———. (1992b). Is pain sensitivity associated with occupational fears in police recruits? *Behavior Research and Therapy, 30,* 407–09.

Grushka, M., & Sessle, B. J. (1984). Applicability of the McGill Pain Questionnaire to the differentiation of "toothache" pain. *Pain, 19,* 49–57.

Gryll, S. L., & Katahn, M. (1978). Situational factors contributing to the placebo effect. *Psychopharmacology, 57,* 253–61.

Hayes, S. C. (2004). Acceptance and commitment therapy, relational frame theory, and the third wave of behavioral and cognitive therapies. *Behavior Therapy, 35,* 840–68.

Holland, G. R. (2001). Management of dental pain (pp. 211–20). In J. P. Lund, F. J. Lavigne, R. Dubner, & B. J. Sessle (eds.), *Orofacial Pain: From Basic Science to Clinical Management.* Chicago: Quintessence.

Jerremalm, A., Jansson, L., & Ost, L. G. (1986). Individual response patterns and the effects of different behavioral methods in the treatment of dental phobia. *Behavior Research and Therapy, 34,* 587–96.

Kaakko, T., Horn, M. T., Weinstein, P., Kaufman, E., Leggott, P., & Coldwell, S. E. (2003). The influence of sequence of impressions on children's anxiety and discomfort. *Pediatric Dentistry, 25,* 357–64.

Kanfer, F. H., & Goldfoot, D. A. (1966). Self-control and tolerance of noxious stimulation. *Psychological Reports, 18,* 79–85.

Kanfer, F. H., & Seidner, M. L. (1973). Factors enhancing tolerance of noxious stimulation. *Journal of Personality and Social Psychology, 25,* 381–89.

Keefe, F. J., Lumley, M., Anderson, T., Lynch, T., & Carson, K. L. (2001). Pain and emotion: new research directions. *Journal of Clinical Psychology, 57,* 587–607.

Kent, G. (1984). Anxiety, pain and type of dental procedure. *Behavior Research and Therapy, 22,* 465–69.

Kent, G., & Blinkhorn, A. S. (1991). *The Psychology of Dental Care.* 2d ed. New York: Wright.

Kleinknecht, R. A., & Bernstein, D. A. (1978). The assessment of dental fear. *Behavior Therapy, 9,* 626–34.

Klepac, R. K. (1975). Successful treatment of avoidance of dentistry by desensitization or by increasing pain tolerance. *Journal of Behavior Therapy and Experimental Psychiatry, 6,* 307–10.

Klepac, R. K., McDonald, M., Hauge, G., & Dowling, J. (1980). Reactions to pain among subjects high and low in dental fear. *Journal of Behavioral Medicine, 3,* 373–84.

Lang, P. J. (1985). The cognitive psychophysiology of emotion: fear and anxiety. In A. H. Tuma & J. D. Maser (eds.), *Anxiety and the Anxiety Disorders.* Hillsdale, NJ: Lawrence Erlbaum.

LeResche, L. (2000). Epidemiology of orofacial pain (pp. 15–25). In J. P. Lund, G. J. Lavigne, R. Dubner, & B. J. Sessle (eds.), *Orofacial Pain: From Basic Science to Clinical Management.* Carol Stream, IL: Quintessence.

Law, A., Logan, H., & Baron, R. S. (1994). Desire for control, felt control, and stress inoculation training during dental treatment. *Journal of Personality and Social Psychology, 67,* 926–36.

Lethem, J., Slade, P. D., Troup, J. D. G., & Bentley, G. (1983). Outline of a fear-avoidance model of exaggerated pain perception-I. *Behavior Research and Therapy, 21,* 401–8.

Liddell, A., & Locker, D. (1997). Gender and age differences in attitudes to dental pain and dental control. *Community Dentistry and Oral Epidemiology, 25,* 314–18.

Lipton, J. A., & Marbach, J. J. (1984). Ethnicity and the pain experience. *Social Science Medicine, 19,* 1279–98.

Logan, H., Baron, R. S., Keeley, K., Law, A., & Stein, S. (1991). Desired control and felt control as mediators of stress in a dental setting. *Health Psychology, 10,* 352–59.

Ludwick-Rosenthal, R., & Neufeld, R. J. (1988). Stress management during medical procedures: an evaluative review of outcome studies. *Psychological Bulletin, 104,* 326–42.

Maggirias, J., & Locker, D. (2002). Psychological factors and perceptions of pain associated with dental treatment. *Community Dentistry and Oral Epidemiology, 30,* 151–59.

McCracken, L. M., Zayfert, C., & Gross, R. T. (1992). The Pain Anxiety Symptoms Scale: development and validation of a scale to measure fear of pain. *Pain, 50,* 67–73.

McNeil, D. W., & Berryman. M. L. (1989). Components of dental fear in adults? *Behavior Research and Therapy, 27,* 233–36.

McNeill, C., & Dubner, R. (2001). What is pain and how do we classify orofacial pain? (pp. 3–14). In J. P. Lund, F. J. Lavigne, R. Dubner, & B. J. Sessle (eds.), *Orofacial Pain: From Basic Science to Clinical Management.* Chicago: Quintessence.

Melzack, R. (1975). The McGill Pain Questionnaire: major properties and scoring methods. *Pain, 1,* 277–99.

Merskey, H., & Bogduk, N. (1994). *Classification of Chronic Pain.* 2d ed. Seattle: IASP Press.

Milgrom, P., Weinstein, P., Kleinknecht, R., & Getz, T. (1985). *Treating Fearful Dental Patients.* Reston, VA: Reston Publishing Company.

Miller, S. M. (1995). Monitoring versus blunting styles of coping with cancer influence the information patients want and need about their disease. *Cancer, 17,* 167–77.

Miller, S. M., Combs, C., & Stoddard, E. (1989). Information, coping and control in patients undergoing surgery and stressful medical procedures. In A. Steptoe & A. Appels (eds.), *Stress, Personal Control, and Health.* New York: Wiley & Sons.

Mowrer, O. H. (1939). A stimulus-response analysis of anxiety and its role as a reinforcing agent. *Psychological Review, 46,* 553–66.

Norton, P. J., & Asmundson, G. J. G. (2003). Amending the fear-avoidance model of chronic pain: what is the role of physiological arousal? *Behavior Therapy, 34,* 17–30.

Okeson, J. P. (1996). *Orofacial Pain: Guidelines for Assessment, Diagnosis, and Management.* Chicago: Quintessence.

Pau, A. K., Croucher, R., & Marcenes, W. (2003). Prevalence estimates and associated factors for dental pain: a review. *Oral Health & Preventive Dentistry, 1,* 209–20.

Payne, B., & Norfleet, M. A. (1986). Chronic pain and the family: a review. *Pain, 26,* 1–22.

Pickering, T. G., & Friedman, R. (1991). The white coat effect: a neglected role for behavioral factors in hypertension (pp. 35–49). In P. M. McCabe, N. Schneiderman, T. M. Field, & J. S. Skyler (eds.), *Stress, Coping, and Disease.* Hillsdale, NJ: Erlbaum.

Reading, A. E. (1979). The short term effects of psychological preparation for surgery. *Social Science and Medicine, 13,* 641–54.

Reiss, S. (1991). Expectancy theory of fear, anxiety, and panic. *Clinical Psychology Review, 11,* 141–153.

Reiss, S., & McNally, R. J. (1985). Expectancy model of fear. In S. Reis & R. R. Bootzin (eds.), *Theoretical Issues in Behavior Therapy.* Orlando: Academic Press.

Riley, J. L., Gilbert, G. H., & Heft, M. W. (2003). Socioeconomic and demographic disparities in symptoms of orofacial pain. *Journal of Public Health Dentistry, 63,* 166–73.

———. (2004). Oral health attitudes and communication with laypersons about orofacial pain among middle-aged and older adults. *Pain, 107,* 116–24.

Rollman, G. B., Lautenbacher, S., & Jones, K. S. (2000). Sex and gender differences in responses to experimentally induced pain in humans. In R. B. Fillingim (ed.), *Sex, Gender, and Pain: Vol. 17. Progress in Pain Research and Management* (pp. 165–90). Seattle, WA: IASP Press.

Sandell, R., Camner, L. G., & Sarhed, G. (1994). The dentist's attitudes and their interaction with patient involvement in oral hygiene compliance. *British Journal of Clinical Psychology, 33,* 549–58.

Seyrek, S. K., Corah, N. L., & Pace, L. F. (1984). Comparison of three distraction techniques in reducing stress in dental patients. *Journal of the American Dental Association, 108,* 327–29.

Shapiro, D. H., Schwartz, C. E., & Astin, J. A. (1996). Controlling ourselves, controlling our world: psychology's role in understanding positive and negative consequences of seeking and gaining control. *American Psychologist, 51,* 1213–30.

Shepherd, S. (1991). *Francie* [cartoon]. United Feature Syndicate, Inc.

Sinha, P. K., Nanda, R. S., & McNeil, D. W. (1996). Perceived orthodontist behaviors that predict patient satisfaction, orthodontist-patient relationship, and patient adherence in orthodontic treatment. *American Journal of Orthodontics and Dentofacial Orthopedics, 110,* 370–77.

Skevington, S. M. (1995). *Psychology of Pain.* Oxford, England: Wiley.

Sorrell, J. T. (2003). *Effects of Fear of Dental Pain and Information Type on Fear and Pain Responding During Endodontic Treatment.* Unpublished doctoral dissertation, West Virginia University, Morgantown.

Sorrell, J. T., & McNeil, D. W. (2005). Fear of Pain in Dentistry: An Integrated Model. Unpublished manuscript.

Staub, E., Tursky, B., & Schwartz, G. E. (1971). Self-control and predictability: their effects on reactions to aversive stimulation. *Journal of Personality and Social Psychology, 18,* 157–62.

Sullivan, M. J. L., & Neish, N. (1998). The effects of disclosure of pain during dental hygiene treatment: the moderating role of catastrophizing. *Pain, 79,* 155–63.

Taylor, S., Koch, W. J., & McNally, R. J. (1992). How does anxiety sensitivity vary across the anxiety disorders? *Journal of Anxiety Disorders, 6,* 249–59.

Thrash, W. J., Marr, J. N., & Boone, S. E. (1982). Continuous self-monitoring of discomfort in the dental chair and feedback to the dentist. *Journal of Behavioral Assessment, 4,* 273–84.

Turner, J. A., Dworkin, S. F., Manel, L., Huggins, K. H., & Truelove, E. L. (2001). The roles of beliefs, catastrophizing, and coping in the function of patients with temporomandibular disorder. *Pain, 92,* 41–51.

Van Buren, J., & Kleinknecht, R. A. (1979). An evaluation of the McGill Pain Questionnaire for use in dental pain assessment. *Pain, 6,* 23–33.

Vassend, O. (1993). Anxiety, pain and discomfort associated with dental treatment. *Behavior Research and Therapy, 31,* 659–66.

Vlaeyen, J. W. S., & Linton, S. J. (2000). Fear-avoidance and its consequences in chronic musculoskeletal pain: a state of the art. *Pain, 85,* 317–32.

Vlaeyen, J. W. S., de Jong, J., Geilen, M., Heuts, P. H. T. G., & Van Breukelen, G. (2001). Graded exposure in vivo in the treatment of pain-related fear: a replicated single-case experimental design in four patients with chronic low back pain. *Behavior Research and Therapy, 39,* 151–66.

Vowles, K. E., McNeil, D. W., Sorrell, J. T., & Lawrence, S. M. (in press). Which is worse, pain or fear? Investigating the interaction between two aversive states. *Journal of Abnormal Psychology.*

Walker, J. (2001). *Control and the Psychology of Health: Theory, Measurement, and Applications.* Philadelphia, PA: Open University Press.

Weisenberg, M., Kreindler, M. L., Schachat, R., & Werboff, J. (1975). Pain: anxiety and attitudes in Black, White, and Puerto Rican patients. *Psychosomatic Medicine, 37,* 123–35.

Zvolensky, M. J., Eifert, G. H., Lejuez, C. W., Hopko, D. R., & Forsyth, J. P. (2000). Assessing the perceived predictability of anxiety-related events: a report on the perceived predictability index. *Journal of Behavior Therapy and Experimental Psychiatry, 31,* 201–18.

Zvolensky, M. J., Goodie, J. L., McNeil, D. W., Sperry, J. S., & Sorrell, J. T. (2001). Anxiety sensitivity in the prediction of pain-related fear and anxiety in a heterogeneous chronic pain population. *Behavior Research and Therapy, 39,* 683–96.

Zvolensky, M. J., Lejuez, C. W., & Eifert, G. H. (2000). Prediction and control: operational definitions for the experimental analysis of anxiety. *Behavior Research and Therapy, 38,* 653–63.

Chronic Orofacial Pain: Biobehavioral Perspectives

Samuel F. Dworkin and Jeffrey Sherman

Pain: An unpleasant sensory and emotional experience associated with actual or potential tissue damage, or described in terms of such damage.
—Merskey and Bogduk, 1994

This chapter presents current perspectives on assessment and treatment of chronic orofacial pain patients. These perspectives advocate understanding the chronic pain patient as an integration of objectively measured physical and pathologic findings with subjectively reported physical, psychological, and psychosocial conditions. The universally accepted model system for understanding chronic pain from these perspectives is labeled the *biopsychosocial model for pain* (Engel, 1977). Accordingly, the specific objectives of this chapter are:

1. Define chronic pain and the most common chronic orofacial pain conditions confronting dentistry
2. Provide the rationale and description for the biopsychosocial model as applied to chronic orofacial pain
3. Describe the role of the dentist as a biobehavioral clinician whose clinical responsibilities extend to assessing the psychological and psychosocial dimensions of chronic orofacial pain, as well as assessing its physical/pathologic dimensions, and integrating such biobehavioral assessment into evidence-based clinical decisions regarding the comprehensive management of the chronic orofacial pain patient

Introduction

The most prevalent chronic orofacial pain conditions are musculoskeletal (e.g., temporomandibular disorders[TMD]) and neuropathic (e.g., trigeminal neuralgia and atypical odontalgias) pain conditions (LeResche, 2000). As a health-care profession, dentistry is arguably unparalleled in reducing and eliminating acute pain (e.g., toothache, dento-alveolar or periodontal abscess). However, chronic orofacial pain remains, unfortunately for too many patients, more resistant to quick or simple resolution because the amount and even the location of pain experienced and the behaviors of the patient with chronic or persistent pain problems are only poorly related to physical events, making etiology elusive and treatment difficult. Atypical odontalgia, for example, is usually associated with poorly defined pathologic markers inconsistent with expressed pain perception and behavior. Similarly, persistent pain in the masticatory muscles (myalgia) can be a source of minor inconvenience to some patients and for others can become a decades-long major disorganizing force associated with significant depression and disruption of their everyday lives—yet there may be no detectable, let alone diagnosable, physical change to distinguish the two. So, whether persistent pain is experienced as a minor inconvenience or a source of major life stress, chronic orofacial pain and related disability often cannot be understood in terms of diagnosable pathology (Dworkin, 1994).

Musculoskeletal pain, particularly TMD-related pain, is overwhelmingly the most commonly occurring chronic orofacial pain confronting dentistry, with a prevalence of about 10–15% in the United States and around the world (LeResche, 2000). TMD is associated with the same significant psychological and psychosocial issues that are found in all chronic pain conditions, orofacial or otherwise (Von Korff et al., 1988). Much of the remainder of this chapter uses TMD-related pain to elucidate major concepts as well as methods for biobehavioral assessment and management.

Toward a Biopsychosocial Model for Chronic Orofacial Pain

Neurophysiology and cognitive neuroscience now provide a biologic basis for understanding how emotional, thought, and behavioral processes can become linked and stored as integrated neural circuits, or neuromatrices, preserving memories and belief systems that influence the subjective pain experience and guide actions we take to cope with pain. The complex interaction of these multiple dimensions of pain are also known to be under the influence of genetic and reproductive hormonal factors (Mogil, Seltzer, & Devor, 2004). However, pain is always subjective.

Each individual learns the application of the word through experiences related to injury in early life. Biologists recognize that those stimuli that cause pain are liable to damage tissue. Accordingly, pain is that experience we associate with actual or potential tissue damage (Merskey, Bogduk, & Eds, 1994). It is unquestionably a sensation in a part or parts of the body, but it is also always unpleasant and therefore also an emotional experience. Alternatively, activity induced in the nociceptor and nociceptive pathways by a noxious stimulus, in the absence of the subjective self-report, is not pain.

That patients often report pain in the absence of detectable tissue damage or pathophysiological cause can lead a well-meaning practitioner to attribute the pain to psychological rather than organic etiology. We find such a distinction of little practical value for chronic pain because there is usually no way to distinguish the two etiologies. If the patient regards his experience as pain and if he reports it in the same ways as pain caused by tissue damage, it should be accepted as pain and treated accordingly. This definition avoids tying pain to the stimulus and avoids the potential pitfall of attributing a patient's subjective report as reflective of real or imagined pain. Instead, a more useful (and palatable for patients) view is that pain report in the absence of discernible tissue damage can potentially arise from *multiple reasons* (e.g., physical, psychological, social, and/or cultural processes) that invoke physiologic activity, which can be experienced subjectively as pain.

The Biopsychosocial Model

Mechanistic, biomedical views of pain as originating in the body and arising or maintained solely from objectively measurable pathophysiology are now considered scientifically inadequate to fully explain a chronic pain patient's presentation. It is now understood that health care providers have an inherent need to rely on patients as the only reliable source for knowing whether or not pain is present. We simultaneously recognize that the subjective pain report is the result of many co-occurring factors, ranging from pathobiology to prior experience to social context. Hence, the biomedical model of pain has been outgrown because of its too exclusive emphasis on physical factors.

It has been succeeded by a biopsychosocial model system (discussed more fully below), which clarifies how physical events in the body or in the environment often can give rise to not readily predicted pain experiences and behaviors that can be dependably shown to be related to patients' past pain history, gender, ethnicity, and (most critical for dentistry) factors in the environment that are equated with pain or the potential for pain. The term "biopsychosocial" has been applied to the most widely used model system developed to capture how information processing of painful events implicates psychological, behavioral, and psychosocial factors that interact with the physical events. The resultant of this complex interactive process is the wide range of pain expression, which dentists struggle to incorporate into their overall approach to management of dental and orofacial pain.

A model for integrating presumed physiologic activity associated with ongoing pain experience appears in figure 8.1 in schematic form. The model depicts that successively higher levels of central processing by the brain integrate the nociceptive or harmful stimuli present in the pain transmission system so they may emerge in consciousness as pain. Higher-order central processing assigns meaning to the pain for each individual, which then mobilizes patients to act within the social context of permissible behaviors, in response to their uniquely defined pain state. Because the model system seeks to integrate physiologic or pathophysiologic activity with associated

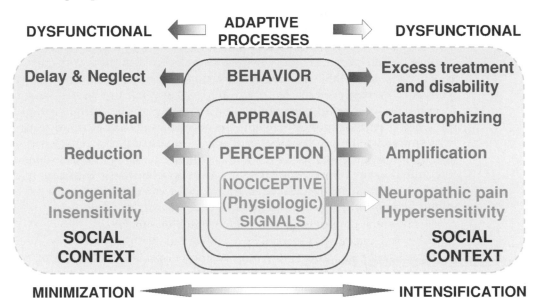

Fig. 8.1. Biopsychosocial model for pain. The model's five-stage processes integrate physiologic or pathophysiologic activity with associated psychological states and socially and culturally determined behavior. (Modified from Dworkin et al., 1992.)

psychological states and socially and culturally determined behavior, the model is labeled a "bio-psycho-social model"—that is, a model integrating biologic, psychologic, and social components of the pain experience (Dworkin, Von Korff, & LeResche, 1992).

The stages of the pain experience offered by this model system all reflect normal or adaptive mechanisms by which individuals come to experience pain and then attempt to make sense of the pain and adapt appropriately. These same higher-order processes are subject to distortions and maladaptive responses as well. Some examples are given for each level at which it is possible to analyze complex expressions of pain using this biopsychosocial model:

- *Nociception:* Physiologic events in the pain transmission system that, among other things, provide pain information to higher centers dealing with attention, memory, emotions, decision making, and motor preparedness.
- *Perception:* The initial stage of forming a subjective pain response, self-identifying the *physical* qualities of the pain experience, which include *sensory* (e.g., sharp, dull, throbbing), *spatial* (e.g., highly localized to an specific anatomic site, as in acute toothache, or diffuse, as in many cases of TMD pain), and *temporal* (e.g., acutely arising, recent onset, as in toothache, or recurrent and persistent over time, as in chronic TMD pain qualities.
- *Appraisal:* Higher order integrative mental operations attaching cognitive and emotional meaning to the painful sensations being perceived. The appraisal level is crucial for attaching attitudes, beliefs, expectations, and

emotional arousal to those pain sensations—in a word, meaning is attributed to the physical experience. Inappropriate attribution of meaning, influenced by interaction of nociceptive activity with attention and memory, may yield cognitive thought processes and emotional states that show themselves as pain-related catastrophizing thoughts, fear, anxiety, or depression.

- *Behavior:* Observable pain behaviors that are either contributory (e.g., bruxism) or the result of pain (verbal and nonverbal expressions of pain, inactivity, diet modification). Fordyce's introduction of the notion of "chronic pain behavior" into the rehabilitation of chronic pain patients was a revolutionary concept that called attention to the possibility for chronic pain conditions to become associated with maladaptive behavioral patterns of work or social avoidance, and that chronic pain treatment should not focus exclusively on uncovering difficult-to-observe pathophysiology but should focus heavily on behaviorally based methods for returning the pain patient to a more productive lifestyle.

- *Sick Role:* Cultural and societal factors shape the pain experience by defining roles for pain patients that may sanction disability, and providing specific forms of pain-related health care and medications. Sanctioning of different sick roles for men and women in response to pain is an important example of the influence that social factors can play in determining observable manifestations of pain. Options for treatment of dental and orofacial pain are often constrained by factors dictated by social or cultural factors, such as availability of health insurance and governmental regulation of narcotic analgesics. However, the sick role for a significant minority of patients experiencing chronic pain is associated with heavy use of health care services and demand for narcotic pain medications, both examples of pain behaviors that can run counter to social norms in many parts of the world.

In summary, the biopsychosocial model, as its name implies, reflects our growing understanding that illnesses and cures are indeed complex, that to understand how and when we experience pain and to understand whether or not we will respond to treatment, a host of factors in addition to biology must be considered. The biopsychosocial model does not seek to compete with, let alone replace, scientifically derived biologic models or current clinical practices. Rather, the model is an integrative one, which conceives that biologic processes and environmental factors, in the broad sense defined earlier, are equipotent for explaining not only pain conditions but also responses to treatment for the alleviation of pain.

A Dual-Axis Approach to Assessment of Dental and Orofacial Pain

Based on the above discussion, it is not surprising that currently no chronic pain problem is conceived of as either solely physical or mental, biologic or psychologic—either in the body, hence "real," or in the mind, hence "imagined." Instead of trying to force a particular patient with pain onto one end or the other of a single psychologic-versus-somatic continuum, the biopsychosocial perspective suggests, as figure 8.2 depicts, that at least two axes be

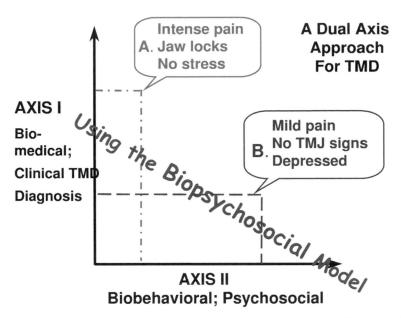

Fig. 8.2. Dual-axis schematic for pain assessment. Axis 1 comprises the status of a patient's physical/clinical factors that may yield a biologically based diagnosis; Axis 2 comprises an assessment of the patient's psychological, emotional, and behavioral status.

conceptualized for characterizing patients in pain. That is, each patient is located on Axis 1, reflecting the status of physical/clinical factors that may yield a biologically based diagnosis, and Axis 2, reflecting psychological, emotional, or behavioral and psychosocial status (Dworkin & LeResche, 1992). The Research Diagnostic Criteria for Temporomandibular Disorders (RDC/TMD) (Dworkin et al., 1992) uses such a dual-axis approach for the diagnosis and assessment of TMD patients. The Axis 2 components have been found to be reliable and valid as screening measures for depression, anxiety, and psychosocial disability. These measures are freely available at the website of the International Consortium for TMD Research (http://www.rdc-tmdinternational.org).

Assessing Psychological and Psychosocial Factors

As a guide to assessing pain patients with regard to the contribution of Axis 2 psychological and psychosocial factors, four domains of such biobehavioral assessment are recommended:

1. Pain history and response to prior treatment
2. Parafunctional oral behaviors (e.g., assessment of bruxism, pernicious oral habits)
3. Psychological screening
4. Interference with usual psychosocial functioning

From a practical treatment perspective, it should be noted that the assessment of these biobehavioral domains is possible largely through routine history and examination methods, supplemented with reliable and valid measures that are relatively easy for dentists to use and interpret.

Pain and Treatment History

Pain and treatment history are typically gathered as part of any new dental patient assessment. It is now strongly recommended that dentists gather data on intensity of pain through the use of 0–10 visual analogue or verbal descriptor scales, where patients simply mark a 10-cm line, anchored at one end with "no pain at all" and the other end with "the most intense pain imaginable" or respond to a verbal question using the same anchors. Such scales are used to assess average or typical pain intensity, worst pain, and current pain intensity. With regard to treatment history, it is important to record extent of prior treatment for chronic pain and degree of success or failure of such past treatments. Repeated bouts of treatment failure often reflect high risk for the failure of the next treatment.

Parafunctional Jaw Behaviors

The RDC/TMD includes a measure for assessing potentially excessive jaw behaviors such as clenching and/or grinding (bruxism) of the jaws. These behaviors are viewed as a significant risk factor by many for the initiation and maintenance of TMD-related orofacial chronic pain, although there has not yet emerged any clear scientific evidence to confirm the etiologic role that jaw parafunctional behaviors may play. This measure and others in widespread use (Stegenga et al., 1993) are straightforward and easy for dentists to use, interpret, and incorporate into their routine history protocols.

Psychological Status

Included here is recommended screening assessment for *depression, anxiety,* and the presence of *multiple nonspecific physical symptoms,* referred to in psychiatry as *somatization.* Formal assessment of psychological status requires specialized measurement instruments and/or diagnostic interview schedules beyond the training and expected clinical expertise of most dentists. However, the inclusion of relatively straightforward measures such as the SCL-90 (Derogatis & Cleary, 1977; Derogatis, 1983) in a clinical database, used routinely with all patients, minimizes resistance to the perception that attention is being unduly given to psychological factors when the patient feels that a physical pain problem is being presented.

Items included in this commonly used symptom checklist to detect anxiety, depression, and somatization are provided in tables 8.1–8.3. Such measures, although representing well-established psychological tests with excellent reliability and validity, are appropriate only as screening aids for psychological disturbance. As emphasized in the RDC/TMD Axis 2, these psychological measures are not intended to be diagnostic of psychopathology. Rather, they allow dentists treating chronic-orofacial-pain patients to obtain a clearer understanding of the psychological status of the chronic-pain patient and to evaluate the need for more specialized psychological assessment. This information will also help the dentist to be able to formulate a treatment plan that has a reasonable chance of succeeding, a plan that is appropriate to the state of the person as well as the state of the organ system in which physical pathology is presumed to reside.

Anxiety and panic are emotional disturbances not only seen in phobic dental patients but also increasingly recognized as concomitant psychological factors of chronic orofacial pain as well. These states are commonly seen during the acute phase of the orofacial pain problem when uncertainty over the meaning and future course of pain and any physical disease or other pathology that might underlie the pain is a dominant concern. Often as the pain becomes more chronic, depression becomes a more prevalent co-occurring problem as fear and anxiety give way to hopelessness about the future and helplessness about finding a cure. Similarly, somatization, the subjective reporting of widespread, nonspecific physical symptoms, is present to an excessive degree in a significant minority of TMD patients, and is associated with such diverse consequences as presenting an important risk factor for poor TMD treatment outcome and for potentially confounding the accurate diagnosis of particular chronic orofacial pain conditions (McCreary et al., 1992). The presence of these psychological disturbances can be assessed with items found in the RDC/TMD and shown in tables 8.1, 8.2, and 8.3.

Psychosocial Status
Included here is RDC/TMD Axis 2 Graded Chronic Pain Scale (GCP) to assess current level of psychosocial function (Von Korff et al., 1992). The GCP

Table 8.1 Depression Scale Items

Feeling lonely	Worrying too much
Low energy/slowed	Everything an effort
Feeling blue	Feeling caught/trapped
Crying easily	No interest in things
Trouble falling asleep	Hopeless about future
Restless or disturbed sleep	Worthlessness
Loss of sexual interest	Feelings of guilt
Poor appetite	Blaming self
Overeating	Thoughts of death or dying
	Thoughts of ending your life

Note: Screening for depression, from SCL-90.

Table 8.2 Anxiety Scale Items

Spells of terror or panic	Nervous or shaky inside
Trembling	Feeling tense or keyed up
Feeling something bad is going to happen to you	Suddenly being scared for no reason
Thoughts or images of a frightening nature	Heart pounding or racing
Feeling so restless can't sit still	Feeling fearful

Note: Screening for anxiety, from SCL-90.

Table 8.3   Somatization Scale Items

Headaches	Trouble breathing
Pains in heart/chest	Hot/cold spells
Pains in lower back	Numbness/tingling
Nausea/gastric upset	Lump in throat
Muscle soreness	Weakness in body
Faintness/dizziness	Heaviness in limbs

Note: Screening for anxiety, from SCL-90.

has been used primarily in conjunction with Axis 2 assessment of chronic orofacial pain patients to assess, in a single index, both the severity of pain and the extent of pain-related interference with activities of daily living and extent of health-care utilization. The seven items of the GCP are shown in table 8.4. Prognosis is more guarded when self-reported activity limitations due to chronic pain are high and when pain interferes appreciably with ability to discharge responsibilities at home, school, or work and/or limits socializing activities.

Additional Useful Measures of Psychosocial Functioning

Multidimensional Pain Inventory (MPI)
The MPI is an important and widely used instrument to assess psychosocial function in chronic pain patients (Kerns, Turk, & Rudy, 1985). The MPI is much longer than the simple GCP but provides somewhat more information

Table 8.4   Graded Chronic Pain Scale (7-Item Visual Analog Scales)

Pain intensity rating (visual analog scales)
On a 0 to 10 scale, where 0 is "no pain" and 10 is "pain as bad as could be," how would you rate your facial pain:
    1. Present pain?
    2. Worst pain, past six months?
    3. Average pain, past six months?

Pain interference (visual analog scales)
On a 0 to 10 scale, where 0 is "no change" and 10 is "extreme change," in the past six months, how would you rate how much pain has interfered with your ability to:
    4. Take part in recreational, social, and family activities?
    5. Work?

On a 0 to 10 scale, where 0 is "no interference" and 10 is "unable to carry on any activities," in the past six months, how much has pain interfered with:
    6. Daily activities?

Days lost
How many days in the past six months has pain kept you from your usual activities:
    7. _____ (0–180) days

for those who find it helpful in their clinical management and research to have a more detailed measure of psychosocial function. The MPI assesses pain impact (severity, interference), responses of others, and activities, and enables patients to be classified into dysfunctional, interpersonally distressed, and adaptive-coper subgroups. Such categorization has also proven useful in treatment planning because studies have shown that dysfunctional patients improved more when treatment of depression was added to standard appliance and biofeedback therapy, and acute TMD pain patients who were found to be dysfunctional and distressed on the MPI have been shown to be more likely to develop chronic TMD pain, while the dysfunctional profile also has been shown to predict treatment failure.

Substance Abuse

Substance abuse, principally with alcohol and narcotics, is frequently reported in the chronic pain and TMD literature to be more common than in the general population. Dentists may wish to consider the Alcohol Use Disorders Identification Test (AUDIT-C) as a brief screen for these problems. It uses three questions (How often do you have a drink containing alcohol? How many drinks containing alcohol do you have on a typical day when you are drinking? How often do you have six or more drinks on one occasion?). An even briefer screen for both alcohol and drug abuse is the two-item conjoint screening test (TICS) (In the last year, have you ever drunk or used drugs more than you meant to? Have you felt you wanted or needed to cut down on your drinking or drug use in the last year?). These brief measures have been shown to have good sensitivity and specificity for detecting current substance use disorders (Bush et al., 1998).

Sleep Disturbance

Disturbed sleep is a potent dysregulator of homeostatic bodily processes, and sleep disturbance is consistently reported to be higher among chronic pain and patients than in the population at large. The Pittsburgh Sleep Quality Inventory (Buysse et al., 1995) is a widely used measure of sleep disturbance. Supplementing it with a single question, "How is your sleep overall?" may serve as an adequate screen to detect the possible presence of a sleep disturbance warranting further pursuit. There are therapeutic modalities available to enhance sleep hygiene, which range from medications to brief cognitive-behavioral therapy interventions.

Assessing Post-Traumatic Stress Disorder, Physical and Sexual Abuse

In addition to the more commonly assessed psychological and psychosocial factors discussed above, there are a number of other issues that seem to have direct relevance for at least some chronic TMD pain patients.

Post-Traumatic Stress Disorder (PTSD)

PTSD is a psychiatric disorder that can occur following the experience or witnessing of life-threatening events such as military combat, natural disasters, serious accidents, or violent personal assaults like rape. People who suffer from PTSD often relive the experience through nightmares and flashbacks, have difficulty sleeping, and feel detached or estranged. These symptoms can be severe enough and last long enough to significantly impair the person's daily life. We have shown that in addition to being highly prevalent in chronic orofacial pain, patients with TMD and PTSD present with a more complicated clinical picture that includes more intense pain and functional impairment when compared to those without PTSD (Sherman et al., 2005).

There is good evidence supporting a synergy between chronic pain, including chronic TMD pain, and PTSD, but what remains unknown to date is the predictive value of routinely assessing PTSD in such TMD pain patients. However, it seems reasonable that screening measures be used in cases where PTSD is suspected. This can be done using the Clinician Administered PTSD Scale (CAPS) or the PTSD Checklist (Blake et al., 1990).

Physical and Sexual Abuse (Domestic Violence)

The literature contains numerous accounts of the frequent occurrence of physical and sexual abuse in chronic TMD pain patients. The lifetime prevalence of such domestic violence is estimated to be about 16% of the American population. While women are the most common target of such abuse, men, the very young, and the elderly are also targets.

Because the consequences can be so grave, and because the overwhelming tendency is to hide or deny any experience of abuse, it seems appropriate to recommend to clinicians treating patients where persistent pain is a dependable part of the clinical picture, that sensitive screening for issues of physical and sexual abuse be undertaken after a secure dentist-patient relationship has been obtained. The recommended assessment process in the so-called AVDR model: Ask about abuse, provide Validating messages, Document presenting signs and symptoms, Refer victims to domestic violence specialists (Blake et al., 1990).

The Dentist as Biobehavioral Clinician: Guidelines for Obtaining and Using Biobehavioral Assessment Data

As previously mentioned, it is recommended that biobehavioral assessment be conducted for screening purposes on all dental patients reporting persistent pain. When such psychological and psychosocial measures are incorporated into a routinely administered battery of history questionnaires, it is unusual to find resistance to these inquiries—instead many patients express gratitude for the clinician's interest in getting a comprehensive understanding of their total pain-related experiences.

As a general rule, biobehavioral assessment is conducted before the clinician encounters the patient, through the use of baseline history questionnaires. When resistance is met ("why are you asking me such personal questions" or "why do you need to know that"), it is recommended that the clinician accept the patient's hesitancies and allow the patient not to answer any or all questions deemed sensitive or irrelevant. Again, this rarely occurring resistance is best responded to with empathy and support, together with a brief explanation of how the desired information allows the clinician to better understand how patients are coping with this condition, and that such questions do not imply that the cause of their problem is psychologically related.

The label "biobehavioral" has gained acceptance as a collective term to refer to treatment approaches for chronic pain derived from applying behavioral science theories and methods to changing the perception and appraisal of pain and ameliorating or eliminating the personal suffering and psychosocial dysfunction that often accompany persistent pain conditions (National Institutes of Health, 1995). The biobehavioral pain management modalities are drawn more specifically from cognitive-behavioral therapy (CBT) as well as educational approaches; these psychologically based therapies include biofeedback, relaxation, imagery, and hypnosis.

Substantial evidence has emerged over the past two decades that such modalities are safe and effective in the management of chronic pain conditions (Vlaeyen & Morley, 2005). These biobehavioral treatments (National Institutes of Health, 1995; Turk & Meichenbaum, 1989; Turk, 1990)constitute a component of virtually every chronic pain treatment program and the management of chronic orofacial pain, notably TMD, has benefited from such biobehavioral interventions as well. Overwhelmingly, these methods emphasize as their common objectives self-management and the acquisition of self-control over not only pain symptoms but also cognitive attributions or meanings given to those symptoms and, most important, to maintaining a productive level of psychosocial function, even if pain is not totally absent (Turner et al., 1990). Our own and others' research has shown in repeated randomized clinical trials how CBT, including use of education, relaxation, and relapse-prevention strategies may be applied in general or specialty dental offices, by dentists or, in many cases of chronic TMD-related pain, by qualified members of the dental office staff (Dworkin et al., 2001; Turk, Zaki, & Rudy, 1993). Alternatively, the dentist may elect to refer to mental health professionals (psychiatrists, clinical psychologists, and qualified psychiatric social workers) those chronic orofacial pain patients who have been identified by biobehavioral screening as burdened with heightened psychological or psychosocial disability (Dworkin et al., 2002).

By and large, when biobehavioral treatments are employed in the management of chronic orofacial pain, effects are virtually always positive and in the hypothesized beneficial direction, though often effects are moderate in size. However, these biobehavioral methods, especially those subsumed under the label "cognitive-behavioral," appear to have the potential for producing long-lasting benefits that exceed those observed with usual clinical treatment for TMD. Increasingly, it should be noted, conservative, noninvasive approaches to TMD management are being advocated as the preferred overall treatment approach for this hard-to-understand chronic pain problem (Greene, 1992). These so-called conservative treatments generally incorporate many of the same elements (i.e., relaxation, stress-education, habit behavior modification, etc.) found in cognitive-behavioral and biobehavioral therapies for TMD. Thus, both usual clinical treatment for TMD and biobehavioral treatment employ multimodal approaches, and it does not yet appear possible to disengage which of the multiple therapeutic components are most efficacious. If one method had to be singled out, relaxation seems to emerge consistently as an effective method for chronic pain management across a wide variety of pain conditions and over a wide variety of clinical settings. In any event, of the combined biobehavioral methods commonly used in clinical practice and in research, one method has as yet failed to emerge as superior to another.

It is important to note that much the same situation obtains with regard to biomedically based TMD treatments. Little is known about the superiority of any one of the multiple methods commonly employed to biomedically manage TMD—there is no strong scientific evidence to substantiate invasive versus noninvasive treatments or pharmacological treatments emphasizing analgesics versus those stressing antidepressants or muscle relaxants. It is the absence of compelling evidence to the contrary that has led many clinical researchers to advocate conservative, reversible therapies for the largest number of TMD patients.

Summary

Psychological and psychosocial factors are universally accepted as prominent features among patients seeking treatment for amelioration of chronic orofacial pain, including, TMD. Indeed, for a significant number of chronic TMD pain patients, these pain-related emotional and behavioral factors may represent the major burden their condition imposes, putting an important stamp on the clinical presentation. While definitive information is not yet available regarding whether such emotional and behavioral factors are causes or effects of TMD pain, it is nevertheless widely accepted that comprehensive management of such patients requires attention to these issues. In practical terms, this means assessing levels of psychological and psychosocial disturbance in order to determine whether treatment decision making should also include recommendations for incorporating psychological and/or behavioral management into comprehensive TMD treatment. In terms of clinical utility for biomedical clinicians seeking to provide the most comprehensive treatment for their chronic TMD pain patients, four domains of psychological and psychosocial assessment are recommended: (1) pain; (2) mandibular function and behaviors; (3) psychological status—principally, depression, and somatization; and,(4) psychosocial level of function as related to quality of life and use of health-care services or medications.

The RDC/TMD offers a battery of reliable and valid measures that have gained wide acceptance and use. Psychological domains worthy of assessment but not incorporated into the RDC/TMD include anxiety, substance abuse, and sleep disturbance. Additional domains seemingly relevant to a comprehensive assessment of the TMD patient include physical/sexual abuse and PTSD. Finally, the major thrust of this chapter has been to persuade the reader that a biopsychosocial approach—the model system that guides all major multidisciplinary pain centers—should be used by all clinicians treating TMD patients. Current scientific evidence overwhelmingly confirms that this approach enhances both the understanding and the management of all chronic orofacial pain conditions.

References

Blake, D., Weathers, F., Nagy, L., Kaloupek, D., Gusman, F., & Charney, D. (1990). A clinician rating scale for assessing current and lifetime PTSD: The CAPS-1. *Behavior Research and Therapy, 13,* 187–88.

Bush, K., Kivlahan, D., McDonell, M., Fihn, S., & Bradley, K. (1998). The AUDIT alcohol consumption questions: an effective brief screening test for problem drinking. *Archives of Internal Medicine, 158,* 1789–95.

Buysse, D., Reynolds, C. I., Monk, T., Berman, S., & Kuofer, D. (1995). Pittsburgh Sleep Quality Index (PSQI). In N. Schutte & J. Malouff (eds.), *Sourcebook of Adult Assessment* (pp. 349–58). New York: Plenum Press.

Derogatis, L. R. (1983). *SCL-90-R: Administration, Scoring and Procedures Manual—II for the Revised Version.* Towson, MD: Clinical Psychometric Research.

Derogatis, L. R., & Cleary, P. A. (1977). Confirmation of the dimensional structure of the SCL-90: a study in construct validation. *Journal of Clinical Psychology, 33,* 981–89.

Dworkin, S. F. (1994). Behavioral, emotional, and social aspects of orofacial pain. In C. S. Stohler & D. S. Carlson (eds.), *Biological and Psychological Aspects of Orofacial Pain* (pp. 93–112). Ann Arbor: The University of Michigan.

Dworkin, S. F., & LeResche, L. (1992). Research diagnostic criteria for temporomandibular disorders: review, criteria, examinations and specifications, critique. *Journal of Craniomandibular Disorders: Facial & Oral Pain, 6,* 301–55.

Dworkin, S. F., Huggins, K. H., Wilson, L., Mancl, L., Turner, J. A., Massoth, D. L., et al. (2001). A randomized clinical trial using research criteria for temporomandibular disorders-axis II to target clinic cases for a tailored self-care treatment program. *Journal of Orofacial Pain, 16,* 48–63.

Dworkin, S. F., Turner, J. A., Mancl, L., Wilson, L., Massoth, D., Huggins, K. H., et al. (2002). A randomized clinical trial of a tailored comprehensive care treatment program for temporomandibular disorders. *Journal of Orofacial Pain, 16,* 259–76.

Dworkin, S. F., Von Korff, M., & LeResche, L. (1992). Epidemiologic studies of chronic pain: a dynamic-ecologic perspective. *Annals of Behavioral Medicine, 14,* 3–11.

Engel, G. (1977). The need for a new medical model: a challenge for biomedicine. *Science, 196,* 129–36.

Greene, C. S. (1992). Temporomandibular disorders: the evolution of concepts. In B. G. Sarnat & D. M. Laskin (eds.), *The Temporomandibular Joint: A Biological Basis for Clinical Practice* (4th ed., pp. 298–315). Philadelphia: W. B. Saunders Company.

Kerns, R. D., Turk, D. C., & Rudy, T. E. (1985). The West Haven-Yale Multidimensional Pain Inventory (WHYMPI). *Pain, 23,* 345–56.

LeResche, L. (2000). Epidemiology of orofacial pain (in press). In J. P. Lund, G. Lavigne, R. Dubner, & B. Sessle (eds.), *Orofacial Pain: From Basic Science to Clinical Management* (pp. 1–11). Carol Stream, IL: Quintessence Publishing Co.

McCreary, C. P., Clark, G. T., Oakley, M. E., & Flack, V. (1992). Predicting response to treatment for temporomandibular disorders. *Journal of Craniomandibular Disorders: Facial & Oral Pain, 6,* 161–69.

Merskey, H., Bogduk, N., & eds. (1994). *Classification of Chronic Pain, Second Edition.* Seattle: IASP Press.

Mogil, J. S., Seltzer, Z., & Devor, M. (2004). Gene-environment interactions affecting pain phenotype. In J. S. Mogil (ed.), *The Genetics of Pain, Progress in Pain Research and Management, vol. 28* (pp. 257–81). Seattle: IASP Press.

National Institutes of Health. (1995). *Integration of behavioral and relaxation approaches into the treatment of chronic pain and insomnia: National Institutes of Health Technology Assessment Conference Statement, October 16–18, 1995.* Bethesda, MD: NIH Office of the Director.

Sherman, J., Carlson, C. R., Wilson, J. F., Okeson, J. P., & McCubbin, J. A. (2005). Post-traumatic stress disorder among patients with orofacial pain. *Journal of Orofacial Pain*. In Press.

Stegenga, B., de Bont, L. G. M., de Leeuw, R., & Boering, G. (1993). Assessment of mandibular function impairment associated with temporomandibular joint osteoarthrosis and internal derangement. *Journal of Orofacial Pain, 7*, 183–95.

Turk, D. C. (1990). Customizing treatment for chronic pain patients: who, what, why. *Clinical Journal of Pain, 6*, 255–70.

Turk, D. C., & Meichenbaum, D. (1989). A cognitive behavioral approach to pain management. In P. D. Wall & R. Melzack (eds.), *Textbook of Pain* (2d ed., pp. 1001–9). London: Churchill Livingstone.

Turk, D. C., Zaki, H. S., & Rudy, T. E. (1993). Effects of intraoral appliance and biofeedback/stress management alone and in combination in treating pain and depression in patients with temporomandibular disorders. *Journal of Prosthetic Dentistry, 70*, 158–64.

Turner, J. A., Clancy, S., McQuade, K. J., & Cardenas, D. D. (1990). Effectiveness of behavioral therapy for chronic low back pain: a component analysis. *Journal of Consulting and Clinical Psychology, 58*, 573–79.

Vlaeyen, J. W., & Morley, S. (2005). Cognitive-behavioral treatments for chronic pain. *Clinical Journal of Pain, 21*, 1–8.

Von Korff, M., Dworkin, S. F., LeResche, L., & Kruger, A. (1988). Epidemiology of temporomandibular disorders: TMD pain compared to other common pain sites. In R. Dubner, G. F. Gebhart, & M. R. Bond (eds.), *Pain Research and Clinical Management* (pp. 506–11). Amsterdam: Elsevier Science Publishers.

Von Korff, M., Ormel, J., Keefe, F. J., & Dworkin, S. F. (1992). Grading the severity of chronic pain. *Pain, 50*, 133–49.

Chairside Techniques for Reducing Dental Fear

Ronald W. Botto

How, when, or why it happened is a mystery to me, but somehow I've developed a dental phobia so extreme as to keep me away from a dental office most of my adult life. Just mentioning the word "dentist" made me cringe. Hearing an orthodontic or toothpaste commercial on radio or TV made me run from the room.
—Adult Female

I don't know, just the word "dentist" does something to me. So after I got in the chair, I asked the dentist if I could go to the bathroom. He said "yes", so I went to the waiting room, grabbed my hat and coat, and ran out.
—Adult Male

The feelings expressed in the quotations above from two different dental patients, although perhaps somewhat extreme, are not uncommon. As other chapters in this book have shown, dental fear is probably one of the most prevalent problems that dentists face in treating patients. Dental fear contributes greatly to avoidance of dental care (Morse, 2002), and if care is sought, fear makes the experience trying for patient, staff, and dentist alike (Moore & Brodsgaard, 2001), and can impact the patient's life negatively (Cohen, Fiske, & Newton, 2000; Locker, 2003). While practitioners and their staff may feel that avoiding the issue and just working fast to get the patient out of the chair is the best approach, not resolving a patient's anxiety can lengthen appointments, exacerbate pain perception, and reinforce negative attitudes, making subsequent appointments even worse.

In this chapter, I provide a "reader's guide" to performing a few of the many different behavioral techniques that can help reduce patient fear. One approach to categorizing the various behavioral interventions is according to the role that relaxation plays in each. Thus, one can identify (1) nonrelaxation-based techniques, (2) "quasi-relaxation"-based techniques, and (3) relaxation-based techniques.

Nonrelaxation-based techniques are those that employ intervention strategies that do not utilize relaxation types of procedures (directly or indirectly) in their implementation. Examples of procedures of this type are communication skills (including the redefining of sensations), distraction, behavior modification, modeling, cognitive restructuring or cognitive behavior modification, stress inoculation, flooding or implosion, and acupressure. Quasi-relaxation-based techniques are those that achieve relaxation indirectly, without employing a formal progressive muscle relaxation procedure. Examples are guided imagery, paced breathing, biofeedback, graduated exposure, and meditation. Relaxation-based techniques incorporate progressive relaxation-type procedures directly as part of the intervention. Included in this category are progressive relaxation, systematic desensitization, and hypnosis.

These techniques vary also in terms of both expediency and the level of training needed to use them effectively, with hypnosis requiring the most formal training to be both safe and effective. Because the degree of complexity varies with these approaches, the technique used should reflect the degree of fear the patient is experiencing. In general, complexity increases from nonrelaxation-based techniques to relaxation-based techniques. In addition, relaxation-based techniques would usually be more appropriate for moderate to high levels of fear than mild levels of fear. For example, using a relaxation procedure on a patient who feels mildly apprehensive would be effective, but would not be an efficient use of either the patient's or practitioner's time. Because of space limitations, only a few representative interventions can be discussed here.

Nonrelaxation-Based Techniques

Communication

First (and foremost) on the list of intervention techniques is that of communication (van der Molen, Klaver, & Duyx, 2004). In many respects, one could argue that effective communication is actually a foundation skill for all of the others, especially listening skills. In interpersonal communication, it is not only critical that the listener does indeed listen, but that the speaker also feels heard. One common cue that the patient is not feeling heard or understood is that the message continues to be repeated.

Before discussing some specific communication skills, the question of whether or not to even communicate needs to be addressed. Some practitioners hold the belief that discussing fear with the patient "will make it worse," including concern over employing Corah's Dental Anxiety Scale. Dailey , Humphris, & Lennon (2002) assessed the impact of patients' completing the scale and sharing the results with the dentist. The results clearly showed that patients preferred to have the dentist aware of their fear. The problem is generally not with patients expressing their fears, but what the practitioner does with that information.

The practitioner or staff will commonly attempt to "reassure" the patient by stating something along the lines of "Don't worry; everything will be fine," or "There's nothing to be afraid of." Although well-intentioned, reassurance is ineffective, causing the patients to feel that their concerns are being dismissed or diminished (Chambers & Abrams, 1992). A quick affirmation of this concept can be experienced by the reader by simply taking a couple of minutes to reflect on something he or she considers very threatening and then imagining someone saying "Don't worry, everything will be all right," and seeing how much it diminishes the perceived threat. Instead of attempting to directly reassure the patient, it is more effective to listen empathetically and teach interventions that resolve the patient's apprehension. In other words, reassurance is the outcome, not the intervention.

The first step in communicating with patients about their fears is to determine whether or not the patient is fearful. As mentioned above, patients who are fearful want the dentist to know how they feel. While many different assessment tools exist for this task, formal quantification is more critical for research purposes than for clinical treatment. The practitioner will usually find it sufficient to simply ask each patient "How apprehensive or fearful are you about having dental work done?" If the patient answers "Not at all," nothing else needs to be discussed on this topic and the patient will appreciate the practitioner's being sensitive and caring enough to ask. If the patient answers anything greater than that—even "A little"—then the practitioner needs to gather more information regarding what types of things bother the patient and how anxious each activity makes him or her, and then let the patient know that there are a number of things that the practitioner can do to help the patient feel more comfortable. This discussion should normally be part of the initial diagnostic interview with each patient.

It is important in the above discussion that the practitioner state clearly to the patient that he/she understands the patient's fears rather than evaluate their "validity." This is simply accomplished by stating, "I understand," and then stating back to the patient what the practitioner understands the patient to be saying. This reflection can include both the content and feelings that the practitioner perceives the patient to be expressing.

There may not always be concordance among the various ways that fear can be expressed (verbal, behavioral, physiological), called "response desynchrony." A patient may say that he is relaxed, yet be gripping the chair, tense, sweating profusely, and/or breathing shallowly. The opposite could also occur, in that the patient may say that he is anxious, but show no other signs of fear. A simple rule of thumb is to address any messages that might be associated with apprehension, whether they are verbal, behavioral, or physiological. A simple method to remember the preceding communication points is to think about them as the "Three A's of Anxiety":

1. *Ask* how anxious they are
2. *Acknowledge* what you have heard
3. *Address* the fears by offering solutions

Other communication guidelines include the careful choice of terms used. Anxiety-producing terms or phrases such as "give a shot," "cut down a tooth," "pull your tooth," "have a root canal," or "this may hurt a bit," should be avoided. Instead, terms such as "get the area numb," "remove the tooth," "shape the tooth," "endodontic treatment," or "pinch or sting a little," are preferable. In addition, avoid describing the instruments used. Telling a patient about using needles, syringes, files, scalpels, or forceps is not going to comfort them. Finally, only make promises that can be backed. Although this may seem obvious, it is not uncommon to hear the following statement, "Before we start, we will numb you up so you won't feel anything." Local anesthesia rarely renders the patient devoid of sensation. As a result, the sensations that are perceived (e.g., movement, pressure) are often interpreted by the patient as indicating insufficient anesthesia, and therefore often are perceived as painful. Instead, let the patient know what sensations will be perceived following anesthesia (e.g., "You will feel pressure and vibration").

A final communication "rule" to be mentioned is to ensure that the patient has a means of communicating while the practitioner is working and the patient's mouth is open. In spite of the recurring comic parodies of a dentist conversing with a patient whose mouth is open and full of instruments, patients at times feel reduced to this form of "communication." A more effective way for the patient to communicate when verbal methods are impaired is to signal the practitioner when the discomfort gets too great, or if she or he wishes the practitioner to stop. This approach has the added benefit of giving the patient the perception of being in control during the procedure, thereby reducing fear and playing an important role as an antecedent to, and consequence of, the patient's dental experience (Milgrom, Weinstein, & Getz, 1995).

One easily implemented signal is to tell the patient to raise the hand opposite the practitioner. It is important that the practitioner honor the guidelines that he or she has set, and cease working when the patient signals discomfort. Extremely anxious patients, especially children, may "test" the practitioner by raising their hands before any procedure actually occurs. It is important that the dentist stop as promised. At the same time, the practitioner needs to address the patient's testing and let the patient know that she or he must be accurate when signaling and use it only when too uncomfortable to continue. Also, when administering local anesthesia, discomfort primarily occurs while inserting the needle and when injecting the anesthetic. When the patient raises his/her hand, the practitioner can acknowledge the signal by stopping the injection process, saying "OK," but not removing the needle. After a brief pause, the process can be continued. In this way, although there may be a number of pauses, the process will be completed and the patient will feel more at ease.

Distraction

Distraction is an easily utilized method of reducing a patient's apprehension during the occurrence of uncomfortable sensations. Most commonly taught and used is the jiggling of the patient's cheek during the administration of local anesthesia. Another technique commonly used with children is asking them to hold their leg up in the air. While both of these can be helpful, they can have limited utility.

The purpose of distraction techniques is to refocus the patient's attention away from the potentially painful stimulus or procedure. Distraction techniques can be grouped into two main categories: physical methods and mental methods. Both are effective and can be employed separately or in combination.

Physical methods include the aforementioned cheek jiggling and leg raising. Other methods include listening to music or recorded books through earphones, playing video games, watching movies, or other recorded programs on monitors or specially constructed glasses, rubbing the cheek of the patient or massaging the gums (during injections), or simply asking the patient to count the holes in the acoustic tiles in the ceiling over the operatory.

One particularly easy and effective physical distraction method is the use of breath control. In this method, the patient is asked to breathe according to the practitioner's directions. Have the patient place hands on stomach, and then direct the patient to breathe according to the following pattern:

1. Take a deep breath, hold it briefly, and then let it out slowly.
2. Take a normal slow breath.
3. Take another deep breath, hold it briefly, then let half out, hold it, then let the rest out.
4. Take a normal breath.
5. For successive breaths, let breath out a third at a time, a quarter at a time, a fifth at a time, etc.

Between each paced breath, have the patient take a slow normal breath. This helps the patient relax in a couple of ways. First, it distracts the patient by placing the focus on the stomach rising and falling and the task of controlling breathing. Second, it slows down respiration, and by inducing deep diaphragmatic breathing, it will stimulate the parasympathetic nervous system, which is associated with relaxation.

Mental methods of distraction include various mental exercises that the patient can engage in while the practitioner is performing particularly stressful parts of a procedure. Examples include having the patient count backwards to themselves from one hundred by threes, then fours, saying the alphabet backwards, solving mathematical long division or multiplication problems in their head, or thinking about different events such as holidays or birthday celebrations (assuming the patient considers them positive and nonstressing).

Quasi-Relaxation-Based Techniques

As stated earlier, these are referred to as quasi-relaxation-based techniques because they employ relaxation indirectly. For example, when using biofeedback, the patient is not routinely instructed in formal progressive relaxation, but simply is asked to relax and reduce the muscle tension in the measured area. It is not uncommon for the patient to relax all the muscles in the body while relaxing the frontalis or masseter muscles. In paced breathing, similar to the breath-control method mentioned above, the patient is taught to regulate breathing in a rhythmic fashion, which is timed to a signal, often a metronome. This regulation of breathing results in the same type of physiological reaction discussed above.

Guided Imagery

Guided imagery is a more elaborate version of the mental distraction technique discussed above involving the patient thinking about positive events. In guided imagery, ask the patient about particularly pleasant, relaxing scenes he or she would like to imagine. Tell the patient to remember as much detail as possible because after the dental procedure is over, you want to hear a description. Once the patient identifies the specific scene(s) he or she would like to imagine (e.g., relaxing on a particular familiar beach, sitting in a park at a particular season), the patient is asked to get relaxed, close his/her eyes, engage in slow regular breathing, and begin imagining the scene in as much detail as possible. The patient's imagery should incorporate as many senses as possible (sight, sound, smell, touch, taste), and again, be as specific as possible. Directions by the practitioner such as "notice the color of the sky; listen to the children playing in the distance, smell the ocean" can be used. The practitioner can periodically reinforce the patient's imagery work by telling the patient to "continue to imagine yourself enjoying relaxing [wherever the scene is]" or, if more than one scene was suggested by the patient, by suggesting that the patient switch scenes. After the dental procedure is over, the dentist should discuss the experience with the patient, asking for a description of what the patient was imagining, how well it worked, and what would enhance its effectiveness.

There are a number of variations of guided imagery, which vary in complexity. In the above method, the patient is simply asked to relax before engaging in the imagery (Milgrom et al., 1995). Other versions include a fifteen- to twenty-minute formal relaxation procedure prior to the imagery (Geboy, 1985). In this case, the procedure would be included in the next category of relaxation-based techniques and entail more time.

Relaxation-Based Procedures

These methods employ a formal progressive muscle relaxation (or, as in the case of hypnosis, a relaxation-like) procedure as part of the method, or as the intervention itself. The methods most commonly employed in this category are *progressive relaxation, systematic desensitization*, and *hypnosis*. Of these, hypnosis should only be used after formal training. Systematic desensitization involves first training the patient in relaxation, then gradually introducing the patient to the feared stimulus in a highly structured fashion. While it does not require the degree of formal training that hypnosis does, it can be fairly time-consuming. As a result, both systematic desensitization and hypnosis are often recommended primarily for extremely anxious or phobic patients, and are often accomplished in the office of a mental health practitioner to whom the patient has been referred. It should be noted, however, that formal training in hypnosis for dentists is available.[1] After completing training, the dentist can effectively use hypnosis in the dental office (Patel, Potter, & Mellor, 2000; Finkelstein, 2003).

Traditional formal progressive deep muscle relaxation can also be a rather lengthy procedure and can require multiple sessions of training. In its traditional format, it can be even more time-consuming than many hypnosis procedures. As such, it is not very adaptable to the dental office or clinic. Typically, it involves the patient reclining comfortably, closing his/her eyes, and focusing on various groups of muscles, which are alternately tensed and relaxed, while breathing in a regular paced fashion. This process continues with each of the major muscle groups of the body until all muscles are relaxed and the patient is at ease. Each session can take anywhere from twenty or thirty minutes to one hour, depending on the practitioner. Because of the time involved with relaxation procedures, they are usually recommended for, and effective with, those patients who express moderate to high levels of fear (Berggren, Hakeberg, & Carlsson, 2000). They can also be effective with phobic patients who can at least enter the dental office, since by relaxing in the dental chair, they will, in effect, be accomplishing "in vivo" desensitization.

A brief relaxation procedure developed by the author, which can be read to the patient in approximately twelve to fifteen minutes, will be discussed here. It not only incorporates bodily relaxation and breath control, but also includes a brief guided imagery segment, and specific suggestions regarding relaxation and personal control. As a result, it combines many of the advantages of both guided imagery and hypnosis with those of progressive relaxation without most of the disadvantages of each. In addition, it lends itself to audio recording so that it can be performed in a "generic" version for all patients. Audio recordings, however, are more effective when made specifically for each patient when first administered, and then taken home by the patient to practice. The patient can then arrive at the office highly skilled in the procedure and self-administer it during successive dental appointments.

To best understand the usefulness of this specific procedure, a classification system first introduced by Davidson and Schwartz is helpful (Davidson & Schwartz, 1976). They discussed two main components of anxiety: somatic and cognitive. Somatic anxiety is that which is experienced predominantly in a bodily fashion, while cognitive anxiety is that which is experienced predominantly in a mental fashion. Fear and anxiety can be high or low on both or either of the two continuums (fig. 9.1).

An example of anxiety that is low on the cognitive continuum but high on the somatic continuum is when someone is feeling fidgety or shaky but has no particular thoughts in mind. An example of the opposite, high-cognitive anxiety but low-somatic anxiety, is when a person is physically relaxed, but his or her mind is racing with anxious thoughts. One can also classify anxiety reduction procedures in a similar fashion. Thus, procedures such as distraction or paced breathing are most effective with low to moderate cognitive and/or somatic anxiety. Procedures such as systematic desensitization and hypnosis are most effective with high levels of somatic and/or cognitive anxiety. Techniques that focus predominately on physical relaxation such as biofeedback and traditional relaxation are most effective for somatic anxiety; techniques that involve a strong mental component such as guided imagery

Somatic Anxiety[*]

		Moderate	High
	Mod.	Paced Breathing Distraction Meditation Graduated Exposure Rehearsal	Progressive Relaxation Biofeedback
Cognitive Anxiety	High	Guided Imagery Cognitive Restructuring Stress Inoculation Thought Stopping	Guided Imagery + Relaxation Systematic Desensitization Hypnosis Botto Brief Relaxation

[*] Adapted from Davidson & Schwartz, 1976

Fig. 9.1.   Somatic and cognitive orientation of various relaxation methods. (Adapted from Davidson & Schwartz, 1976.)

or cognitive restructuring (the changing of irrational thinking) are most effective for cognitive anxiety. The brief relaxation procedure discussed here includes both cognitive components (imagery and suggestion) and somatic components (muscle relaxation and deep breathing). As a result, as with systematic desensitization and hypnosis, it is effective with both high-somatic and cognitive anxiety.

The procedure involves four main phases:[1] rapport, relaxation, suggestion, and mental imagery.[2] In the preparation phase, the patient is educated about the procedure and how it works. The main purpose of this phase is to set expectations regarding the procedure's efficacy. This phase is critical. The same detailed relaxation procedure has been shown to both raise and lower anxiety depending on the expectations of the individual (Botto, 1981). In addition, the practitioner is directed to answer patient questions and elicit information regarding the patient's preference of a scene for the imagery phase of the procedure, much in the same way as discussed above in the guided-imagery technique. Finally, information regarding any particular area of the body where the patient tends to feel especially tense is identified.

The relaxation phase of the procedure consists of three steps: (1) selecting a group of muscles and relaxing those muscles, (2) taking two deep breaths, and (3) suggestions to feel "calm, controlled, and relaxed." The script starts by having the patient tense and then relax the muscles of the feet to experience "the contrast between tension and relaxation." After that, muscle groups are not tensed. The patient is simply asked to focus on tension present in each muscle group and then relax each group. An example of the "patter" used for each muscle group is:

> Now think about the muscles in your back and shoulders. Concentrate on the muscles in your lower and upper back, your shoulders, and any tension in them. Think about them . . . think about them . . . now relax them. Relax them and feel the tension draining down . . . down from your shoulders and back . . . down from your legs . . . down

from your feet . . . down and away. All the tension draining down, draining away. Letting your muscles go limp, limp, heavy and limp. Breathing deep . . . and slow. Deep . . . and slow. Feeling relaxed and comfortable; relaxed and at ease; calm, controlled, relaxed, and at ease. By being relaxed, you have better control over your thoughts, feelings, and actions.

Six different muscle groups are included: the feet, legs (lower and upper legs), back and shoulders, stomach and chest, arms and hands, and head and neck. If the patient indicated any particular areas in which tension tends to be felt, those areas would also be identified.

Once the muscle groups are relaxed, suggestions to maintain relaxation are given and the relaxation is reinforced. At this time, the mental-imagery phase begins and a detailed picture of the patient's scene is "painted" for the patient. The description, as with Geboy's guided imagery, appeals to each of the five senses. By being relaxed, the patient is more suggestible and better able to engage in visualizing the scene.

That completes the relaxation procedure, and the practitioner is directed to begin the dental procedures, periodically reinforcing the patient's relaxation, especially if the patient starts to become tense, or during a particularly difficult treatment phase. Once the dental procedure is completed, if necessary, directions for removing the relaxation can be given. Afterward, the practitioner conducts a debriefing with the patient, reinforcing the patient's performance as well as soliciting feedback regarding the experience (e.g., how did the patient feel about it, what worked particularly well, what, if anything, would the patient like changed the next time). Finally, the patient is directed to continue to practice the relaxation procedure at home.

One final word about the use of behavioral interventions compared to pharmacological interventions: although the latter are more common (e.g., premedication, N$_2$O, IV sedation), the major problems with their use are twofold. First, they carry potential danger in both their direct effects and side effects. Second, their amelioration of patient fear tends to be short term (Johren et al., 2000; Thom, Sartory, & Johren, 2000). Each time the patient experiences dental procedures, the agent must be readministered, taking time, adding cost, and exposing the patient and sometimes staff to risk. In contrast, behavioral procedures help the patient "unlearn" his or her fears and resolve them (Hakeberg, Berggren, & Carlsson, 1990; Hakeberg et al., 1993). Eventually, the fear subsides and the patient can experience dentistry more comfortably. In addition, patients attribute their success to themselves rather than a drug. This self-attribution is very empowering for the patient in gaining control over fear (Liddell & Locker, 2000). Finally, practitioners will find that taking the time to show the patients that they care about their comfort and well-being will result in highly satisfied patients and strong practices. In the words of the first patient quoted at the beginning of this chapter:

And best of all, my bottom teeth, at least the ones I have left, feel so clean and smooth. Why I waited all these years to get this work done is beyond me. It probably has something to do with the fact that as a child, I can remember having cavities drilled without anesthesia, and numbing shots administered without any topical. All of this from way back in the dark ages of dentistry. You've come a long way baby!

Notes

1. The interested reader should contact the American Society for Clinical Hypnosis, or the Society for Clinical and Experimental Hypnosis regarding training workshops.

2. Due to space limitations, the procedure will be outlined here. Copies of the entire script, including directions, may be obtained from the author.

References

Berggren, U., Hakeberg, M., & Carlsson, S. G. (2000). Relaxation vs. cognitively oriented therapies for dental fear. *Journal of Dental Research, 79(9)*, 1645–51.

Botto, R. W. (1981). The efficacy of relaxation training in coping with dental stress as a function of expectation of success. *Missouri Psychologist, 39*, 10–16.

Chambers, D. W., & Abrams, R. G. (1992). *Dental communication.* Sonoma, CA: Ohana Group.

Cohen, S. M., Fiske, J., & Newton, J. T. (2000). The impact of dental anxiety on daily living. *British Dental Journal, 189(7)*, 385–90.

Dailey, Y. M., Humphris, G. M., & Lennon, M. A. (2002). Reducing patients' state anxiety in general dental practice: a randomized controlled trial. *Journal of Dental Research, 81(5)*, 319–22.

Davidson, R. J., & Schwartz, G. E. (1976). The psychobiology of relaxation and related states: a multi-process theory. In D. I. Mostofsky (ed.), *Behavior Control and Modification of Physiological Activity.* Englewood Cliffs, NJ: Prentice-Hall, Inc.

Finkelstein, S. (2003). Rapid hypnotic inductions and therapeutic suggestions in the dental setting. *International Journal of Clinical Hypnosis, 51(1)*, 77–85.

Geboy, M. J. (1985). *Communication and behavior management in dentistry.* Baltimore: Williams & Wilkins.

Hakeberg, M., Berggren, U., & Carlsson, S. G. (1990). A 10-year follow-up of patients treated for dental fear. *Scandinavian Journal of Dental Research, 98(1)*, 53–59.

Hakeberg, M., Berggren, U., Carlsson, S. G., & Grondahl, H. G. (1993). Long-term effects on dental care behavior and dental health after treatments for dental fear. *Anesthesia Progress, 40(3)*, 72–77.

Johren, P., Jackowski, J., Gangler, P., Sartory, G., & Thom, A. (2000). Fear reduction in patients with dental treatment phobia. *British Journal of Oral Maxillofacial Surgery, 38(6)*, 612–16.

Liddell, A., & Locker, D. (2000). Changes in levels of dental anxiety as a function of dental experience. *Behavior Modification, 24(1)*, 57–68.

Locker, D. (2003). Psychosocial consequences of dental fear and anxiety. *Community Dental Oral Epidemiology, 31(2)*, 144–51.

Milgrom, P., Weinstein, P., & Getz, T. (1995). *Treating Fearful Dental Patients: A Patient Management Handbook* (2d ed., rev. ed.). Seattle: University of Washington Continuing Dental Education.

Moore, R., & Brodsgaard, I. (2001). Dentists' perceived stress and its relation to perceptions about anxious patients. *Community Dental Oral Epidemiology, 29(1)*, 73–80.

Morse, Z. (2002). Despite the remarkable advances in oral health care, pain and anxiety continue to be significant deterrents for seeking dental services. *Journal of Dental Education, 66(6)*, 689.

Patel, B., Potter, C., & Mellor, A. C. (2000). The use of hypnosis in dentistry: a review. *Dental Update, 27(4)*, 198–202.

Thom, A., Sartory, G., & Johren, P. (2000). Comparison between one-session psychological treatment and benzodiazepine in dental phobia. *Journal of Consulting Clinical Psychology, 68(3)*, 378–87.

van der Molen, H. T., Klaver, A. A., & Duyx, M. P. (2004). Effectiveness of a communication skills training programme for the management of dental anxiety. *British Dental Journal, 196(2)*, 101–7.

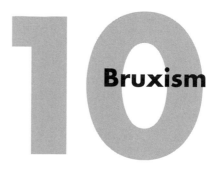

Bruxism

Alan G. Glaros

Bruxism is the nonfunctional contact of the teeth during sleep. In this chapter, I will review the definition of bruxism, describe the prevalence of the disorder, and discuss its effects on teeth and other systems. I will present two main etiological theories of bruxism and also discuss the relationships between personality traits and bruxism and between stress and bruxism. Methods for diagnosing and treating the disorder will conclude the chapter.

Definition

As measured by sleep electromyographic (EMG) recordings, at least two distinctly different nonfunctional behaviors occur during sleep: (1) high-amplitude, brief rhythmic EMG bursts that can vary in total duration, and (2) arrhythmic, high-amplitude activity, typically of short duration (Wruble, Lumley, & McGlynn, 1989). The first is associated with grinding, gnashing, or tapping behaviors of the teeth, and the second is associated with clenching. Grinding is most likely to occur at night, whereas clenching occurs during both the day and night.

A considerable proportion of the published literature does not make a distinction between nocturnal grinding and diurnal/nocturnal clenching, and it can be difficult to know whether nocturnal grinding alone, nighttime clenching, daytime clenching, or some combination of these contributes to the effects of bruxism (Lobbezoo & Lavigne, 1997). To the extent possible, this chapter will focus primarily on data obtained from individuals who have clear evidence of nighttime grinding. When primary sources do not make a distinction between grinding and clenching, I will note this by referring to nocturnal parafunctions.

Prevalence

Nighttime parafunctional behaviors can begin in early childhood and last throughout adulthood. Tooth grinding can occur as soon as teeth erupt and often increases in frequency during early and middle childhood (Magnusson, Carlsson, & Egermark, 1993). Bruxism is a relatively common, intermittent problem in children, often associated with other oral parafunctions (Wanman & Agerberg, 1986). A small proportion of childhood bruxers will continue these behaviors into adolescence and adulthood (Egermark, Magnusson, & Carlsson, 2003). Twenty-year follow-up records of orthodontically treated children suggest that wear in adults can be predicted with considerable accuracy from measures of wear observable from the same individuals at the point of mixed dentition during childhood (Knight et al., 1997).

Sleep bruxism is common in the general population and is considered to be the third most common parasomnia (sleep-related disorder). According to a study of approximately 13,000 adults living in the United Kingdom, Germany, and Italy (Ohayon, Li, & Guilleminault, 2001), teeth grinding occurring at least weekly was reported by 8.2% of subjects, and half of these also reported muscle discomfort on awakening and a need for dental work as a consequence of their grinding. A study of nearly 28,000 19-year-old Korean men showed that 8.4% reported nocturnal grinding (Choi et al., 2002), and a sample of 2,019 Canadian adults showed that 8% of subjects reported tooth grinding (Lavigne & Montplaisir, 1994). Sleep bruxism is more likely to occur in a supine position (Miyawaki et al., 2003). Adults who reported obstructive sleep apnea, snoring, daytime sleepiness, heavy alcohol use, use of caffeinated beverages, smoking, stress, and anxiety appeared to have higher risks for nocturnal parafunctions (Ohayon et al., 2001).

Twin studies indicate no substantial heritability of oral parafunctions (Michalowicz et al., 2000). Monozygotic twins (MZ) are no more similar than dizygotic twins on oral parafunctions, and reared-together MZ twins are no more similar than reared-apart MZ twins.

Effects of Bruxism

The most common correlate of grinding appears to be occlusal wear, but diet and harsh environmental and climatic conditions may also contribute to wear (Kaidonis, Richards, & Townsend, 1993). Hypertrophy of the masticatory muscles may be observed in patients who report bruxism.

Pain may accompany both clenching and grinding (Sari & Sonmez, 2002), although the evidence linking nocturnal parafunctions with facial and temporomandibular joint (TMJ) pain and other temporomandibular disorders (TMD) is mixed. Some investigators have concluded that the link is weak (Lobbezoo & Lavigne, 1997), while others have reported a dose-response relationship between severity of parafunctions and pain in the masticatory muscles and TMJ (Molina et al., 1999). An association between pain and parafunctional activity may be present in children as young as four to six years of age (Widmalm et al., 1995), and children with headache may have higher rates of nocturnal parafunctions (Aromaa et al., 1998).

Nocturnal grinding may include bilateral mandibular excursions, small lateral movements, and unilateral excursions (Chung, Kim, & Kim, 2000). The amount of force exerted during nocturnal bruxing behaviors can be considerable and may exceed amplitudes generated during maximum voluntary bite force (Ohayon et al., 2001). Parafunctional activity may contribute to a number of TMJ pathologies, including condylar bony change, disk displacement (including cartilage degradation), and biochemical and biomechanical abnormalities.

Mechanical stimulation increases mercury (Hg) release from dental amalgam fillings, and increased Hg exposure and bodily uptake may accompany grinding. Greater plasma concentrations of Hg may be present in patients who grind their teeth, but the magnitude of the increase appears to be less than from the use of chewing gum (Isacsson et al., 1997).

Increased health-care expenses are a societal cost of nocturnal parafunctions. Patients with these conditions have a larger number of visits to dentists, physicians, and other health-care providers (Molina et al., 2000) than nonparafunction controls. They use more medications than controls. The individual social costs of nocturnal parafunctions cannot be estimated with great accuracy, but they may include decreased productivity at work or school, strained relationships with bed partners, and pain-related irritability affecting colleagues, friends, and family. Those who suffer from bruxism-related chronic pain have a greater likelihood of being depressed.

Etiological Theories of Bruxism

There are two main etiological models of bruxism (Glaros & Rao, 1977): (1) a local, mechanical theory that focuses primarily on occlusion, and (2) a centrally mediated theory that views bruxism as a sleep-related disturbance (e.g., Lobbezoo & Naeije, 2001). The local, mechanical theory hypothesizes that occlusal interferences predispose an individual to brux.

The view that bruxism is a sleep-related disorder (parasomnia) was first proposed by Broughton (1968). The hypothesis advanced by Broughton was that bruxism was part of a family of sleep parasomnias such as sleepwalking, sleep talking, and enuresis. Studies that have examined this connection have shown that individuals with bruxism are indeed more likely to report other parasomnias (Lavigne & Montplaisir, 1994; Weideman et al., 1996). Consistent with this view are data showing that those who have severe parasomnias are also likely to have bruxism (Ohayon, Caulet, & Priest, 1997).

Nocturnal parafunctions typically occur during stage 2 sleep (the most common sleep stage), during REM sleep, and in the transition from deeper to shallower levels of sleep (Bader et al., 1997). Teeth grinding may also be associated with abnormalities in autonomic function, particularly in sympathetic vasoconstrictor function, K-complexes in the EEG, tachycardia, and gross body movements (Wruble et al., 1989).

More recent work has confirmed that bruxismlike activity occurs secondary to sleep-related arousal. In one study (Kato et al., 2003), polygraphic recordings were taken from eight bruxists and eight matched controls. While sleeping, vibrotactile or auditory stimuli were used to induce arousal without causing awakening. All the bruxist subjects but only one of the controls responded with rhythmic masseter muscle activity to the presentation of the stimuli. There are differences in the microstructure of sleep between sleep bruxists and normal controls. However, the macrostructure is similar between the two groups, and bruxists often report good sleep. Indeed, nighttime grinders may be unaware of nocturnal grinding and report astonishment when bed partners complain of wakening caused by grinding sounds.

The alternative viewpoint focuses most intensely on occlusal variables. In this model, high restorations and other local irritants, malocclusions, or traumas induce the nervous system to engage in nocturnal grinding. When the local irritant is removed, grinding will then cease. The logical implication of this perspective has led dentists to perform occlusal adjustments in an attempt to remove occlusal disharmonies and eliminate nocturnal parafunctions.

Evidence for this perspective is mixed. Deliberate creation of occlusal disharmonies is generally well tolerated in both bruxing and nonbruxing patients (Shiau & Syu, 1995). Pain, a potential indicator of nocturnal parafunctions, may decrease during orthodontic treatment (Egermark & Thilander, 1992). This may be interpreted as evidence of the importance of occlusion for understanding nocturnal parafunctions, and it can also mean that orthodontically moved teeth are sensitive to contact, resulting in a reduction of oral parafunctions. Studies have reported bruxism to be associated with Class II and III occlusions, deep bite, and overjets (Vanderas & Manetas, 1995). However, the ability to predict or modify nocturnal parafunctions from occlusal contacts has not received consistent support in the scientific literature (Clark et al., 1999).

Personality studies of grinders suggest that they are shy, stiff, cautious, and aloof. They may have difficult expressing themselves and be prone to worrying (Fischer & O'Toole, 1993). Similar findings have been reported in other studies (see Glaros and Rao, 1977, for a review). Other studies suggest that bruxism is not associated with psychological disturbance as measured by the Minnesota Multiphasic Personality Inventory (Harness & Peltier, 1992). Bruxism (and teeth-baring) has also been linked to aggressiveness in primates and other mammals. It is difficult to know if these psychological traits are etiologically related to grinding or whether they are a response to the social embarrassment of having significantly eroded teeth and an unattractive smile or are a consequence of chronic pain and discomfort.

Bruxism has been linked to stress, but like the personality trait studies, it is difficult to know if stress precedes, is coexistent with, or follows bruxism (Pierce et al., 1995). Studies carried out with mammals suggest that the deliberate creation of occlusal dysharmonies can increase plasma and urinary cortisol levels associated with stress and central catecholaminergic activity (Areso et al., 1999). Urinary catecholamines are significantly correlated with bruxism in children (Vanderas et al., 1999). The combination of Type A behavior patterns (e.g., sense of time urgency, impatience, easily aroused hostility, frequent and intense feelings of anger) and stress may be a good predictor of nocturnal parafunctions (Pingitore, Chrobak, & Petrie, 1991). Other researchers have argued that nonfunctional masticatory activity is a stress-control mechanism affecting central catecholaminergic neurotransmission (Gomez et al., 1999). These studies suggest that psychological stress may have physiological correlates that may, in turn, influence nighttime sleep patterns.

Diagnosis

The "gold standard" for diagnosing bruxism is sleep polysomnography. Among the measures that might be obtained during sleep are electroencephalographic activity, electromyographic activity, electrooculographic activity (to record eye movement), respiration, pulse oximetry, electrocardiogram, blood pressure, and body temperature. Multiple recording sessions may be needed to obtain sufficiently accurate and reliable data, although fewer sessions will probably be sufficient for moderate to severe bruxers (Lavigne et al., 2001). Sleep polysomnography is expensive and time-consuming, although polysomnographic diagnostic criteria for bruxism can accurately diagnosis sleep bruxism (or its absence) in over 80% of those who undergo this procedure (Lavigne, Rompre, & Montplaisir, 1996).

An alternative to polysomnography is the Bruxcore monitoring device, fabricated from four thin layers of colored plastic laminated to a total thickness of 0.02 inches, with microdots printed on the top surface. The dots are 1/180 inches in diameter and one square inch contains 14,400 dots. The plastic is molded into a mouth guard and worn at night. As grinding occurs, the microdots on the top surface are worn away; severe grinding can expose colored layers underneath the top, white surface. The severity of grinding can be computed as the number of dots missing, multiplied by the color of any exposed layer. For example, the number of missing dots on the top layer are summed and multiplied by one, the number of missing dots that expose the next layer (orange) are counted and multiplied by two, and so forth. The total score reflects the severity of grinding. Forgione (1974) has suggested that Bruxcore scores of 1–400 indicate mild parafunction, 401–600 moderate parafunction, and >600 severe parafunction.

Both polysomnography and Bruxcore plates require considerable effort and time and may not be useful to a clinician in practice. Many clinicians examine teeth for evidence of excessive attrition or atypical wear facets and use evidence obtained this way as *prima facie* evidence of bruxism. Unfortunately, attrition is an historical record and may not be reliable as evidence of current bruxism. A report from bed partners of rhythmic tooth noises that occur during sleep may signify ongoing grinding.

Clenching, on the other hand, is not associated with noise and may not be accompanied by excessive attrition or atypical facets. Patients who engage in nocturnal parafunctions may complain of pain, soreness, or TMJ stiffness upon awakening. Some evidence has suggested that parafunctions are associated with a higher incidence of mandibular tori (Kerdpon & Sirirungrojying, 1999). Advances in miniaturization of electronic instruments have led to the development of nighttime EMG monitoring devices to detect bruxism (e.g., Amemori et al., 2001). A variety of devices is available for purchase, but their operation, user-friendliness, and ability to distinguish clenching from grinding can vary substantially.

Because bruxism consists of at least two behaviors, providers must utilize multiple sources of information to properly diagnose the condition. Evidence of grinding may take several forms (e.g., attrition, noise), and evidence of diurnal and nocturnal clenching may take different forms (e.g., pain, stiffness). Reliance on attrition alone will be insufficient to diagnose the condition properly.

A thorough evaluation of a bruxing patient therefore requires inquiry into nondental domains as well as dental domains (Winocur et al., 2003). Various medications may be implicated in the onset or exacerbation of bruxism. These include methylphenidate as a treatment for attention deficit hyperactivity disorder (Gara & Roberts, 2000) and supplemental serotonin reuptake inhibitors for depression (Lobbezoo et al., 2001). For example, individuals with various dystonias may report high levels of bruxism. Rett syndrome and its variants (Ribeiroet al., 1997) are associated with bruxism. Oral parafunctions may be more prevalent among drug addicts (Winocur et al., 2001).

Treatment

There is broad consensus that interocclusal appliances ("splints," mouth guards) are a safe and effective treatment for limiting the attrition to teeth caused by grinding (Dao & Lavigne, 1998). There is considerably less consensus on how the device should be constructed. Interocclusal appliances can be made from acrylic and considerably softer materials. They can cover the maxillary or mandibular teeth. The devices can present a relatively flat plane to the opposing dentition or may be designed to place the teeth and jaws into a specific occlusal pattern. In any case, the evidence in favor of a particular design or material is either of poor quality or inconsistent.

There is no clear evidence that interocclusal appliances permanently or temporarily reduce grinding (Holmgren, Sheikholeslam, & Riise, 1993. Clinicians should therefore view the use of such appliances as strictly preventive (with respect to tooth damage), not curative (Hartmann, 1994). Few studies on the long-term effects of appliances have been carried out. Some investigators have suggested that long-term use of mandibular advancement appliances or appliances that do not make contact with the opposing occlusion can create severe and irreversible complications (Widmalm, 1999). Patients should therefore be monitored closely for signs of untoward changes.

Occlusal equilibration and other occlusal therapies have been utilized as more permanent treatments for bruxism and myofascial pain. It is relatively common for nonblinded treatments to report considerable success with this approach (e.g., Kerstein & Farrell, 1990). However, more controlled trials show no particular benefit to occlusal adjustments as a treatment for nocturnal grinding (Tsukiyama, Baba, & Clark, 2001).

The data regarding interocclusal appliances and clenching are considerably less clear. Individuals who report parafunction-related pain often experience reduction in pain while an appliance is used. The presence of the appliance may alter clenching behaviors associated with pain (Kreiner, Betancor, & Clark, 2001). Some patients may experience long-term reduction in oral parafunction-related pain, while others will experience a return of pain.

An alternative to interocclusal appliances are nocturnal alarms. These devices typically monitor masseter EMG activity (or noises produced during grinding) while a patient sleeps. When EMG activity exceeds a threshold for specified length of time, an alarm sounds. Generally, the alarm continues until the patient actively engages in a behavior that terminates the alarm. Studies suggest that becoming fully awake enhances the efficacy of this approach (Cassisi, McGlynn, & Belles, 1987).

Nocturnal alarms can reduce the frequency and intensity of bruxing behavior while the alarm is in use (Cassisi et al., 1987). Removal of the device often results in a return of these behaviors and may even produce a rebound effect in which bruxing behaviors occur at a higher rate than at baseline. Monitoring EMG activity requires placement of surface electrodes on the face. Patients may not be reliable in their technique for preparing the skin or for placing the electrodes in the proper location. Surface electrodes are relatively small, but they can be a source of discomfort when patients sleep on their sides.

Several other approaches have been used to treat nocturnal parafunctions. The NTI clenching suppression device (Nissani, 2000), for example, is designed to reduce parafunctions using taste aversion. In this approach, a removable wire-frame appliance is fabricated with liquid-filled capsules installed in the area of the molars. The capsules are filled with a small quantity of a mildly noxious liquid. When a patient exerts pressure on the capsules, they break open, spilling the liquid into the mouth, waking the subject, and ending the oral parafunction.

Pharmacologic approaches to the treatment of bruxism are appearing with increased frequency. Perhaps the most common pharmacologic approach involves botulinum toxin (Botox) injections. Several reports have suggested that this approach has merit in the treatment of bruxism patients, although controlled trials of its efficacy have not been published. Several other drugs have been tested as treatment for bruxism, such as amitriptyline (Raigrodski et al., 2001) and bromocriptine (Lavigne et al., 2001). None has yet emerged as a consistently effective alternative to interocclusal appliances.

Summary

Bruxism consists of at least two separate behaviors, grinding and clenching. These behaviors can begin in early childhood and last throughout adulthood. It is a relatively common disorder affecting about 8% of the adult population. The most common effect of grinding is tooth wear, but a variety of other symptoms may also occur, including pain and personal distress. There is reasonably good evidence that bruxism is a sleep-related disorder; the evidence favoring an occlusal approach is considerably weaker. Bruxism may be linked to stress through a number of mechanisms, and psychological traits may also be related to bruxism.

Occlusal wear and possibly reports of pain on awakening may be evidence of bruxism, but polysomnographic studies are the "gold standard" for diagnosis. Unfortunately, polysomnography is both expensive and time-consuming, while attrition is an historical record of wear and not evidence that bruxism is currently a problem. A thorough evaluation of a patient suspected of having bruxism must include strategies other than evaluation of the teeth. Treatment via interocclusal appliances is primarily designed to prevent damage to the teeth. Other approaches may temporarily reduce bruxism. There are no dental, behavioral, or pharmacological treatments that permanently eliminate the behavior.

Considerably more work needs to be done to identify the behavioral and biological mechanisms that influence, and are influenced by, nocturnal parafunctions. Similarly, more work needs to be carried out to develop and test interventions that reduce and eliminate nocturnal parafunctions. By their nature, studies of nocturnal parafunctions are difficult to conduct, especially when sleep recordings are obtained from patients. However, work carried out in this area provides an excellent example of the ways in which both dental and nondental professionals contribute to our knowledge of this common and complex disorder.

Note

Preparation of this chapter was aided by a grant from the National Institutes of Health, DE13563.

Bibliography

Amemori, Y., Yamashita, S., Ai, M., Shinoda, H., Sato, M., & Takahashi, J. (2001). Influence of nocturnal bruxism on the stomatognathic system. Part I: a new device for measuring mandibular movements during sleep. *Journal of Oral Rehabilitation, 28*, 943–49.

Areso, M. P., Giralt, M. T., Sainz, B., Prieto, M., Garcia-Vallejo, P., & Gomez, F. M. (1999). Occlusal disharmonies modulate central catecholaminergic activity in the rat. *Journal of Dental Research, 78*, 1204–13.

Aromaa, M., Sillanpaa, M. L., Rautava, P., & Helenius, H. (1998). Childhood headache at school entry—a controlled clinical study. *Neurology, 50*, 1729–36.

Bader, G. G., Kampe, T., Tagdae, T., Karlsson, S., & Blomqvist, M. (1997). Descriptive physiological data on a sleep bruxism population. *Sleep, 20*, 982–90.

Broughton, R. J. (1968). Sleep disorders: disorders of arousal? *Science, 159*, 1070–78.

Cassisi, J. E., McGlynn, F. D., & Belles, D. R. (1987). EMG–activated feedback alarms for the treatment of nocturnal bruxism: Current status and future directions. *Biofeedback & Self Regulation, 12*, 13–30.

Choi, Y. S., Choung, P. H., Moon, H. S., & Kim, S. G. (2002). Temporomandibular disorders in 19–year–old Korean men. *Journal of Oral & Maxillofacial Surgery, 60*, 797–803.

Chung, S. C., Kim, Y. K., & Kim, H. S. (2000). Prevalence and patterns of nocturnal bruxofacets on stabilization splints in temporomandibular disorder patients. *Cranio, 18*, 92–97.

Clark, G. T., Tsukiyama, Y., Baba, K., & Watanabe, T. (1999). Sixty-eight years of experimental occlusal interference studies: what have we learned? *Journal of Prosthetic Dentistry, 82,* 704–713.

Dao, T. T., & Lavigne, G. J. (1998). Oral splints: the crutches for temporomandibular disorders and bruxism? *Critical Reviews in Oral Biology & Medicine, 9,* 345–61.

Egermark, I., & Thilander, B. (1992). Craniomandibular disorders with special reference to orthodontic treatment: an evaluation from childhood to adulthood. *American Journal of Orthodontics & Dentofacial Orthopedics, 101,* 28–34.

Egermark, I., Magnusson, T., & Carlsson, G. E. (2003). A 20-year follow-up of signs and symptoms of temporomandibular disorders and malocclusions in subjects with and without orthodontic treatment in childhood. *Angle Orthodontist, 73,* 109–15.

Fischer, W. F., & O'Toole, E. T. (1993). Personality characteristics of chronic bruxers. *Behavioral Medicine, 19,* 82–86.

Forgione, A. G. (1974). A simple but effective method of quantifying bruxism behavior. *Journal of Restorative Dentistry, 53,* 127.

Gara, L., & Roberts, W. (2000). Adverse response to methylphenidate in combination with valproic acid. *Journal of Child & Adolescent Psychopharmacology, 10,* 39–43.

Glaros, A. G., & Rao, S. M. (1977). Bruxism: a critical review. *Psychological Bulletin, 84,* 767–81.

Gomez, F. M., Giralt, M. T., Sainz, B., Arrue, A., Prieto, M., & Garcia-Vallejo, P. (1999). A possible attenuation of stress-induced increases in striatal dopamine metabolism by the expression of non-functional masticatory activity in the rat. *European Journal of Oral Sciences, 107,* 461–67.

Harness, D. M., & Peltier, B. (1992). Comparison of MMPI scores with self-report of sleep disturbance and bruxism in the facial pain population. *Cranio, 10,* 70–74.

Hartmann, E. (1994). Bruxism. In M. H., Kryger, T. Roth, W. C. Dement (eds.), *Principles and practice of sleep medicine* (2d ed., pp. 598–601). New York: W. B. Saunders.

Holmgren, K., Sheikholeslam, A., & Riise, C. (1993). Effect of a full-arch maxillary occlusal splint on parafunctional activity during sleep in patients with nocturnal bruxism and signs and symptoms of craniomandibular disorders. *Journal of Prosthetic Dentistry, 69,* 293–97.

Isacsson, G., Barregard, L., Selden, A., & Bodin, L. (1997). Impact of nocturnal bruxism on mercury uptake from dental amalgams. *European Journal of Oral Sciences, 105,* 251–57.

Kaidonis, J. A., Richards, L. C., & Townsend, G. C. (1993). Nature and frequency of dental wear facets in an Australian aboriginal population. *Journal of Oral Rehabilitation, 20,* 333–40.

Kato, T., Montplaisir, J. Y., Guitard, F., Sessle, B. J., Lund, J. P., & Lavigne, G. J. (2003). Evidence that experimentally induced sleep bruxism is a consequence of transient arousal. *Journal of Dental Research, 82,* 284–88.

Kerdpon, D., & Sirirungrojying, S. (1999). A clinical study of oral tori in southern Thailand: Prevalence and the relation to parafunctional activity. *European Journal of Oral Sciences, 107,* 9–13.

Kerstein, R. B., & Farrell, S. (1990). Treatment of myofascial pain-dysfunction syndrome with occlusal equilibration. *Journal of Prosthetic Dentistry, 63,* 695–700.

Knight, D. J., Leroux, B. G., Zhu, C., Almond, J., & Ramsay, D. S. (1997). A longitudinal study of tooth wear in orthodontically treated patients. *American Journal of Orthodontics & Dentofacial Orthopedics, 112,* 194–202.

Kreiner, M., Betancor, E., & Clark, G. T. (2001). Occlusal stabilization appliances: evidence of their efficacy. *Journal of the American Dental Association, 132,* 770–77.

Lavigne, G. J., & Montplaisir, J. Y. (1994). Restless legs syndrome and sleep bruxism: prevalence and association among Canadians. *Sleep, 17,* 739–43.

Lavigne, G. J., Guitard, F., Rompre, P. H., & Montplaisir, J. Y. (2001). Variability in sleep bruxism activity over time. *Journal of Sleep Research, 10,* 237–44.

Lavigne, G. J., Rompre, P. H., & Montplaisir, J. Y. (1996). Sleep bruxism: validity of clinical research diagnostic criteria in a controlled polysomnographic study. *Journal of Dental Research, 75,* 546–52.

Lavigne, G. J., Soucy, J. P., Lobbezoo, F., Manzini, C., Blanchet, P. J., & Montplaisir, J. Y. (2001). Double-blind, crossover, placebo-controlled trial of bromocriptine in patients with sleep bruxism. *Clinical Neuropharmacology, 24,* 145–49.

Lobbezoo, F., & Lavigne, G. J. (1997). Do bruxism and temporomandibular disorders have a cause-and-effect relationship? *Journal of Orofacial Pain, 11,* 15–23.

Lobbezoo, F., & Naeije, M. (2001). Bruxism is mainly regulated centrally, not peripherally. *Journal of Oral Rehabilitation, 28,* 1085–91.

Lobbezoo, F., van Denderen, R. J., Verheij, J. G., & Naeije, M. (2001). Reports of SSRI-associated bruxism in the family physician's office. *Journal of Orofacial Pain, 15,* 340–46.

Magnusson, T., Carlsson, G. E., & Egermark, I. (1993). Changes in subjective symptoms of craniomandibular disorders in children and adolescents during a 10-year period. *Journal of Orofacial Pain, 7,* 76–82.

Michalowicz, B. S., Pihlstrom, B. L., Hodges, J. S., & Bouchard, T. J., Jr. (2000). No heritability of temporomandibular joint signs and symptoms. *Journal of Dental Research, 79,* 1573–78.

Miyawaki, S., Lavigne, G. J., Pierre, M., Guitard, F., Montplaisir, J. Y., & Kato, T. (2003). Association between sleep bruxism, swallowing-related laryngeal movement, and sleep positions. *Sleep, 26,* 461–65

Molina, O. F., dos Santos, J., Nelson, S. J., & Nowlin, T. (1999). A clinical study of specific signs and symptoms of CMD in bruxers classified by the degree of severity. *Cranio, 17,* 268–79.

———. (2000). Profile of TMD and bruxer compared to TMD and nonbruxer patients regarding chief complaint, previous consultations, modes of therapy, and chronicity. *Cranio, 18,* 205–19.

Nissani, M. (2000). Can taste aversion prevent bruxism? *Applied Psychophysiology & Biofeedback, 25,* 43–54.

Ohayon, M. M., Caulet, M., & Priest, R. G. (1997). Violent behavior during sleep. *Journal of Clinical Psychiatry, 58,* 369–76.

Ohayon, M. M., Li, K. K., & Guilleminault, C. (2001). Risk factors for sleep bruxism in the general population. *Chest, 119,* 53–61.

Pierce, C. J., Chrisman, K., Bennett, M. E., & Close, J. M. (1995). Stress, anticipatory stress, and psychologic measures related to sleep bruxism. *Journal of Orofacial Pain, 9,* 51–56.

Pingitore, G., Chrobak, V., & Petrie, J. (1991). The social and psychologic factors of bruxism. *Journal of Prosthetic Dentistry, 65,* 443–46.

Raigrodski, A. J., Christensen, L. V., Mohamed, S. E., & Gardiner, D. M. (2001). The effect of four-week administration of amitriptyline on sleep bruxism. A double-blind crossover clinical study. *Cranio, 19,* 21–25.

Ribeiro, R. A., Romano, A. R., Birman, E. G., & Mayer, M. P. (1997). Oral manifestations in Rett syndrome: a study of 17 cases. *Pediatric Dentistry, 19,* 349–52.

Sari, S., & Sonmez, H. (2002). Investigation of the relationship between oral parafunctions and temporomandibular joint dysfunction in Turkish children with mixed and permanent dentition. *Journal of Oral Rehabilitation, 29,* 108–12.

Shiau, Y. Y., & Syu, J. Z. (1995). Effect of working side interferences on mandibular movement in bruxers and non-bruxers. *Journal of Oral Rehabilitation, 22,* 145–51.

Tsukiyama, Y., Baba, K., & Clark, G. T. (2001). An evidence-based assessment of occlusal adjustment as a treatment for temporomandibular disorders. *Journal of Prosthetic Dentistry, 86,* 57–66.

Vanderas, A. P., & Manetas, K. J. (1995). Relationship between malocclusion and bruxism in children and adolescents: A review. *Pediatric Dentistry, 17,* 7–12.

Vanderas, A. P., Menenakou, M., Kouimtzis, T., & Papagiannoulis, L. (1999). Urinary catecholamine levels and bruxism in children. *Journal of Oral Rehabilitation, 26,* 103–10.

Wanman, A., & Agerberg, G. (1986). Mandibular dysfunction in adolescents. I. Prevalence of symptoms. *Acta Odontologica Scandinavica, 44,* 47–54.

Weideman, C. L., Bush, D. L., Yan-Go, F. L., Clark, G. T., & Gornbein, J. A. (1996). The incidence of parasomnias in child bruxers versus nonbruxers. *Pediatric Dentistry, 18,* 456–60.

Widmalm, S. E. (1999). Use and abuse of bite splints. *Compendium of Continuing Education in Dentistry, 20,* 249–54.

Widmalm, S. E., Gunn, S. M., Christiansen, R. L., & Hawley, L. M. (1995). Association between CMD signs and symptoms, oral parafunctions, race and sex, in 4–6-year-old African-American and Caucasian children. *Journal of Oral Rehabilitation, 22,* 95–100.

Winocur, E., Gavish, A., Voikovitch, M., Emodi-Perlman, A., & Eli, I. J. (2003). Drugs and bruxism: a critical review. *Journal of Orofacial Pain, 17,* 99–111.

Winocur, E., Gavish, A., Volfin, G., Halachmi, M., & Gazit, E. (2001). Oral motor parafunctions among heavy drug addicts and their effects on signs and symptoms of temporomandibular disorders. *Journal of Orofacial Pain, 15,* 56–63.

Wruble, M. K., Lumley, M. A., & McGlynn, F. D. (1989). Sleep-related bruxism and sleep variables: a critical review. *Journal of Craniomandibular Disorders, 3,* 152–58.

11

Stress, Coping, and Periodontal Disease

Gernot Wimmer and Rudolf O. Bratschko

Introduction

Periodontal diseases are opportunistic infections caused by specific peri-opathogenic microorganisms and their metabolic products (Socransky & Haffajee, 1992). Epidemiological studies indicate several so-called risk factors that may be closely related to the emergence and progression of periodontitis (Genco, 1996). On the one hand, susceptibility to the disease may be increased by inherent biological conditions and, on the other hand, factors influencing the disease may be acquired in the course of one's life and render a primarily resistant individual susceptible to the disease (Genco & Löe, 1993). Of the immanent factors, mainly genetic factors like polymorphisms and gene mutations are those that influence the immune system and are associated with a harmful progression of the disease (Kornman et al., 1997). In addition to systemic disease, unfavorable forms of behavior such as smoking or individual oral hygiene may be related to the pathogenesis and development of periodontal disease.

Following some earlier research by Giddon (Goldhaber & Giddon, 1964; Giddon, 1966) and his more recent summary of prior studies (Giddon, 1999), it has been assumed that psychological stresses and psychosocial factors play a role in the development of periodontal disease. It is also suspected that stress enhances the individual's susceptibility to periodontitis (overview studies by Ballieux, 1991; Monteira da Silva et al., 1995, 1998; Breivik et al., 1996; Solis et al., 2004). The mechanisms by which psychological strains, psychosocial factors, or individual internalized physiological changes and/or behavior in response to stress influence the initiation or progression of periodontitis are nearly unknown and remain hypothetical (Genco et al., 1998).

In this chapter, in particular, the influence of individual stress-coping strategies upon the emergence, progression, and treatment of periodontal disease will be investigated, and clinical implications thereof will be discussed.

Studies on Stress Coping

The majority of stress-relevant studies dealing with the impact of stress on oral conditions tries to establish an association between the influence of various psychological and psychosocial stresses and their potential disease-producing outcomes. However, they do not consider individual reactions or responses to such stresses. The mode of confronting stressors and dealing with them or the efforts made to overcome difficulties, stress, and stressful situations is termed "coping." The manner in which individuals cope with stressful events is, according to Lazarus (1966), more important for their psychological and physical well-being than the frequency and severity of the stressors as such. Either consciously or unconsciously, individuals use coping measures as a response to stress in order to reduce its intensity or to overcome stress altogether. In a large cross-sectional study, Genco and coworkers (1999) found that psychosocial stress factors in conjunction with financial worries are significant risk indicators for adult periodontal disease. Furthermore, the authors point out that adequate coping behaviors as evidenced by high levels of problem-based coping may reduce the stress-associated risk. The results of this study justify the assumption that the individual concept of stress coping is especially significant, and that inadequate stress-coping strategies might modulate the impact of stress on periodontal disease.

Coping with Stress: Its Influence on Periodontal Disease

Using a stress-coping questionnaire, the coping patterns used by patients with existing periodontal disease to react to specific stressful situations were determined. That is, do patients with periodontitis have specific stress-coping strategies that differ from the coping strategies of periodontally intact controls (Wimmer et al., 2002)? For a psychodiagnostic registration of data concerning stress coping, all persons answered a stress-coping questionnaire (SVF) consisting of 114 questions, which included a total of 19 actional and intrapsychic stress-coping modes (Janke, Erdmann, & Kallus, 1985). Each of these 19 subtests was optionalized with 6 questions. Activity-related coping included behaviors that signify attack, escape, social contact, withdrawal, and so on, that is, all strategies that aim to actively alter the stressful situation or one's own reaction to it. Intrapsychic strategies are processes such as perception, thinking, imagination, and all motivational-emotional processes (e.g., distraction, devaluation, denial, and overestimation of one's own resources).

The test instrument (stress questionnaire) had the following three features:

1. The 19 subtests provided a very detailed documentation of stress-coping measures, which made the test different from other instruments that at-

tempt to study stress coping on the basis of a single dimension or a few dimensions.

2. The questionnaire also contained questions about "stress-enhancing" strategies such as "social isolation," as it is assumed that the measures used by the individual not only "reduce" stress but also may aggravate it.

3. The questionnaire did not address cognitive strategies alone, but also recorded behavior-oriented strategies such as "escape," "avoidance," and "pharmaceutical drugs."

The respondent was repeatedly confronted with the same statement: "When I am thwarted, inwardly upset or made to lose my balance by something or someone." These statements were followed by various items like "I visit pleasant friends or acquaintances" or "what I'd like to do most is run away." The five-point Likert-scale answers ranged from "0 = not at all" to "4 = very likely". T-transformed scale values were then calculated from raw data to permit comparisons with the random sample used for standardization. Using a factor analysis, five factors that strongly correlated with each other were extracted from the 19 subtests (table 11.1).

Factor 1 was termed "resigned coping" and included the following subtests: avoidance, escape, social withdrawal, resignation, self-pity, and rumination. Factor 2 comprised the subtests response control, situation control, positive self-instruction, and minimization; and was termed "active coping." A similar degree of charge was found for the subtests in the extracted factor 3, which was termed "distractive coping." The subtests for this factor were distraction, search for self-affirmation, substitute gratification, and need for social support. Factor 4 was termed "defensive coping" and included the following subtests: averting blame, accusation of self, and playing down in comparison with others. For the subtests aggression and drug use, no association with other factors was found. Therefore, these two variables were summarized as factor 5 and designated accordingly. Factors 1 and 2 describe active problem-oriented coping strategies while the factor groups 3 and 4 (5) describe passive emotion-oriented coping.

Table 11.1 Extracted Factors After Factor Analysis

Factors	Subtests
Factor 1 = Resigned coping	Avoidance, escape, social withdrawal, resignation, self-pity, rumination
Factor 2 = Active coping	Response control, situation control, minimization, positive self-instruction
Factor 3 = Distractive coping	Distraction, search for self-affirmation, substitute gratification, need for social support
Factor 4 = Defensive coping	Averting blame, accusation of self, playing down in comparison with others
Factor 5 = Coping with aggression and drug use	Aggression, drug-use

Statistical evaluation revealed that, in the present study, the stress-coping behavior of patients with periodontitis differed from that of controls in regard to stress-coping strategies. Patients had significantly less loading for factor 2 (active coping) than did controls. In other words, patients used active stress-coping strategies to a lesser extent than did controls. On the other hand, patients had a higher loading for factor 3, namely "distractive coping," than did controls. Thus, when patients lose their equilibrium, they tended to be distracted, to reward themselves with substitute gratification, or to seek support from others. Patients with periodontitis also had the highest correlation with factor 4, defensive coping. That is, patients tended to cope with stress situations by "averting blame." "I have done no harm" is a typical item for this strategy. Accordingly, "accusation of self" was less pronounced. "Playing down in comparison with others" ("I take such situations more lightly than others do") sums up the image of an extenuating coping pattern that only provides temporary relief. The last extracted factor, factor 5, consists of two subtests: "drug use and aggression." This category of behavior was treated as a separate factor in the present study, as neither of these aspects could be assigned to the other factors. This factor permits the cautious conclusion that the test group members tended to counteract their aggressive irritation by means of tranquilizers more than the control group.

The potential effect of different coping strategies on attachment loss within patients with periodontitis was then evaluated. The amount of clinical attachment loss (CAL) was used to classify the severity of periodontal disease. The mean loss of clinical attachment was calculated for each patient. According to their CAL, the patients were divided into two groups: slight = 1 or 2 mm CAL and moderate = 3 or 4 mm CAL constituted patient group 1; severe = $\geq$ 5 mm constituted patient group 2. An evaluation of the association between individual coping styles and the severity of disease showed that factor 4, "defensive coping," played an important role.

Periodontitis patients with a defensive coping style had significantly greater clinical attachment loss. This finding was further emphasized by an increasing factor value in conjunction with increasing CAL. Thus, in stressful situations, these patients were more inclined to decline all responsibility and tended to compare themselves with others with a view to enhancing their own importance ("others would not digest it so easily," "I have much better control over that than others do in the same situation," "I'm still able to calm down and take control of myself much faster than others," "I'm glad I'm not as sensitive as others"). At the same time, they tended to reject self-accusation much more than control persons ("I can't help it," "That situation is not my responsibility," "I've done no wrong").

This coping style is indicative of a strongly defensive attitude and a marked resistance to agitation and risks caused by external factors, which, in terms of a psychoanalytical defense mechanism, are a major threat for the individual's personality. The threat is perceived with fear and must be warded off, which causes the person not to experience nervous agitation in the first place. In a stress situation created in the laboratory by way of a lecture in front of alleged language experts, the subtest "playing down" (reducing in importance) correlated negatively with subjective stress reactions. In the repression-sensitization stress concept (Krohne & Rogner, 1982), it is assumed that individuals who are of the repressor type tend to ward off threatening information and stimuli because of a marked tendency toward fearfulness, while sensitizers need more stimuli. It is these features of coping that are of immense importance in guiding the patient, educating him or her about the disease, and administering therapy and posttreatment.

In summary, the results of the present study showed that patients with periodontal disease confront stressful problems in different ways. Compared to healthy controls, they use a number of different coping strategies. Patients used active problem-oriented coping styles significantly less often; rather, they employed passive emotional stress strategies like distractive coping and defensive coping to resolve problems. The study also showed that the progression of disease, measured by the clinical attachment loss (CAL), was correlated with these inadequate coping strategies. In other words, periodontitis patients with a defensive coping style had significantly more clinical attachment loss. Furthermore, the tendency toward an increasing CAL was emphasized by concomitant increasing values in coping strategies.

Coping with Stress: Its Influence on Periodontal Therapy

The role of inappropriate coping styles as a risk to the general health of an individual is considered to be important for the emergence of disease and its progression. The same is true for the impact of such coping styles on the severity of disease. To investigate such a modulating effect on therapy and the course of disease, the influence of the patients' individual coping behavior (which had been recorded by psychodiagnostic procedures as described above) on a nonsurgical periodontal treatment and the subsequent course of the disease for two years was tested (Wimmer et al., 2005). The clinical and psychodiagnostic data of the first investigation were used as baseline data and compared with clinical as well as new psychodiagnostic data obtained after the completion of periodontal therapy and posttreatment two years later. During this period, all patients underwent identical nonsurgical periodontal therapy and posttreatment maintenance.

The analysis of data indicates a negative influence of that coping strategy, which correlated with the extent of disease at the initial investigation. Defensive, suppressive coping was statistically significant correlated with clinical attachment loss. Periodontitis patients with a defensive coping style had significantly greater attachment loss at the two-year evaluation compared to patients with other coping behaviors. Furthermore, the percentage reduction of CAL 4 mm was significantly less in defensive copers. The less the patients used these presumably inadequate coping strategies, the greater was the percentage increase in sites with attachment loss below 4 mm, that is, improvement of the disease (fig. 11.1). Conversely, an increase in defensive suppressive coping was associated with a lesser reduction in the number of severe disease sites. Patients who largely used this inadequate "poor" coping strategy had a greater percentage of sites with advanced clinical attachment loss; thus the improvement of the disease was inhibited. In addition, patients with a defensive coping style had significantly more sites with severe attachment loss. Thus, patients who belong to the group of the "more strongly defensive and suppressive copers" were at greater risk of experi-

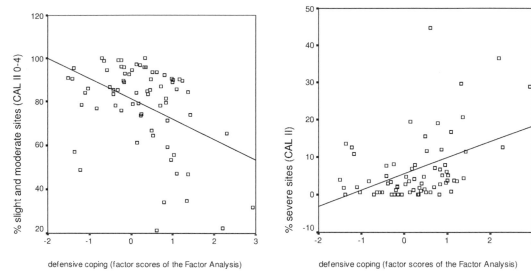

Fig. 11.1. Significant correlations (p = 0.0001) between defensive coping (factor 4), reduced number of slight and moderate sites (AV 0-4), and increased number of severe sites. Solid boxes denote severe smokers.

encing more clinical attachment loss after two years compared to those using other stress-coping strategies. If the response to nonsurgical treatment was the same, one would expect a similar percentage reduction of deep pockets among patients with different coping strategies. These correlations of different stress-coping strategies with the extent of periodontal destruction from the first and the second investigation may be interpreted as follows: a defensive suppressive coping style may have a negative impact on the development of the disease as well as its course and treatment.

In this context, the relation of the results for the nineteen individual subtests of the SVF (table 11.1), those addressing stress-coping measures indicated by responses to six questions each, or changes in these subtests over time, to changes in periodontal status was determined. By doing so, an attempt was made to identify the different strategies used by patients in stressful situations and the outcome of such strategies. Very few strategies were altered during the study period. Most remarkably, the subtest drug use was highly significantly correlated with the CAL. Drug use in the baseline survey as well as changes of the subtest drug use were correlated with less improvement in clinical parameters.

In addition to drug use, averting blame and playing down in comparison with others also showed changes, although not to such a significant degree. Averting blame, playing down in comparison with others, and drug use are coping strategies that do not permit active confrontation of the stressful situation. A habitual preference for a nonconfronting stress-coping style is possibly responsible for an unfavorable course of the treatment and the disease in the long term. High factor values in the subtest of drug use are indicative of strategies to indirectly avoid or reduce the stressful situation or reaction.

In stressful situations, patients tend to use pharmaceutical agents, such as

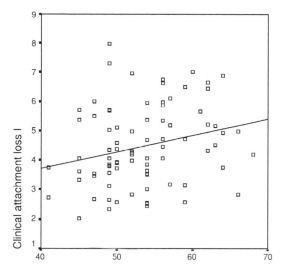

Fig. 11.2. An increase in t-values for the subtest drug use (pharmaceutical drugs) reveals a significant increase of CAL. The greater the abuse, the poorer were the clinical values. Solid boxes denote severe smokers.

drugs, psychotropic stimulants, or so-called substitute gratification to a greater extent. The typical items of this subtest are: "I tend to smoke much more or start smoking again," "I take tranquilizers," "I tend to get drunk," "I first drink a glass of beer, wine or schnapps," "I take sleeping tablets," "I tend to take medication of some kind." Substitute gratification also includes nicotine, alcohol, or drug abuse.

Smoking is considered to be one of the most important predisposing behavior-oriented risk factors for the development of periodontal disease (Rivera-Hidalgo, 2003). Smoking also impairs healing after nonsurgical therapy (Preber, Linder, & Bergstrom, 1995). In the present study, smoking was found to have no statistical impact on the course of the disease in the patient group. However, the number of smokers in the group was small (n = 15), which was possibly the reason why the results were not statistically significant. However, it should be noted that nearly all heavy smokers in those patient groups with advanced forms of the disease (fig. 11.1) also had negative correlations between the disease and so-called substitute gratification, as indicated by the subtest of drug use (fig. 11.2).

Even excessive alcohol intake (Pitiphat et al., 2003) in association with a specific lifestyle (Sakki et al., 1995; Shizukuishi et al., 1998) is considered to exercise a harmful effect on periodontal disease. A passive stress-coping strategy that directly supports the risk factor is predominant in those seeking substitute gratification, especially smoking. In such cases, it is absolutely necessary to intervene. Therefore, the dental team, in particular the periodontal one, should confront the challenge of smoking prevention and cessation. The fact that some of the health professionals most commonly visited by patients are the dentist and oral hygienist offers a very important opportunity for counseling about smoking cessation (Giddon & Anderson 2005). The stress-coping strategy, as a behavior variable, plays a very important role especially in cases of failure or relapse. In addition to general measures (Miller, 1990), the modification of patient behavior in regard to drug intake, as well as by more active than passive confrontation coping behavior, could simultaneously influence these risk factors of smoking, alcohol, drug abuse, and possibly diabetes and related obesity (Suls & Fletcher, 1985).

The results of this study show that passive coping strategies were more pronounced in advanced disease as well as in cases of poor response to a nonsurgical periodontal treatment. In contrast, patients with active coping modes had milder disease and a more favorable course of treatment. Thus, maladaptive behavior, especially in association with behavior-related risk factors such as smoking, as determined by the medical history are of great importance in the medical history, treatment, and maintenance of patients with periodontal disease.

Conclusion

Although it is impossible to conclusively state whether stress is a cause, a risk factor, or even a consequence of disease, studies such as those reported here are necessary as well as future large longitudinal studies, randomized interventional studies, and animal experiment studies, which directly investigate the influence of stress on periodontitis. It has already been established that stress weakens the immune system and facilitates the emergence of disease (Kiecolt-Glaser, 1999). Furthermore, as noted earlier, the available knowledge on this subject indicates that stress, psychological and psychosocial pressures, and inadequate coping are significant risk indicators for periodontal disease.

As noted by many authors, both intrapsychic (depression, anxiety) and psychosocial (life events, professional and family situations) factors relative to the individual's stress-coping strategies should be noted and evaluated in the patient's history. Although such inquiries into personal coping strategies will often be difficult for the treating dentist, this information must be assessed because, as demonstrated in the studies reported here, coping strategies usually influence the individual's risk behavior for periodontitis. Economical screening instruments for the deleterious behavior noted earlier would be desirable for the treating dentist to use when counseling the patient, as well as when identifying patients at risk and optimizing patient compliance.

Obviously, some patients who are evaluated as being under stress may best be referred to appropriate specialists for psychological-psychiatric support, stress management, or addiction counseling.

Acknowledgments

The authors thank Mag. M. Janda, Mag. G. Köhldorfer, and Dipl. Ing. I. Mischak, who participated in the investigations presented here. The authors also acknowledge support from the Austrian Society of Dentistry, Subsidiary Styria for these investigations.

References

Ballieux, R. E. (1991). Impact of stress on the immune response. *Journal of Clinical Periodontology, 18,* 427–30.

Breivik, T., et al. (1996). Emotional stress effects on immunity, gingivitis and periodontitis. *European Journal of Oral Science, 104(4),* 327–34.

Genco, R. J. (1996). Current View of Risk Factors for Periodontal Diseases. *Journal of Periodontology, 67 (Supp.),* 1041–49.

Genco, R. J., & Löe, H. (1993). The role of systemic conditions and disorders in periodontal disease. *Periodontology 2000, 2,* 98–116.

Genco, R. J., et al. (1998). Models to evaluate the role of stress in periodontal disease. *Annals of Periodontology, 3(1),* 288–302.

———. (1999). Relationship of stress, distress, and inadequate coping behaviors to periodontal disease. *Journal of Periodontology, 70,* 711 23.

Giddon, D. B. (1966). Psychophysiology of the oral cavity. *Journal of Dental Research, 45,* 1627–36.

———. (1999). Mental-dental interface: window to the psyche and soma. *Perspectives in Biology and Medicine, 43(1),* 84–97.

Giddon, D. B., & Anderson, N. K. (2005). Attitudes toward expanded roles for paramedical personnel. *American Journal of Health Studies, 19(4),* 220–25.

Goldhaber, P., & Giddon, D. B. (1964). Present concepts concerning the etiology and treatment of acute necrotizing ulcerative gingivitis. *International Dental* Journal, *14,* 468–96.

Janke, W., Erdmann, G., & Kallus, W. (1985). *The Stress Coping Questionnaire (SVF) Manual* (in German). Göttingen: Verlag für Psychologie, Dr. C. J. Hogrefe.

Kiecolt-Glaser, J. K. (1999). Stress, Personal relationships, and immune function: health implications. *Brain, Behavior, and Immunity, 13(1),* 61–72.

Kornman, K. S., et al. (1997). The interleukin-1 genotype as a severity factor in adult periodontal disease. *Journal of Clinical Periodontology, 24(1),* 72–77.

Krohne, H. W., & Rogner, J. (1982). Repression-sensitization as a central construct in coping research. In H. W. Krohne & L. Laux (eds.), *Achievement, Stress and Anxiety.* Washington: Hemisphere Publishing.

Lazarus, R. S. (1966). *Psychological Stress and the Coping Process.* New York: McGraw-Hill.

Miller, S. M. (1990). To see or not to see: cognitive informational styles in the coping process. In M. Rosenbaum (ed.), *Learnt Resourcefulness.* New York: Springer.

Monteiro da Silva, A. M., et al. (1998). Psychosocial factors, dental plaque levels and smoking in periodontitis patients. *Journal of Clinical Periodontology, 25(6),* 517–23.

Monteiro da Silva, A. M., Newman, H. N., & Oakley, D. A. (1995). Psychosocial factors in inflammatory periodontal diseases: a review. *Journal of Clinical Periodontology, 22,* 516–23.

Pitiphat, W., et al. (2003). Alcohol consumption increases periodontitis risk. *Journal of Dental Research, 82(7),* 509–13.

Preber, H., Linder, L., & Bergstrom, J. (1995). Periodontal healing and periopathogenic microflora in smokers and non-smokers. *Journal of Clinical Periodontology, 22(12),* 946–52.

Rivera-Hidalgo, F. (2003). Smoking and periodontal disease. *Periodontology 2000, 32,* 50–58.

Sakki, T. K., et al. (1995). Association of lifestyle with periodontal health. *Community Dentistry and Oral Epidemiology, 23,* 155–58.

Shizukuishi, S., et al. (1998). Lifestyle and periodontal health status of Japanese factory workers. *Annals of Periodontology, 3,* 303–11.

Socransky, S. S., & Haffajee, A. D. (1992). The bacterial etiology of destructive periodontal disease: current concepts. *Journal of Periodontology, 63(4 Supp),* 322–31.

Solis, A. C., et al. (2004). Association of periodontal disease to anxiety and depression symptoms, and psychosocial factors. *Journal of Clinical Periodontology, 31,* 633–368;

Suls, J., & Fletcher B. (1985). The relative efficacy of avoidant and nonavoidant coping strategies: a meta-analysis. *Health Psychology, 4,* 249–88.

Wimmer, G., et al. (2002). Coping with stress: its influence on periodontal disease. *Journal of Periodontology, 73,* 1343–51.

——. (2005). Coping with stress: its influence on periodontal therapy. *Journal of Periodontology, 76,* 90–98.

Health Behavior and Helping Patients Change

Anne Koerber

Importance of Behavior Change to Oral Health and Dentistry

The management of caries and periodontal disease, like other chronic diseases, is seriously affected by lifestyle behaviors, such as plaque removal, diet, and tobacco use. In addition, other chronic physical conditions and their treatments that are affected by lifestyle issues, such as diabetes or cancer, can have significant effects on oral health. As a result, maintaining oral health requires patient participation and cooperation, and requires a practitioner who can facilitate patient participation and cooperation. The purpose of this chapter is to describe and discuss counseling skills that dental and dental hygiene students and practitioners may use to facilitate their patients in making proper choices to improve the health of their mouths and the rest of their bodies.

The dental professions have been at the forefront in recognizing the importance of prevention in oral diseases, beginning with the professions' endorsements and promotions of fluoride to control dental caries. Furthermore, dentists and hygienists have long recognized that patient involvement is essential in controlling caries and periodontal disease. The education of dentists and hygienists has included training them to teach their patients about plaque removal and other methods of controlling oral diseases. This has been recognized by *Dental Education at the Crossroads* (Field, 1995).

However, increasing a patient's knowledge is often not enough to cause patients to make the necessary changes to maintain their own oral health. For example, research shows that plaque-control programs usually result in increased knowledge, but only short-term improvements in plaque removal (Brown, 1994; Kay & Locker, 1998). Similar difficulty has been experienced

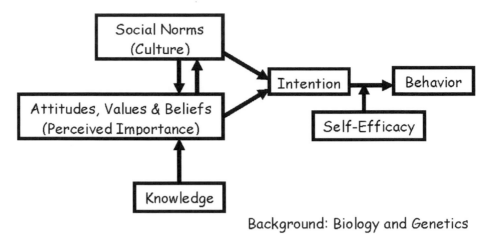

Fig. 12.1. Theory of Planned Action with Modifications.

in encouraging mothers to practice feeding habits that are healthy for their children's teeth (Tinanoff et al., 1999; Benitez, O'Sullivan, & Tinanoff, 1994). The medical profession also has difficulty in helping patients lose weight, improve their diets, increase their exercise, or cease addictive behaviors. Something more than knowledge or education is needed to help patients improve their oral health.

A Model of Health Behavior

In order to help patients choose more healthy behavior, practitioners must understand the determinants of health behavior. Over the decades, models have been developed that have clarified our understanding of health behavior considerably. These models were summarized by Inglehart and Tedesco, who proposed the comprehensive *Model for the New Century* for oral health behavior (Inglehart & Tedesco, 1995). This chapter will use the simpler model proposed by Ajzen (1985), the *Theory of Planned Action*, with modifications suggested by other models (Inglehart & Tedesco, 1995; Miller & Rollnick, 2002b), to illustrate the factors that affect health behavior. The model is shown in figure 12.1.

The theory of planned action has been supported as explaining many health behaviors, including oral health behaviors (Kneckt et al., 1999; Stewart, Strack, & Graves, 1997; Syrjala, Kneckt, & Knuuttila, 1999; Tedesco, Keffer, & Fleck-Kandath, 1991). This model illustrates three important components of health behavior: social norms, personal beliefs/attitudes/values, and self-efficacy. Social norms are those aspects of behavior that people engage in because that is how they were brought up, because that is what they assume is "normal" without necessarily giving it much thought. It also includes patients' perceptions of what is expected of them by the people around them. The next component, beliefs/attitudes/values, includes a person's beliefs about illness and health, what causes illness and what alleviates it, along with considerations of importance or value. Finally, self-efficacy covers perceptions of whether a patient is capable of doing the desired behavior, and this includes whether the patient feels she (or he) has the resources to engage in the behavior.

Note that knowledge is not directly a determinate of behavior. Knowledge is important only insofar as it affects beliefs and values. Knowledge might affect norms or self-efficacy, but that is indirectly through changing a person's attitudes. In order for knowledge to change behavior, at least three steps must occur. First, the person's attitudes and values must change, such that the patient comes to believe the behavior to be worthwhile. Second, the person's new attitude toward the behavior must be strong enough to offset any preconceived ideas from the surrounding social and cultural norms. Third, the person must see herself as capable of doing the behavior.

The theory of planned action can be applied to health behaviors as serious as quitting smoking, and as comparatively innocuous as selecting a toothbrush. Let's understand this model by using flossing as an example. For a dental patient, John, to start flossing regularly, he must see flossing as worthwhile. This falls in the beliefs/attitudes/values realm. The dentist or hygienist can explain the importance of removing plaque for oral health—that is, strive to improve the knowledge realm—but if "oral health" is not a priority for John, he is not going to do it, regardless of his level of knowledge. John is more likely to accept flossing if he values his teeth, either functionally or esthetically, and if he sees a link between flossing and keeping his teeth or nice smile. The link between the desired behaviors and the patient's values is important. Thus, if the practitioner wants John to floss, the most direct way is to link flossing to John's *preexisting* values and beliefs. Many practitioners, perhaps without realizing it, try to change the patient's value system. They spend time trying to convince the patient that oral health is important, instead of learning what the patient considers important and linking the behavior to that.

John is also more likely to accept flossing if the people he knows also floss; that is, if it fits into his cultural norms. Similarly, if flossing is not in his cultural experience, he might be dubious about doing it, even if it were recommended by a dental professional. Even if the people he knows are aware of flossing but do not engage in it, then John is less likely to floss himself. This addresses the social norms part of the model in figure 12.1, which is the set of cognitions that have to do with cultural, family, and individual norms and expectations.

The dental practitioner is usually not in a position to change a person's social norms directly. A patient's perception of what is normal or expected depends on her background and the people around her. Examples of interventions that affect social norms are changes in school environments, such as children brushing their teeth together in class; influencing the family of a child to change a child's diet; or societal changes such as laws against smoking in public places. Most often, changes in norms occur without the dentist's knowledge or participation, such as John's girlfriend insisting that he floss.

A practitioner could affect John's perceived norms indirectly by influencing his attitudes and value system. If John's norms are not congruent with flossing, he will only start flossing if his attitudes toward flossing can overcome his social and background situation. This illustrates the greater difficulty of influencing a patient whose social norms differ from the practitioner's. The practitioner's task is then to help the patient engage in the desired behavior in spite of social norms and peer pressure; in other words, help strengthen those patient values that move the patient to floss in spite of his background.

The third part of the model is self-efficacy. John will not floss if he doesn't know how, or if he feels incompetent at it. He will also not floss unless he perceives himself as having "what it takes" to floss. For example, he must feel he can afford floss. He must feel that he can get floss when he needs it. He must feel he has the time to floss. All these might be summed by the word "resources." Self-efficacy is used in this chapter to include all the patient's perceptions of whether he or she has the skills, self-confidence, and resources needed to engage in a particular behavior. Dental practitioners can affect self-efficacy through skills training, and through helping a patient think through difficulties to find a way to engage in the desired behavior.

When this model is used, the task of encouraging healthy patient behavior is put in the context of the whole patient. It becomes clear why simple knowledge doesn't have much effect on behavior change, especially if it conflicts with well-entrenched beliefs, values, or norms. If a behavior change is congruent with norms and beliefs, and if self-efficacy is present, the change is highly likely to take place, and simple education will suffice to initiate it. The practitioner's task is made easier if she links the desired behavior with preexisting values of the patient instead of trying to change the values.

How People Change

If knowledge doesn't directly change health behavior, what can a practitioner do to help people change? The model in figure 12.1 implies several strategies:

- Link the desired behavior change with the patient's personal value system.
- Don't assume that oral health is an important value to the patient.
- Don't assume that increasing patient knowledge will change the patient's value system; instead, try to work within the patient's frame of reference.
- When a behavior change is difficult for a patient, facilitate the *patient's* finding solutions to the difficulty. The patient understands her situation better than the practitioner. Any solutions coming from the practitioner run the risk of not fitting with the patient's norms or values.
- Support a patient's self-confidence and mustering of resources to promote change.
- Offer a *menu* of alternatives as opposed to recommending one particular action, to increase the chance that one of them will fit in with the patient better than the others.

Prochaska and DiClemente proposed a model of how people change behavior, called the *Trans-Theoretical Model of Behavior Change* (DiClemente & Prochaska, 1998), shown in figure 12.2, which includes an understanding of how relapse fits into the change process.

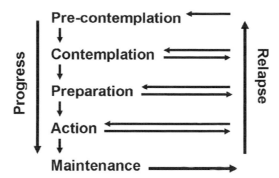

Fig. 12.2. Transtheoretical Model of the Stages of Change. (After Prochaska & DiClemente, 1986.)

At the precontemplation stage, the person is unaware of or uninterested in change. At the contemplation stage, the person has begun to accept that change might be beneficial, but has not committed to it. At the preparation stage, the person has committed to change and is deciding how to make it happen. At the action stage, the person is implementing the change. Finally, at the maintenance stage, the person is working to maintain the changes. A person who is making a change moves through the stages, but not always in a forward direction. Often, difficult changes such as smoking cessation are characterized by cycling back and forth between stages, as the patient quits, relapses, and works up to quitting again.

This suggests that different interventions are more effective at different stages, and also highlights the ambivalence of motivation. The dental practitioner would be making a mistake to characterize John as either "motivated" or "not motivated" to floss. Most people can see the benefits of change but are also aware of the difficulties. A practitioner is most helpful if he (or she) recognizes the ambivalence, identifies John's stage of readiness, and adopts an intervention appropriate to his stage.

Readiness to Change

Rollnick and Miller suggested that there are two dimensions to readiness to change: the patient's perception of the *importance* of change, and the patient's *self-confidence* to carry out the change (Miller & Rollnick, 2002b; Rollnick, Mason, & Butler, 1999). These dimensions are compatible with the model in figure 12.1: importance lies in the realm of attitudes/beliefs/values, and self-confidence lies in the realm of self-efficacy. These dimensions of readiness to change help us understand which interventions are most effective at which stages of change. When a patient is in the precontemplative stage, importance is usually the issue to be addressed, and later on, self-confidence becomes more important, although it is important to assess both dimensions throughout the intervention.

To increase the patient's perception of the importance of the change, the practitioner should consider two steps: first, give the patient brief factual advice concerning the change, allowing the patient to ask questions. Second, link the behavior change to an outcome that is important to the patient. To increase the patient's self-confidence, support the patient's self-efficacy by encouraging the patient to come up with solutions and keep adapting the solutions until they work. Brief, factual advice about how change works may also be useful.

Let us now consider giving advice.

The Role of Advice and Education in Facilitating Change

The risk a practitioner runs when giving advice is to arouse resistance in a patient. This is human nature. When any of us are told we need to change something basic and important to us, our instinct is to resist or oppose it, especially if no symptoms are being experienced and the gain is in some hypothetical future. Yet, the practitioner has an obligation to give the patient the necessary information. The trick is to provide advice and information in a manner least likely to arouse resistance, and most likely to help the patient be interested in the change.

Rollnick recommends that advice be brief, be given after asking permission to give the advice, and be neutral in tone (Rollnick et al., 1999). Elaborate discussions of the problems and solutions should be postponed until the patient has time to assimilate the basic information, or until the patient requests more information. Argumentation and pressure should be avoided. The patient should not be labeled or characterized in any way. Instead, the facts should be presented, and the treatment recommended in a neutral manner, that is simultaneously clearly applicable to this patient but avoids characterizing the patient. For example, instead of saying to John, "You aren't keeping your mouth clean, and you should start to floss regularly," instead say, "There is plaque on your teeth, which is causing an infection in the gums. This kind of infection gets better with thoroughly removing the plaque from the teeth. I'd really like to know what you think about that." This series of statements explain the problem factually, links it to John without characterizing him as unclean or negligent, and states the desired behavior. It also asks permission to go further in the discussion, and elicits the patient's reaction. Table 12.1 provides more examples contrasting advice that might cause resistance with advice that should minimize resistance.

If the patient indicates unwillingness to hear the advice, in some circumstances the practitioner may feel impelled to give it regardless. In this case, the information should still be given in a neutral, factual manner, but the practitioner should make it clear that she has a stand on the issue. For example, a practitioner could say, "I recommend you quit smoking. I understand you don't want to talk about it now, but when you are ready, I might be able to help." See the chapter "Ethical Considerations" in Miller and Rollnick's text for a further discussion of this issue (Miller & Rollnick, 2002a).

This section has discussed how advice can be given in a way to minimize resistance. Giving advice in the prescribed manner is one way of influencing a patient's rating of the importance of a recommended change. The second technique that can facilitate a patient considering change is to link the requested change with the patient's value system.

Table 12.1   Contrasts Between Statements That Might Arouse Resistance, with Statements That Facilitate Change

Statements More Likely to Arouse Resistance	Statements More Likely to Facilitate Change
You aren't brushing well enough.	There is more plaque on your teeth than the last time you came in. Do you have any concerns about that?
Your smoking is making your gum disease worse.	Studies have shown that smoking makes gum disease worse. I'd like to know what your feelings about that are.
You should quit smoking.	Could we talk a bit about smoking? *Or* It is a fact that gum disease gets worse when people smoke, and gets better when they stop. Can you tell me your reaction to that?
Stop giving your child a bottle to sleep with at night.	Scientists have found that putting your child to bed with a bottle of formula or even milk can cause cavities. I'd like to know what you think about that.
Just don't give your children as many sugary foods, cut out the soda, and don't give them candy.	I wonder what steps you could take that would work in your situation to help your children eat less sugar?
Why don't you brush and floss while you watch the evening news, so you don't forget to do it?	Since your problem seems to be remembering to brush and floss, I wonder what tricks you could use to remember?
Stay away from your smoking friends, because they will just make you want to smoke more.	In my experience, people often need to make plans about how they will handle social situations after they stop smoking. What have you done in the past? What has worked before?

Linking Requested Behavior Change to the Patient's Values

Linking change to values can be done either directly by the practitioner, or the practitioner can elicit it from the patient. An example of making the link directly would be, "John, you originally came here because you had a missing tooth. You have been willing to invest time and money in getting a bridge. My experience indicates that when people clean the bridge and the rest of their teeth after each meal, they reduce their risk of losing the bridge or losing their other teeth. I'd like to know your reaction to that." This type of intervention assumes that the bridge is important to the patient, because the patient chose to get the bridge. This is probably the shortest way to give advice and link the advice with the patient's values. However, many times, that link isn't obvious. If John has just come in for a routine dental visit, and the dentist discovers by the way that he has periodontitis, there is no obvious link to John's value system.

A more effective approach would be to elicit from John the link between the behavior (flossing) and his goals and values. This requires somewhat more skill and time from the practitioner, but could be done with only a small investment in time. Using the previous example, the practitioner might ask John, "Can you see any reason for flossing your teeth after each meal?" This elicits the reasons for change from John's perspective. Another method is to ask patients what they value about their mouth and their health. The patient might reply something like, "I don't want to lose my teeth," or, "My teeth have always caused me a lot of trouble. I just want them to stop causing me problems." Then the practitioner uses that information and invites the patient to make the link, by saying something like, "Can you see any way that flossing after each meal might help you [keep your teeth?] or [avoid future problems with your teeth]?"

Often this means the practitioner must limit the goals for a particular session. The goal of any session should be to provide assistance as the patient moves back and forth through the stages of change. The practitioner will only be disappointed if she expects the patient to change a behavior as a result of a single intervention.

Motivational Interviewing

The above discussion about how to give brief advice and how to link the advice with the patient's value system are techniques from a counseling method called Motivational Interviewing (MI) (Rollnick et al., 1999; Rollnick et al., 2002). MI is a patient-centered mode of counseling that is designed to help patients approach change by maximizing intrinsic motivation and minimizing resistance. It was originally developed to help patients deal with addictions (including alcohol and tobacco), but has also been used to help medical patients make difficult lifestyle changes, such as dietary changes, increased exercise, and weight loss (Resnicow et al., 2002). Formal MI is a form of psychotherapy, designed for 30–45-minute sessions and requiring training, and so is probably not cost-effective for most dental practitioners. However, an understanding of the principles of MI can help a practitioner understand how to make her time with a patient more effective, even with limited time and training.

Principles of MI

The principles of MI are expression of empathy, development of discrepancy between where the patient is and where she wants to be, rolling with resistance, and supporting self-efficacy. These are further elaborated in table 12.2.

Full training in MI develops the practitioner's skills and techniques in each of these areas, and is beyond the scope of this chapter. However, if less time is available, the practitioner could still adopt an attitude or manner of approaching a patient that focuses on eliciting the patient's motives to make the change instead of exhorting the patient to change. The practitioner does NOT tell the patient what to do, but instead makes recommendations. The

Table 12.2   Principles of Motivational Interviewing

MI principle	Explanation/elaboration	Possible interventions
Expression of empathy	Acceptance of the patient as she is facilitates change. Reflective listening skills are fundamental. Ambivalence is normal.	Ask permission to discuss the subject. Ask open-ended questions about the patient's attitude toward the subject, and listen. Ask the patient to discuss both sides of the ambivalence.
Development of discrepancy	The patient rather than the counselor should provide the arguments for change. Your goal is to help the patient discover goals or values of her own that will be facilitated by the behavior change.	Ask the patient to list the reasons for and against change. Do not list them for her. Through summarizing and reflective listening, highlight the discrepancy between the patient's goals and her current situation.
Roll with resistance	Avoid arguing for change or "selling" change. Invite new perspectives, but do not impose them. The patient is the primary resource for finding solutions. Resistance is a signal for the practitioner to respond differently.	Instead, acknowledge both sides of the ambivalence. See examples in table 12.1. Acknowledge that it is up to the patient whether or not she wants to make the change.
Support self efficacy	The patient's belief in the possibility of change is an important motivator. The patient, not the practitioner, is responsible for choosing and carrying out change. The counselor's own belief in person's ability to change becomes a self-fulfilling prophecy.	Encourage the patient to consider what has and hasn't worked in the past. Encourage the patient to list the needed changes and plan for the difficulties. Trust the patient to find her own solutions. Be positive and optimistic.

Source: Adapted from Miller & Rollnick, 2002.

practitioner asks the patient to consider how he might incorporate the recommended change into his life.

Evidence Basis of MI

The evidence basis of MI is reviewed in Miller and Rollnick's latest text and summarized here (Burke, Arkowitz, & Dunn, 2002). Adaptations of MI have been shown to be effective, even with only three or four sessions in studies of alcohol abuse treatment, and the treatment effects have been shown to last over a year. However, when MI was tested against other treatments, all treatments were better than no treatment, and MI was only as effective as the other treatments. This was possibly because of validity issues; that is, the interventions were not defined clearly with manuals, and checks were not made to insure the therapists were adhering to the definitions of the contrasting treatments. However, Miller was able to establish a direct correlation between therapist confrontations in alcohol treatment programs and the frequency of drinking alcohol at one year follow-up, which is support for avoiding a confrontational approach (Miller, 1996).

Burke et al., concluded there is evidence to support the use of brief MI with hypertension, diabetes, and eating disorders. However, for cigarette smoking, brief adaptations of MI may help patients improve in some areas—such as more quit attempts, smoking fewer cigarettes, and increased delay for the first cigarette of the day—but there was no difference from more authoritarian counseling methods in rates of quitting for more than a week (Butler et al., 1999). Cigarette smoking is a particularly difficult addiction to treat, and may require both use of nicotine replacement therapy and formal counseling by professional counselors. However, the dental practitioner can still play an important role by helping to motivate a patient to seek such counseling.

Uses of MI in Oral Health Settings

A review of the literature revealed few studies of MI in oral-health settings. Weinstein showed that MI in a public health clinic setting was effective in convincing Bengali immigrants to adopt more appropriate nursing habits for their children, using a Bengali lay educator who spoke the language of the participants. Since other studies have had difficulty in accomplishing the same task (Tinanoff et al., 1999; Benitez et al., 1994), this is an important finding. Another study showed that MI training was effective in changing the counseling behavior of dental students (Koerber, Crawford, & O'Connell, 2003). However, there have been no studies of the efficacy of MI techniques at the chairside in dentistry for nutritional counseling, oral hygiene, or smoking cessation. This is a promising area for research.

Summary

This chapter has attempted to explain the determinants of health behavior to help the dental and dental hygiene student and practitioner better understand the patient's perspective when attempting to change the patient's behavior. In addition, suggestions were made concerning how to phrase interventions to maximize the patient's ability to hear and accept the intervention through the use of motivational interviewing (MI) techniques. Finally, the literature was reviewed on the efficacy of MI in helping patients change.

Acknowledgments

My grateful thanks to Khatija Noorullah, Esther Vega, and Dr. Ron Botto for their insightful comments and help.

References

Ajzen, I. (1985). From decisions to actions: a theory of planned behavior. In J. Kuhl & J. Beckmann (eds.), *Action-Control: From Cognition to Behavior.* New York: Springer.

Benitez, C., O'Sullivan, D., & Tinanoff, N. (1994). Effect of a preventive approach for the treatment of nursing bottle caries. *Journal of Dentistry for Children, 61(1)*, 46–49.

Brown, L. F. (1994). Research in dental health education and health promotion: a review of the literature. *Health Education Quarterly, 21(1)*, 83–102.

Burke, B. L., Arkowitz, H., & Dunn, C. (2002). The efficacy of motivational interviewing and its adaptations. In W. R. Miller & S. Rollnick (eds.), *Motivational Interviewing: Preparing People for Change.* 2d ed. New York: Guilford Press.

Butler, C. C., Rollnick, S., Cohen, D., Russel, I., Bachmann, M., & Stott, N. (1999). Motivational consulting versus brief advice for smokers in general practice: a randomized trial. *British Journal of General Practice, 49*, 611–16.

DiClemente, C. C., & Prochaska, J. (1998). Toward a comprehensive, transtheoretical model of change: stages of change and addictive behaviors. In W. R. Miller & N. Heather (eds.), *Treating Addictive Behaviors.* 2d ed. New York: Plenum Press.

Field, M. J., ed. (1995). *Dental Education at the Crossroads: Challenges and Change/ Committee on the Future of Dental Education.* Washington, DC: Institute of Medicine, National Academy Press.

Inglehart, M., & Tedesco, L. A. (1995). Behavioral research related to oral hygiene practices: a new century model of oral health promotion. *Periodontology 2000, 8*, 15–23.

Kay, E., & Locker, D. (1998). A systematic review of the effectiveness of health promotion aimed at improving oral health. *Community Dental Health, 15*, 132–44.

Kneckt, M. C., Syrjala, A. M. H., Laukkanen, P., & Knuuttila, M. L. E. (1999). Self-efficacy as a common variable in oral health behavior and diabetes adherence. *European Journal of Oral Sciences, 107(2)*, 89–96.

Koerber, A., Crawford, J. M., & O'Connell, K. (2003). The effects of teaching dental students brief motivational interviewing for smoking cessation counseling: a pilot study. *Journal of Dental Education, 67*, 439–47.

Miller, W. R. (1996). Motivational interviewing: research, practice, and puzzles. *Addictive Behaviors, 21(6)*, 835–42.

Miller, W. R., & Rollnick, S. (2002a). Ethical considerations. In W. R. Miller & S. Rollnick, (eds.). *Motivational Interviewing: Preparing People for Change.* New York: Guilford Press.

———. (2002b). *Motivational Interviewing: Preparing People for Change.* 2d ed. New York: Guilford Press.

Prochaska, J., & DiClemente, C. C. (1986). *The Transtheoretical Approach: Crossing the Traditional Boundaries of Therapy.* Homewood, IL: Dow Jones Irwin.

Resnicow, K., DiIorio, C., Soet, J. E., et al. (2002). Motivational interviewing in medical and public health settings. In W. R. Miller & S. Rollnick (eds.), *Motivational Interviewing: Preparing People for Change.* New York: Guilford Press.

Rollnick, S., Allison, J., Ballasiotes, S., et al. (2002). Variations on a theme: motivational interviewing and its adaptations. In W. R. Miller & S. Rollnick (eds.), *Motivational Interviewing: Preparing People for Change.* New York: Guilford Press.

Rollnick, S., Mason, P., & Butler, C. (1999). *Health Behavior Change: A Guide for Practitioners.* Edinburgh: Churchill Livingstone.

Stewart, J. E., Strack, S., & Graves, P. (1997). Development of oral hygiene self-efficacy and outcome expectancy questionnaires. *Community Dentistry and Oral Epidemiology, 25(5)*, 337–42.

Syrjala, A. M. H., Kneckt, M. C., & Knuuttila, M. L. E. (1999). Dental self-efficacy as a determinant to oral health behavior, oral hygiene and HbA1$_c$ level among diabetic patients. *Journal of Clinical Periodontology, 26(9)*, 616–21.

Tedesco, L. A., Keffer, M. A., & Fleck-Kandath, C. (1991). Self-efficacy, reasoned action, and oral health behavior reports: a social cognitive approach to compliance. *Journal of Behavioral Medicine, 14(4)*, 341–55.

Tinanoff, N., Daley, N. S., O'Sullivan, D. M., & Douglass, J. M. (1999). Failure of intense preventive efforts to arrest early childhood and rampant caries: three case reports. *Pediatric Dentistry, 21(3)*, 160–63.

Changing Behaviors

Behavior Management in Dentistry: Thumb Sucking

Raymond G. Miltenberger and John T. Rapp

Thumb and finger sucking (hereafter called thumb sucking) is common in early childhood. Studies of the prevalence of thumb sucking show that one-quarter to one-half of children ages three to six years suck their thumbs (e.g., Gutermuth-Foster, 1998; Troster, 1994; Widmalm, Christiansen, & Gunn, 1995). Interestingly, studies conducted in other countries have shown that the prevalence of thumb sucking is substantially lower (e.g., Kharbandaet al., 2003; Vignarajah & William, 1992), suggesting that thumb sucking may be influenced by cultural practices.

Although there is very little empirical support for the notion that thumb sucking is symptomatic of psychological disturbance or psychopathology in children (e.g., Friman, Larzelere, & Finney, 1994; Tryon, 1968), a number of physical problems are correlated with thumb sucking if it persists beyond the age of four or five. Thumb sucking may contribute to malocclusion (e.g., Afzelius-Alm et al., 2004; Reid & Price, 1984), digital deformities (e.g., Malek, Oger, & Rivet-Forsans, 1994; Rankin et al., 1988; Reid & Price, 1984), temporomandibular disorders (e.g., Sari & Sonmez, 2002; Widmalm et al., 1995), altered facial-muscle activity (Ahlgren, 1995), and increased susceptibility to toxins (e.g., Cowie, Black, & Fraser, 1997). In addition to physical problems, Friman et al. (1993) found that first-graders who engaged in thumb sucking received lower ratings of social acceptance from their non-thumb-sucking peers. Thus, children who continue to suck their thumb beyond the age of four may require behavioral intervention. This chapter discusses behavioral assessment and intervention for thumb sucking.

Assessment of Thumb Sucking

Behavioral assessment of thumb sucking is necessary to document the severity of the problem and to evaluate the effects of treatment. Behavioral assessment will involve direct observation and recording of the behavior as it occurs in the child's natural environment.

Because the length of time the thumb is in the child's mouth is the most important aspect of the behavior, a duration measure often is chosen for recording thumb sucking. However, time sample recording can also be used. With duration recording, an observer records the length of time thumb sucking is observed throughout the observation period and reports the percentage of time in which the behavior occurred (duration of thumb sucking divided by the duration of the observation period; Long, Miltenberger, & Rapp, 1999b; Rapp et al., 1999). With time-sample recording, an observer records the occurrence of the behavior during periodic observations and reports the percentage of observations in which thumb sucking was observed (e.g., Ellingson et al., 2000). For example, a parent might observe the child once every ten to fifteen minutes while the child is watching television and record whether thumb sucking is occurring or not occurring during each observation.

Because thumb sucking often occurs only when the child is alone, it may be necessary to observe the behavior surreptitiously while the child is alone (e.g., via video, through an observation window, or during unannounced checks; Friman, Barone, & Christopherson, 1986; Long et al., 1999b; Rapp et al., 1999). For example, Rapp et al. (1999) placed a video camera in the family room of the child's home to record thumb sucking because the parents reported that the child typically sucked his thumb while watching television there.

Functional Assessment of Thumb Sucking

Various forms of social reinforcement from the parent often are found to maintain child problem behaviors (e.g., positive reinforcement involving attention from parents, negative reinforcement involving escape from aversive tasks), and, thus, treatment involves modifying parental responses to the behavior. However, thumb sucking is a behavior that typically is not maintained by social consequences but through some reinforcing outcome produced by the behavior itself. The reinforcing outcome of thumb sucking is thought to consist of arousal reduction or modulation (automatic negative reinforcement; Friman, Boyd, & Oskol, 2001) or some form of sensory stimulation such as oral or digital stimulation (automatic positive reinforcement; Ellingson et al., 2000; Stricker et al., 2002). Thus, the reinforcer for thumb sucking typically is not under the parents' control.

Even though thumb sucking is likely to be automatically reinforced, it is nonetheless important to conduct a functional assessment to identify or rule out any possible social reinforcement for the behavior. A functional assessment, typically conducted through interview or direct observation, identifies the antecedents and consequences associated with the behavior (Lennox & Miltenberger, 1989; O'Neill et al., 1997).

In a functional assessment interview the therapist asks the parents to identify all of the situations in which thumb sucking occurs (antecedents) and asks the parents how they or other caregivers typically respond to the behavior (consequences). If thumb sucking is automatically reinforced, it most often occurs when the child is alone, or occurs across situations, with no consistent reaction from the parent. In many cases, thumb sucking occurs mainly when the child is alone due to a history of punishment for the behavior (e.g., scolding) when it has occurred in the parents' presence (Rapp et al., 1999). If thumb sucking is socially reinforced, it will be more likely to occur in the presence of the parents or other persons who provide reinforcing consequences. Possible reinforcing consequences for thumb sucking include attention (e.g., expressions of concern, reprimands, or emotional responses contingent on thumb sucking), the provision of other reinforcers (e.g., receipt of a pacifier, candy, or another item to suck on contingent on thumb sucking), or escape from aversive activities or situations (e.g., being removed from an activity or event contingent on thumb sucking).

In addition to conducting a functional assessment through an interview and direct observation of the behavior, in some cases, a functional analysis is conducted to identify the reinforcer maintaining thumb sucking (Ellingson et al., 2000; Rapp et al., 1999; Stricker et al., 2002). In a functional analysis, possible reinforcing consequences are manipulated to demonstrate their influence on the target behavior. For example, Rapp et al. (1999) conducted three experimental conditions to determine whether thumb sucking was maintained by social or automatic reinforcement for two five-year-old boys. In one condition, the parents provided attention contingent on thumb sucking (to assess positive reinforcement). In another condition, the parent made requests and allowed the child to escape the requests contingent on thumb sucking (to assess negative reinforcement). Finally, thumb sucking was recorded when the child was alone to determine whether the behavior persisted in the absence of social reinforcement (to assess automatic reinforcement). Rapp et al. found that thumb sucking occurred almost exclusively in the alone condition. Other researchers have found similar results in their functional analyses of thumb sucking (Ellingson et al., 2000; Stricker et al., 2002).

Treatment for Thumb Sucking

Because thumb sucking typically persists in the absence of social reinforcement and often occurs when the child is alone, interventions that alter the antecedents or consequences for the behavior in the absence of the parents or other adults usually are indicated.

Antecedent Intervention

Antecedent interventions exert their effect on a targeted behavior before that behavior is exhibited. Two types of antecedent interventions for thumb sucking have been evaluated; procedures that involved response prevention and procedures that influence thumb sucking by targeting covarying behaviors.

Response Prevention

A variety of apparatuses, such as oral appliances, splints, gloves, and headgear, has been used to physically prevent thumb sucking. Although a number of studies have described the use of oral appliances (e.g., Gawlik, Ott, & Mathieu, 1995; Greenleaf & Mink, 2003; Haskell & Mink, 1991; Viazis, 1991) and headgear (e.g., Taylor & Walker, 1997) as interventions for thumb sucking, few if any of these studies employed an experimental design to empirically evaluate treatment effects. In contrast, a number of behavioral studies have experimentally demonstrated that finger or thumb splints (e.g., Lassen & Fluent, 1978; Watson & Allen, 1993), gloves (Ellingson et al., 2000; Lewis, Shilton, & Fuqua, 1981), or taped cotton (Rolider & Van Houten, 1988) decreased or eliminated daytime and nocturnal thumb sucking.

In a representative study from this category, Ellingson et al. (2000) first conducted a functional analysis and determined that the finger sucking of two children, aged seven and ten years, occurred almost exclusively when each child was alone. In the second phase of the functional analysis, Ellingson et al. found that finger sucking was either greatly reduced or eliminated when adhesive bandages were worn on the fingers, which suggested that finger sucking produced automatic reinforcement in the form of oral or tactile stimulation. Treatment for both participants involved wearing a glove when each was alone (e.g., watching television, lying in bed). For the ten-year-old, the glove immediately eliminated finger sucking. In addition, fading of the glove was accomplished by systematically cutting off pieces over a five-month period. In contrast, the seven-year-old (Sally) continued to suck her finger even when she wore multiple gloves. Ultimately, Sally's finger sucking was eliminated using an awareness enhancement device (AED; see below). Although the glove was only effective for one child, parents of both participants rated the glove intervention as highly acceptable.

One limitation in the use of response prevention strategies should be noted. If the child is able to remove the apparatus (glove, splint, etc.) when the parent is not present, its effectiveness will be diminished. Therefore, the parents will need to monitor the child, perhaps surreptitiously, to insure that the apparatus is not removed.

Response Covariation

A number of studies have shown that thumb sucking is eliminated when the sequence or chain of behavioral events that culminates in thumb sucking is interrupted (e.g., Friman, 1988; 1990; 2000; Watson et al., 2002). Similarly, other studies have shown that eliminating thumb sucking, which appears as the first response in a behavioral chain (i.e., one behavior consistently preceded another), also eliminated hair pulling (e.g., Friman & Hove, 1987; Watson & Allen, 1993; Watson, Dittmer, & Ray, 2000).

Mahalski (1983) reported that as many as 50% of children who display thumb sucking also display attachments to transitional objects such as blankets, pillows, and dolls. In many of these cases, the child obtains one of these objects prior to engaging in thumb sucking. For example, Friman (1988) found that a five-year-old girl displayed thumb sucking only when she was holding a doll; treatment involved simply withholding access to the doll. Follow-up assessment at six months posttreatment showed that thumb sucking suppression was sustained in the absence of the doll.

Watson et al. (2002) also found that two typically developing brothers, ages five and nine years, each engaged in thumb sucking while holding a pillow. Using a reversal design, Watson et al. found that removal of the nine-year-old's pillow decreased and ultimately eliminated thumb sucking for both participants. It appeared that the behavior of the older brother served as a model for the younger brother, whose thumb sucking abated without direct intervention when the older brother's thumb sucking stopped. For both children, the elimination of thumb sucking was maintained at eight weeks posttreatment.

Friman (2000) evaluated the effects of presenting and withholding a transitional object (i.e., a surgical cloth) on the thumb sucking of a three-year-old boy. The results showed that the child displayed thumb sucking only when he had access to the cloth. Treatment involved attaching a pacifier to a cloth swatch. Thereafter, contact with tactile stimulation from the cloth swatch was associated with sucking of the pacifier. However, in the absence of a pacifier, the cloth evoked thumb sucking.

At least two behavioral mechanisms have been cited to account for reductions in thumb sucking following the removal of transitional objects and reductions in hair pulling following the elimination of thumb sucking. Friman and Hove (1987) speculated that decreased hair pulling following the elimination of thumb sucking is the result of interrupting a behavior chain or sequence. Alternatively, results of other studies indicate that some automatically reinforced behaviors may be more likely to occur in the presence of given forms of stimulation (Friman, 2000; Rapp, 2004; Rapp et al., in press). Thus, the stimulation from hair pulling may be more reinforcing when stimulation from thumb sucking is present.

These findings have implications for successful treatment of thumb sucking. In particular, when thumb sucking occurs primarily when an attachment object is present, the most efficient form of treatment may be to remove the object. In addition, if thumb sucking occurs in conjunction with another behavior such as hair twirling or pulling, treatment of one behavior is likely to result in reductions in both behaviors. Therefore, intervention should be directed to the behavior considered easiest to treat or most amenable to change.

Consequent Interventions

Treatment procedures involving the punishment of thumb sucking have assumed two forms; the application of an aversive-tasting substance to the thumb of the child (Friman et al., 1986; Friman & Hove, 1987; Friman & Leibowitz, 1990) or having the child wear a device that delivers auditory stimulation when the child's hand is placed within 10 cm of the head (Ellingson et al., 2000; Stricker et al., 2001; Strickeret al., 2003). Both types of intervention provide consequences for thumb sucking in the absence of a parent or caregiver.

Friman et al. (1986) evaluated the effect of Stop-zit, an over-the-counter substance that was designed to reduce thumb sucking and other oral habits, on the thumb sucking of seven children aged four to twelve years. Parents collected data each night by observing their child for thirty minutes after putting the child to bed. During the treatment, parents applied the solution once in the morning, once in the evening, and after each observed instance of thumb sucking. The treatment rapidly eliminated each child's thumb sucking. Furthermore, the parents of the children rated the intervention as highly acceptable. Likewise, as previously indicated, Friman and Hove (1987) found that thumb sucking and hair pulling of two children, ages two years and five years, were both eliminated using an aversive-tasting substance applied to the thumb. Treatment effects maintained at ten-month and twelve-month follow-up assessments, respectively, without continued application of the aversive-tasting solution. The results of the Friman and Hove study are significant in that treatment of a high probability behavior (thumb sucking) also decreased a low probability, though highly damaging, behavior (hair pulling).

Researchers have also used contingent auditory stimulation via a battery-operated device (AED) to treat thumb or finger sucking. The AED is a two-component apparatus, with one part worn on the wrist and the other part worn on the shirt collar, that delivers a 65-dB tone contingent on the movement of the hand within 10 cm of the head (Rapp, Miltenberger, & Long, 1998). Stricker et al. (2001) rapidly eliminated thumb sucking when using the AED with two typically functioning children. Stricker et al. found that the AED suppressed thumb sucking only when it was "active" (a tone was produced when finger sucking occurred) but not when it was worn but was "inactive" (no tone was produced when finger sucking occurred). As previously noted, Ellingson et al. (2000) found that the finger sucking of one child continued even when she wore two gloves. For this child, the addition of the AED to the glove intervention rapidly suppressed thumb sucking, and the child's parent gave high ratings of social approval for both the glove and AED interventions.

In one other study, Stricker et al. (2003) initially found that the AED was ineffective for decreasing the finger sucking of six-year-old girl. Subsequently, Stricker et al. augmented the effects of the AED by providing a 90-dB stimulus in conjunction with the 65-dB tone from the AED. The child's finger sucking was eliminated when the 90-dB stimulus was activated contingent on the behavior. Thus, although the device is labeled an "awareness enhancement device," it appears that the device achieves its effect through a punishment process; that is, the activation of the auditory stimulus contingent on thumb sucking serves to punish thumb sucking. Nonetheless, it has been rated high in acceptability by the parents of the children with whom it has been used (e.g., Ellingson et al., 2000; Stricker et al., 2003).

Procedures involving the use of contingent aversive stimulation (e.g., taste or auditory) may be limited to the extent that the child can remove AED or the aversive-tasting substance in the absence of adult supervision (see Watson & Allen, 1993). Thus, even though these interventions provide consequences for thumb sucking in the absence of a change agent, supervision is still required to ensure that the integrity of the intervention is not compromised.

Combination Interventions

Several studies have evaluated the effects of habit-reversal procedures alone (e.g., Christensen & Sanders, 1987) and in conjunction with other procedures (Long et al., 1999b; Rapp et al., 1999) to treat thumb sucking in children. In general, habit reversal involves (1) training the individual to detect each occurrence of the target behavior, (2) training the individual to engage in a physically incompatible competing response (e.g., putting hands in your pockets) contingent on the target behavior, and (3) enlisting social support from others to help the individual detect instances of the target behavior and to provide praise for engaging in a competing response. Although Christensen and Sanders (1987) showed that habit reversal substantially reduced thumb sucking for thirty children aged four to nine years, several studies have shown that habit reversal, alone, is ineffective for decreasing the habit behavior of children younger than seven years of age (Long et al., 1999b; Rapp et al., 1999) or individuals diagnosed with cognitive delays (e.g., Long et al., 1999a; Rapp et al., 1998).

Long et al. (1999b) found that habit reversal was ineffective for reducing the thumb sucking and hair pulling of a seven-year-old girl. Subsequently, Long and colleagues implemented differential reinforcement and response cost procedures. While observing the child through a one-way window as she was seated alone in a room watching videos, the therapist entered the room and placed M & Ms in a transparent cup contingent on the absence of thumb sucking at the end of graduated time intervals. When this procedure did not eliminate thumb sucking, the therapist entered the room and removed M & Ms from the cup contingent on instances of the behavior. The combined reinforcement and punishment procedures decreased thumb sucking. However, unlike previous studies (e.g., Friman & Hove, 1987), hair pulling decreased only slightly when thumb sucking was eliminated. Thereafter, the same procedures were implemented to eliminate hair pulling.

Rapp et al. (1999) used habit-reversal procedures to treat the thumb sucking of five-year-old twin brothers. A pretreatment functional analysis indicated that both children engaged in thumb sucking when adults were absent but not when adults were present. The effects of treatment were evaluated in the home of the two children as they watched television without their parents present. Following training, the thumb sucking of one child decreased while the thumb sucking of the other child persisted. Subsequently, remote contingencies were implemented whereby the mother was able to observe her sons' behavior when they were on the lower level of the home through a small monitor that was set up in the kitchen on the upper level. Any time thumb sucking was observed on the monitor, the mother called out for the child to stop sucking his thumb. In this way, the child learned that being alone no longer enabled him to avoid social consequences for thumb sucking. Thus, both children required consequences (i.e., punishment in the form of a verbal reprimand) for engaging in thumb sucking as well as prompts and consequences (i.e., reinforcement in the form of praise from parents) for the use of a competing response.

An important finding from Long et al. (1999b) and Rapp et al. (1999) is that social contingencies can be successful in eliminating thumb sucking even when the behavior occurs exclusively when the child is alone. The child is likely to engage in the behavior while alone due to a history of punishment (scolding, reprimands) for having engaged in the behavior in the presence of the parents. If the scolding or reprimands are now delivered for thumb sucking when the child is alone, the behavior will decrease in this context as well. The implication for successful treatment is that the parent must be able to detect thumb sucking when the child is alone in order to deliver an immediate consequence for the behavior.

Summary and Recommendations for Future Research

Thumb sucking is a common childhood problem that can cause a number of problems when it persists beyond the age of four or five. Intervention for thumb sucking begins with assessment of the behavior in the natural context and, subsequently, evaluation of treatment effectiveness within the same context. Prior to treatment, a functional assessment is conducted to identify or rule out any form of social reinforcement for the behavior. Although thumb sucking typically is maintained by automatic reinforcement (Ellingson et al., 2000; Rapp et al., 1999; Stricker et al., 2001; Stricker et al., 2002), appropriate assessment will help isolate the context(s) in which the behavior occurs with greatest probability. Treatment for thumb sucking generally involves (1) antecedent procedures such as response prevention or treatment of covarying behaviors; (2) consequences such as aversive taste treatment, contingent auditory stimulation, or social punishment in the form of reprimands; or (3) some combination of procedures.

The Ellingson et al. (2000) study illustrates a number of important points regarding the assessment and treatment of finger sucking. First, treatment should be designed to address the function of the behavior when possible. Second, treatment should be implemented in the appropriate context (i.e., when the child is alone). Third, not all children will be equally responsive to intervention; use of more-intrusive procedures should be reserved for those whose behavior persists when less-intrusive procedures are used. Finally, treatment should be acceptable to the child and parent.

There are a number of potential avenues for further research into the assessment and treatment of thumb sucking. Future research should continue to evaluate environmental events that set the occasion for thumb sucking. Given that studies have shown that thumb sucking may increase in the presence of certain objects (e.g., Friman, 1988; 2000; Watson et al., 2002), research on how other forms of stimulation affect thumb sucking is warranted (e.g., Rapp, 2004).

Another area for future research would be further evaluation of the AED. Research should focus on generalization and maintenance of treatment effects produced with the AED, as well as procedures for ensuring that the child continues to wear the device in the absence of parental supervision. In general, many punishment procedures have been understudied (Lerman & Vorndan, 2002), perhaps because punishment generally is viewed as unacceptable (Miltenberger, Lennox, & Erfanian, 1989). However, based on the handful of studies conducted to date, the AED represents an acceptable, mildly aversive, and effective intervention for thumb sucking. Therefore, more research is warranted.

Another avenue for further research on the treatment of thumb sucking is the evaluation of remote contingencies to influence the probability of thumb sucking when the child is alone and, similarly, how parents could implement remote contingencies in the natural environment. Relevant to this discussion is the possible influence of inhibitory stimulus control whereby the presence of a salient environmental stimulus that signals punishment for a specific behavior exerts suppressive control over the target behavior. For example, studies have shown that stimuli, which were present when automatically reinforced problem behavior was punished, can produce at least short-term behavior suppression when punishment is not available (e.g., Piazza, Hanley, & Fisher, 1996; Rapp et al., 1998; Rollings & Baumeister, 1981). Considering these findings, it is possible that providing reinforcement for alternative behavior in the presence of stimuli that inhibit thumb sucking may produce longer-term maintenance of treatment effects. As an example of this approach, a parent could provide praise to a child for keeping his hands in his pockets (a competing response) when he is wearing the "inactive" AED (or another stimulus that is discriminative for punishment).

Future research should also examine the effects of providing potential sources of competing stimulation, frequently referred to as "environmental enrichment," when using response prevention and mild punishment. Although the suppressive effects of environmental enrichment on automatically reinforced problem behavior displayed by individuals with disabilities are supported in the literature (e.g., Goh et al., 1995; Piazza et al., 1998), this intervention, alone or in combination with other procedures, has not been formally evaluated to treat thumb sucking of typically functioning children.

References

Afzelius-Alm, Larsson, E., Lofgren, C. G., & Bishara, S. E. (2004). Factors that influence the proclination and retroclination of the lower incisors in children. *Swedish Dental Journal, 28,* 37–45.

Ahlgren, J. (1995). EMG studies of lip and cheek activity in sucking habits. *Swedish Dental Journal, 19,* 95–101.

Christensen, A. P., & Sanders, M. R. (1987). Habit reversal and differential reinforcement of other behavior in the treatment of thumb-sucking: An analysis of generalization and side-effects. *Journal for Child Psychology and Psychiatry, 28,* 281–95.

Cowie, C., Black, D., & Fraser, I. (1997). Blood levels in preschool children in eastern Sydney. *Australian and New Zealand Journal of Public Health, 21,* 755–61.

Ellingson, S. A., Miltenberger, R. G., Stricker, J., Garlinghouse, M., Roberts, J., Galensky, T. L., & Rapp, J. T. (2000). Functional analysis and treatment of finger sucking. *Journal of Applied Behavior Analysis, 33,* 41–52.

Friman, P. C. (1988). Eliminating chronic thumb sucking by preventing a covarying response. *Journal of Behavior Therapy and Experimental Psychiatry, 19,* 301–4.

———. (1990). Concurrent habits: what would Linus do with his blanket if thumb-sucking were treated? *American Journal of Diseases of Children, 144,* 1316–18.

———. (2000). "Transitional objects" as establishing operations for thumb sucking: a case study. *Journal of Applied Behavior Analysis, 33,* 507–9.

Friman, P. C., & Hove, G. (1987). Apparent covariation between child habit disorders: effects of successful treatment for thumb sucking in untargeted chronic hair pulling. *Journal of Applied Behavior Analysis, 20*, 421–25.

Friman, P. C., & Leibowitz, J. M. (1990). An effective and acceptable treatment alternative for chronic thumb- and finger-sucking. *Journal of Pediatric Psychology, 15*, 57–65.

Friman, P. C., Barone, V. J., & Christophersen, E. R. (1986). Aversive taste treatment of finger and thumb sucking. *Pediatrics, 78*, 174–76.

Friman, P. C., Boyd, M. R., & Oksol, E. R. (2001). Characteristics of oral-digital habits. In D. Woods & R. Miltenberger (eds.), *Tic disorders, trichotillomania and other repetitive behavior disorders: behavioral approaches to analysis and treatment* (pp. 197–222). Boston, MA: Kluwer.

Friman, P. C., Larzelere, H., & Finney, J. W. (1994). Exploring the relationship between thumb-sucking and psychopathology. *Journal of Pediatric Psychology, 19*, 431–41.

Friman, P. C., McPherson, K. M., Warzak, W. J., & Evans, J. (1993). Influence of thumb sucking on peer social acceptance in first-grade children. *Pediatrics, 91*, 784–86.

Gawlik, J. A., Ott, N. W., & Mathieu, G. P. (1995). Modification of the palatal crib habit-breaker appliance to prevent palatal soft tissue embedment. *Journal of Dentistry for Children, 62*, 409–11.

Goh, H., Iwata, B. A., Shore, B. A., DeLeon, I. G., Lerman, D. C., Ulrich, S. M., & Smith, R. G. (1995). An analysis of the reinforcing properties of hand mouthing. *Journal of Applied Behavior Analysis, 28*, 269–83.

Greenleaf, S., & Mink, J. (2003). A retrospective study of the use of the Bluegrass appliance in the cessation of thumb habits. *Pediatric Dentistry, 25*, 587–90.

Gutermuth-Foster, L. (1998). Nervous habits and stereotyped behaviors in preschool children. *Journal of the American Academy of Child and Adolescent Psychiatry, 37*, 711–17.

Haskell, B. S., & Mink, J .R. (1991). An aid to stop thumb sucking: the "Bluegrass" appliance. *Pediatric Dentistry, 13*, 83–85.

Kharbanda, O. P., Sidhu, S. S., Sundaram, K., & Shukla, D. K. (2003). Oral habits in school going children of Delhi: a prevalence study. *Journal of the Indian Society of Pedodonics and Preventive Dentistry, 21*, 120–24.

Lassen, M. K., & Fluent, N. R. (1978). Elimination of nocturnal thumbsucking by glove wearing. *Journal of Behavior Therapy and Experimental Psychiatry, 9*, 85.

Lennox, D., & Miltenberger, R. (1989). Conducting a functional assessment of problem behavior in applied settings. *Journal of the Association for Persons with Severe Handicaps, 14*, 304–11.

Lerman, D. C., & Vorndan, C. M. (2002). On the status of knowledge for using punishment: implications for treating behavior disorders. *Journal of Applied Behavior Analysis, 35*, 431–64.

Lewis, M., Shilton, P., & Fuqua, R. W. (1981). Parental control of nocturnal thumbsucking. *Journal of Behavior Therapy and Experimental Psychiatry, 12*, 87–90.

Long, E. S., Miltenberger, R. G., & Rapp, J. T. (1999b). Simplified habit reversal plus adjunct contingencies in the treatment of thumb sucking and hairpulling in a young child. *Child and Family Behavior Therapy, 21*, 45–58.

Long, E. S., Miltenberger, R. G., Ellingson, S. A., & Ott, S. M. (1999a). Augmenting simplified habit reversal in the treatment of oral-digital habits exhibited by individuals with mental retardation. *Journal of Applied Behavior Analysis, 32*, 353–65.

Mahalski, P. A. (1983). The incidence of attachment objects and oral habits at bedtime in two longitudinal samples of children. *Journal of Child Psychology and Psychiatry, 24*, 283–95.

Malek, R., Oger, P., & Rivet-Forsans, C. (1994). Deformities of the fingers secondary to fingersucking. *Annals of Hand and Upper Limb Surgery, 13*, 269–73.

Miltenberger, R., Lennox, D., & Erfanian, N. (1989). Acceptability of alternative treatments for persons with mental retardation: ratings from institutional and community-based staff. *American Journal on Mental Retardation, 93,* 388–95.

O'Neill, R. E., Horner, R. H., Albin, R. W., Sprague, J. R., Storey, K., & Newton, J. S. (1997). Functional assessment and program development for problem behavior: a practical handbook. Pacific Grove, CA: Brooks/Cole.

Piazza, C. C., Fisher, W. W., Hanley, G. P., LeBlanc, L. A., Worsdell, A. S., Lindauer, S. E., & Keeney, K. M. (1998). Treatment of pica through multiple analyses of its reinforcing functions. *Journal of Applied Behavior Analysis, 31,* 165–89.

Piazza, C. C., Hanley, G. P., & Fisher, W. W. (1996). Functional analysis and treatment of cigarette pica. *Journal of Applied Behavior Analysis, 29,* 437–49.

Rankin, E. A., Jabaley, M. E., Blair, S. J., & Fraser, K. E. (1988). Acquired rotational digital deformity in children as a result of finger sucking. *The Journal of Hand Surgery, 13,* 535–39.

Rapp, J. T. (2004). Effects of prior access and environmental enrichment on stereotypy. *Behavioral Interventions, 19,* 287–95.

Rapp, J. T., Miltenberger, R. G., & Long, E. S. (1998). Augmenting simplified habit reversal with an awareness enhancement device. *Journal of Applied Behavior Analysis, 31,* 665–68.

Rapp, J. T., Miltenberger, R. G., Galensky, T. L., Ellingson, S., & Roberts, J. (1999). Functional analysis and treatment of thumb sucking in fraternal twin brothers. *Child and Family Behavior Therapy, 21,* 1–17.

Rapp, J. T., Vollmer, T. R., Dozier, C. L., St. Peter, C., & Cotnoir, N. (2004). Analysis of response reallocation in individuals with multiple forms of stereotyped behavior. *Journal of Applied Behavior Analysis, 37,* 481–501.

Reid, D. A., & Price, A. H. (1984). Digital deformities and dental malocclusion due to finger sucking. *British Journal of Plastic Surgery, 37,* 445–52.

Rolider, A., & Van Houten, R. (1988). The use of response prevention to eliminate daytime thumbsucking. *Child & Family Behavior Therapy, 10,* 135–42.

Rollings, J. P., & Baumeister, A. A. (1981). Stimulus control of stereotypic responding: Effects on target and collateral behavior. *American Journal of Mental Deficiency, 86,* 67–77.

Sari, S., & Sonmez, H. (2002). Investigation of the relationship between oral parafunctions and temporomandibular joint dysfunction in Turkish children with mixed and permanent dentition. *Journal of Oral Rehabilitation, 29,* 108–12.

Stricker, J., Miltenberger, R., Anderson, C., Tulloch, H., & Deaver, C. (2002). A functional analysis of digit sucking in children. *Behavior Modification, 26,* 424–43.

Stricker, J. M., Miltenberger, R. G., Garlinghouse, M., & Tulloch, H. E. (2003). Augmenting stimulus intensity with an awareness enhancement device in the treatment of finger sucking. *Education and Treatment of Children, 26,* 22–29.

Stricker, J. M., Miltenberger, R. G., Garlinghouse, M. A., Deaver, C. M., & Anderson, C. A. (2001). Evaluation of an awareness enhancement device for the treatment of thumb sucking in children. *Journal of Applied Behavior Analysis, 34,* 77–80.

Taylor, M. B., & Walker, R. A. (1997). A minimally obtrusive, secure mask for prevention of access to the mouth. *Clinical Rehabilitation, 11,* 77–79.

Troster, H. (1994). Prevalence and functions of stereotyped behaviors in nonhandicapped children in residential care. *Journal of Abnormal Child Psychology, 22,* 79–97.

Tryon, A. F. (1968). Thumb-sucking and manifest anxiety. *Child Development, 39,* 1159–63.

Viazis, A. D. (1991). The triple-loop corrector (TLC): a new thumb sucking habit control appliance. *American Journal of Orthodontics and Dentofacial Orthopedics, 100,* 91–92.

Vignarajah, S., & Williams, G. A. (1992). Prevalence of dental caries and enamel defects in the primary dentition of Antiguan pre-school children aged 3–4 years including as assessment of their habits. *Community Dental Health, 9,* 349–60.

Watson, T. S., & Allen, K. D. (1993). Elimination of thumb-sucking as a treatment for severe trichotillomania. *Journal of the American Academy of Child and Adolescent Psychiatry, 32,* 830–33.

Watson, T. S., Dittmer, K. I., & Ray, K. P. (2000). Treating trichotillomania in a toddler: Variations on effective treatments. *Child & Family Behavior Therapy, 22,* 29–40.

Watson, T. S., Meeks, C., Dufrene, B., & Lindsay, C. (2002). Sibling thumb sucking: effects of treatment for targeted and untargeted siblings. *Behavior Modification, 26,* 412–13.

Widmalm, S. E., Christiansen, R. L., & Gunn, S. M. (1995). Oral parafunctions as temporomandibular disorder risk factors in children. *The Journal of Craniomandibular Practice, 13,* 242–46.

Management of Children's Disruptive Behavior During Dental Treatment

Keith D. Allen

The skills required to manage disruptive child behavior during dental treatment are as fundamental to successful treatment as are handpiece skills and knowledge of dental materials. These skills are important because the ability to manage disruptive behavior has direct implications for the quality of dental care. In addition, disruptive child behavior increases delivery time and the risk of injury to the child. Not surprisingly, behavior management with children is a topic of considerable interest for dentists.

Fortunately, there have been significant advances in dental technology, materials, and training that have made the dental experience for children more pleasing and enjoyable. Nevertheless, dentists must still be able to perform precise procedures on children who can sometimes be disruptive (Sheller, 2004). Indeed, distress and disruptions continue to be prevalent and problematic within the child population (Bo, 2004). Although most children seen in clinical practice are good, recent estimates suggest that 20–25% of all children exhibit disruptive problems at the dentist (Raadal et al., 1995; Brill, 2000). In addition, these problems are strongly correlated with age, where younger, preschool-aged children are more challenging than school-aged children (Allen, Hutfless, & Larzalere, 2003). Furthermore, these problems are compounded when invasive procedures are required. For example, data from private practice suggest that the younger the child and the more threatening or invasive the procedure, the more often negative, disruptive behavior is observed (Brill, 2000). Unfortunately, preschool children can be so difficult to manage that many general practitioners are not willing to provide care for them when anything more than an examination or prophylaxis is required (Cotton et al., 2001). This is of particular concern given the recent interest in increasing preschool children's access to dental care (Edelstein, 2000; Grembowski, & Milgrom, 2000; Waldman & Perlman, 1999).

Why Children Are Disruptive

Changing child behavior during dental treatment requires understanding why children might be disruptive and noncompliant during dental treatment and also understanding how to help children learn more cooperative, new behaviors. Many variables have been considered by dentists in trying to understand why children are disruptive. For example, dentists have been increasingly concerned that permissive parenting styles have adversely influenced child behavior in the dental clinic (Casamassimo, Wilson, & Gross, 2002). Previous investigations have also explored general maternal anxiety, maternal dental anxiety, child anxiety, and child temperament as predictors of child disruptive behavior during to treatment (Radis et al., 1994; Quninonez et al., 1997; Johnson & Baldwin, 1969). However, none of these investigations have identified reliable predictors of disruptive behavior in the dental clinic.

Empirical studies have been unable to identify a clear link between parent or child characteristics and disruptive behavior in the clinic. Even when investigators have sought to establish a more direct link between disruptive behavior in the dental clinic with disruptive behavior outside the clinic, none has been found (Dunegan et al., 1994). Finally, Allen et al. (2003) actually looked at parenting style in an effort to predict disruptive behavior in the clinic. They found that the only reliable, good predictor of disruptive behavior was age of the child. Younger children were more disruptive no matter what parenting practices were used. Older children were better, no matter what parenting practices were used. More important, no single parenting style was a predictor.

Although years of speculation have continued to suggest that factors outside the clinic are critically important, years of empirical research have indicated that outside influences do not seem to have reliably strong influences on disruptive behavior in the clinic. This should not suggest that outside or past influences have no impact at all, only that the impact is unpredictable. Perhaps more important is the fact that dentists have almost no control over these purported past or outside influences. One must question whether it is useful to continue to focus efforts on attempts to identify predictors over which dentists have little influence. Furthermore, there is every reason to believe that the variables that have the most direct and significant influence on disruptive behavior lie directly within the dental operatory and are variables over which dentists do have some control.

Consider, for a moment, the experience of a young child undergoing restorative dental work. The child must lie on his back, open his mouth, and have someone wearing a mask and gloves insert sometimes multiple instruments that make unusual noises, create unfamiliar sensations, and sometimes inflict discomfort or pain. Fear would be an expected reaction, especially in young children (two to five years of age) where fear of strangers and strange situations; fear about separation from their caregiver; and fear about noises, masks, and novel stimuli are common experiences (Barrios & O'Dell, 1998). But even in older children, there may be anxiety about a potentially unpleasant situation as children tend to overpredict the discomfort they will experience during treatment (Carlsen et al., 1993). That is, merely the antici- pation of discomfort can evoke anxiety or fear. Furthermore, whether one appeals to anxiety, fear, pain, or a combination of all three, the fact that some children might be interested in escaping the dental treatment environment is not surprising. Of course, there are some children who are neither fearful or anxious, but are merely oppositional because they find it unpleasant to be re- quired to do something they wish not to do.

Although these distinctions are very difficult to make in a brief dental visit (Harper & D'Alessandro, 2004), the distinction may not be critical to success, since the child's motivation remains the same: to escape an unpleas- ant (perceived or real) situation. For most children, efforts to escape involve verbal distress such as crying, moaning, or complaining, and/or behavioral distress such as flinching, blocking, thrashing, or turning away. Neverthe- less, it is the real or even perceived unpleasantness of the situation that gen- erates the motivation to escape, and it is the motivation to escape that gen- erates disruptive behavior. It is not surprising then that there is a strong correlation between threatening invasive procedures and negative, disrup- tive behavior (Brill, 2000) and that these problems are more prevalent in younger children.

Of course, not all children view the dental experience as unpleasant. Still others may view the experience as unpleasant, but have learned to accept some unpleasantness in life without attempts to escape. Nevertheless, those who are disruptive are, in effect, communicating via their behavior that they find the experience unpleasant and that they would rather be elsewhere. The task of the dentist interested in behavior management then ultimately be- comes one of reducing the unpleasantness of the dental experience. Indeed, were the dental experience devoid of unpleasantness (whether from fear, anxiety, discomfort, or demands), the incidence of disruptive behavior would be virtually nil. The goal then becomes one of either reducing the un- pleasantness or increasing the pleasantness of the treatment environment. The following approaches represent both time-honored and innovative methods of reducing the unpleasantness of the dental experience.

Positive Approaches to Behavior Management

Inherent in any behavior management approach is the requirement of time. Regardless of the approach, dentists who wish to learn and implement strategies designed to increase the pleasantness of the dental experience for a child must take time. Unfortunately, dentists are not reimbursed for time spent engaged in behavior management, nor are they reimbursed for learn- ing those skills (Sheller, 2004). In addition, recent research suggests that den- tal schools do not plan to devote any more curricular time to behavior man- agement (Adair, Schafer et al., 2004), so procedures must be easy to teach and learn. Although some leaders in the field have challenged dentists who would be unwilling to spend "a few minutes shaping the behavior" of a disruptive child just because that time is not reimbursable (Sheller, 2004), it is clear that interventions must be cost-effective. That is, dentists are most likely to use procedures that produce the most amount of benefit (i.e., improved behavior) with the least amount of time and effort (i.e., time and effort not associated with actual restorative dentistry).

More recently, dentists have also had to consider the risks associated with behavior management as part of the benefit analysis. Changing standards with respect to what constitutes "reasonable care" means dentists must be increasingly cautious about using behavior management procedures that parents might find objectionable. Thus, while the AAPD does endorse procedures such as "hand-over-mouth" and general anesthesia in some cases where other less-invasive strategies have failed (AAPD, 2003), these procedures come with increased legal risk (e.g., Bross, 2004). So, for example, most advanced programs do not now teach the hand-over-mouth procedure, viewing it as an unacceptable behavior management technique (Adair, Rockman et al., 2004), and by far most pediatric dentists do not employ the technique at all (Adair, Waller et al., 2004). As a result, the focus in this chapter will center on techniques that appear reasonably benign, have some empirical support, and appear to be cost-effective.

Reduction of Discomfort

Certainly one way to reduce management difficulties in children is to explore strategies for reducing the pain and discomfort associated with invasive restorative dental procedures themselves. For example, numerous studies have been conducted in an effort to achieve a painless injection (e.g., Houpt et al., 1997), including the use of topical anesthesia and prolonged injection time (e.g., Maragakis & Musselman, 1996; Mathews, et al., 1997). Prolonged injection time has been pursued as a means of reducing the pain associated with an injection, because it is understood that pain is created, at least in part, by the volume pressure changes exerted by the injected solution on small nerve fibers (e.g., Travell, 1955). Slowing the rate of administration may be one means of controlling the volume pressure. However, it can be technically difficult to achieve when done manually (e.g., Chan, 2001).

Recently, several controlled investigations by Allen and colleagues with school-aged children have been conducted exploring the efficacy of a computerized local anesthetic delivery system, designed to reduce the pain of the injection by delivering anesthetic at a constant rate, pressure, and volume. Three controlled investigations demonstrated that, when used properly, a computerized system for slowing the rate of anesthesia administration and thereby controlling the volume pressure did result in children who were significantly less disruptive and who required less restraint to manage when compared with a traditional manual injection method (Asarch et al., 1999; Gibson et al., 2000; Allen et al., 2002). However, the computerized system took four times longer to administer an injection, and preschool-aged children became restless with the lengthy injection duration. Some dentists may become restless too. Nevertheless, even though restless, the younger children were still significantly less disruptive. Although the computerized system clearly requires an investment in time at the beginning of the session, it may be well worth the time for some dentists given the reduction of child disruptive behavior.

Parent Presence in Operatory

Dentists have long questioned whether having a parent present in the operatory is a reasonable approach to behavior management. Over forty years ago, Frankl put the question to the test. In a nicely controlled scientific investigation, Frankl and colleagues demonstrated that preschool-aged children (3–6) were less distressed and disruptive when their parent remained in the operatory as a passive observer (Frankl, Shiere, & Fogels, 1962). Not surprisingly, this effect was strongest for the youngest children. Separating young children from their parents may introduce separation anxiety and thereby increase the unpleasantness of the visit. Subsequent studies of parental presence during dental procedures have repeatedly shown that parental presence has either no impact or a positive impact (e.g., Venham et al., 1978; Pfefferle et al., 1982) on child behavior. Yet, surveys have demonstrated that many dentists are concerned that parental presence will disrupt the child (e.g., Marcum, Turner, & Courts, 1995). This concern is not entirely unfounded. Research has demonstrated that parents can negatively impact child behavior during injections if the parent frequently draws attention to and offers reassurance about the procedures. However, parents can actually be a help if they are instructed to talk with their child about nonprocedure-related topics (Gonzalez, Routh, & Armstrong, 1993). This might include talking about plans for an upcoming vacation, describing a recent experience with a pet or friend, or discussing favorite toys or activities. Results from these types of studies have led to recommendations that dentists simply need to be sure to tell parents exactly what is expected of them (Harper & D'Alessandro, 2004).

Research to date suggests that parents be instructed to either remain silent or to talk about things unrelated to the ongoing procedures. These recommendations are important because significant numbers of parents want to be with their children, especially young children (e.g., Kamp, 1992; Peretz & Zadik, 1998).

Of course, dentists are concerned not only with the impact of the parent on the child, but also with the impact of the parent on the dentist. A parent in the operatory can create distractions and discomfort for the dentist (Marcum, Turner, & Courts, 1995), who may feel more relaxed and comfortable when parents remain in the waiting room. Because dentists who are more relaxed and comfortable are more likely to perform better, many dentists allow parents in the operatory for the initial visits with a young, preschool-aged child, but subsequently ask that parents remain in the waiting room. This would appear to be a reasonable approach.

Effective Communication

The manner in which a dentist communicates with a child can certainly impact the pleasantness of the dental environment. This requires recognizing that children understand best when language is kept simple and concrete. This has commonly led to recommendations that dentists replace dental terminology with more easily understood words such as "raincoat" for rubber dam, "vacuum cleaner" for suction, and "tooth paint" for sealant (Wright, 2000). Perhaps more important is to recognize that children learn best through experience. That is, children are active learners who learn best through direct interaction with the world. Indeed, the most effective educational programs for young children are ones that communicate concepts and ideas through experience (e.g., Weikart, 2002).

Not surprisingly then, dentists have also traditionally valued communication that incorporates direct interaction and experience. Originally called Tell-Show-Do (Addelston, 1959), this experiential technique involves describing for children, in simple terms, what is about to occur (Tell) and then allowing them to see, feel, explore, and manipulate the tools or instruments (Show), before beginning any procedure (Do). This might involve allowing the child to operate the chair, to squirt the water syringe, to feel the high speed on the back of their hand, or to use the suction to clean up a puddle of water. Although neither of these approaches (i.e., simplifying language, Tell-Show-Do) has been empirically evaluated, each could reasonably be expected to increase the pleasantness of dental experience and both are sensitive to children's developmental communication needs.

In contrast, using the delivery of commands in a loud rather than a normal voice has been tested as a strategy for enhancing communication with children. Dentists who, during operative procedures, delivered commands in a sudden, loud, firm voice (e.g., Stop! Put your hands down.), reduced disruptive behavior more effectively than commands that were delivered in a normal voice (Greenbaum et al., 1990). This "voice control" technique has been described in textbooks for decades. However, caution should be exercised when considering use of this approach to communication. It is not a technique that achieves benefits by making the dental environment more pleasant. Using voice control produces less-disruptive behavior in children, not because the environment has been made more pleasant, but because the environment has, in fact, been made more aversive. Unfortunately, it is the interaction with the dentists that is aversive and children are then motivated to escape or avoid the unpleasant interaction with the dentist. This may lead to improved behavior, but it may come at a cost to the dentist-patient relationship. In fact, voice control could be described as a punishment technique, and it may have "dysfunctional" side effects as a result (Greenbaum et al., 1990). Voice control does have a place in the behavior-management armamentarium of the dentist, but always after more positive, benign approaches have been implemented and failed.

Distraction

A common approach to making the dental environment more pleasant is to distract the child with activities such as watching television, playing video games, or listening to music. This approach probably serves two functions. First, by engaging a child's attention toward alternative activities, the child may be less likely to focus on dental procedures and what she perceives as discomfort she might experience. Second, these alternative activities are typically pleasant or even preferred activities, creating an environment that the child is less likely to wish to escape. Overall, scientific studies looking at the use of distraction procedures in the dental operatory have yielded mixed results (Coombs, 1980; Corah, Gale, & Illig, 1979; Sokol, Sokol, & Sokol, 1985; Venham et al., 1981; Havener et al., 2000). In large part, the differences seem to be related to whether the distractions are active or passive. That is, distracting activities that are passive (e.g., watching TV, having a pet nearby) may not be as effective (i.e., distracting) as those that are more active (e.g., playing a video game). Active distractions may hold the attention of a child better. However, active distractors may also disrupt or interfere with ongoing dental procedures. As a result, several attempts have been made to enhance the distracting potential of more passive activities.

One way to make a passive distraction activity more active is to require that the child must do something to be able to watch or listen to the distractor. For example, Ingersoll and her colleagues found that children's disruptive behavior could be reduced by making access to a distractor dependent upon cooperative behavior, as opposed to providing the child with unlimited access. Children were informed that they could listen to an audiotape or watch TV, but only as long as they remained cooperative. Each time the child became disruptive or uncooperative, the dentist immediately terminated the audio or video presentation and did not reinstate it until the child exhibited cooperative behavior. When dentists used this approach, the children were significantly better than when they had unlimited access. However, this approach required the dentist to control access to the distractors during the dental procedures, which could potentially disrupt or distract the dentist.

Filcheck et al. (2004) used choice as a means of making passive distractions more active. They allowed children, prior to starting treatment, to peruse a large number of CDs and to select two or three CDs containing music and/or stories that they liked. The children wore headphones and then could change music tracks and even change CDs during the appointment with a handheld remote. This allowed the child to remain actively engaged while the dentist worked uninterrupted. In this case, children who had choice-based distraction were less likely to be disruptive and were twice as likely to be considered very cooperative by the dentist (Filcheck et al., in press).

In conclusion, the evidence suggests that providing children with distractors can be effective. Not all distractors, however, are equally effective. Passive distractors that require nothing from the child appear to provide little benefit. More active distractors that require some participation from the child appear to offer significantly more benefit. This might be as simple as allowing children to change the channel on a TV with a remote during treatment. This type of approach is relatively inexpensive and quite easily implemented with little or no disruption of the operative procedures. This makes active distraction one of the most cost-effective options available for improving the pleasantness of the environment and reducing disruptive behavior.

Reinforcement of Good Behavior

It is now widely recognized that children who receive positive feedback about their behavior are more likely to repeat those behaviors again. Feedback can take the form of praise, attention, touch, rewards, treats, or even privileges, and those who regularly work with children often use these strategies to encourage and reinforce children for appropriate behavior. Although some experts have challenged the use of reinforcement, arguing that it may rob children of their intrinsic motivation and teach them to expect rewards for behavior they should be doing anyway, there is little empirical support for this concern. Perhaps more important, reinforcement has been shown to be important for teaching new and desired appropriate behaviors.

Whether it is a parent, teacher, coach, or dentist, the most easily accessed and delivered form of reinforcement is praise. Praise is most effective when it describes very specific behaviors (e.g., "I like how you are sitting so still with your hands in your lap"; "It is such a big help to me when you hold your mouth open like that!"). Using specific praise has been found to be an effective means of promoting good behavior in a wide variety of settings and with a wide variety of providers, including dentists. Specifically, children who receive immediate and specific reinforcement from dentists most consistently show reductions in fear-related disruptive behavior (Weinstein et al., 1982a). Likewise, even physical touch can be an important source of reinforcement and has been found to help reduce fidgeting and disruptive movements and result in children who find the dental visits more pleasant (Greenbaum et al., 1993).

Unfortunately, some children do not offer much good behavior for the dentist to praise or acknowledge. In these cases, finding even small approximations of good behavior to praise and reward is important both for shaping new behaviors and for making the environment positive. Although it is easy to slip into negative reprimands and threats in response to disruptive behavior (Weinstein et al., 1982b), these risk increasing the unpleasantness in the dental operatory and escalating the likelihood that the child will try to escape. Although reprimands and negative verbal feedback cannot always be avoided, investigations of child behavior in other settings such as classroom and clinics suggest that children who experience four positive, reinforcing interactions for every one negative interaction exhibit more cooperative and less disruptive behavior.

Scheduled Breaks

Dentists have long recognized that giving children a sense of control is an important strategy in helping them cope with dental procedures. For example, to allow a child to raise a finger or hand and stop treatment when he experiences discomfort is one way that dentists can give children a sense of control and improve the pleasantness of the dental experience. However, hand raising is not the only behavior that a child might use to gain a sense of control. Disruptive behavior can also give children a sense of control because it too can result in the dentist stopping the dental procedures. This is important to recognize because escape from unpleasant or undesirable situations is one of the most common and powerful sources of motivation for children, and it plays a major role in a wide variety of problem behaviors including tantrums and other disruptive behavior. Efforts to escape unpleasantness (i.e., thrashing, blocking with hands, turning head, crying) are natural responses that are, in fact, much more likely to occur than raising ones hand. Unfortunately, the dentists' natural tendency to stop treatment in response to disruptive behavior, in many cases, may serve to encourage that behavior because of the control it offers.

One recently developed management procedure takes advantage of the powerful motivation that comes with escape. The approach uses escape to teach more cooperative behavior (Allen & Stokes, 1987; Allen et al., 1988; Allen & Stokes, 1989; Allen et al., 1992). It is an adaptation of existing management techniques (e.g., raising the hand) that allows the child some control over the dental routine. In this procedure, brief periods of escape from ongoing dental treatment are provided contingent upon cooperative behavior. Instead of raising a hand, the child can receive brief escape (5–10 seconds) from dental treatment by lying very still and quiet. Any disruptive behavior by the child delays escape until cooperation is regained. Research with very disruptive children has demonstrated that this approach was able to dramatically improve child behavior in a relatively short amount of time. Interestingly, children as young as three years old, considered by some dentists to be "precooperative," were nevertheless able to learn very cooperative behaviors. Observations suggest that early in treatment, when very young children are provided with brief opportunities to escape, it prevents gradually escalating disruptive behavior later on.

This "contingent escape" approach is based on well-established learning principles and is designed not only to diminish undesirable behaviors, but also to increase desirable behaviors. The contingent escape approach provides immediately feedback to children to teach them which "in-chair" behaviors are most likely to lead to breaks from treatment. Children learn how to control the situation by being cooperative, still, and quiet, rather than disruptive and uncooperative, which results in no escape. Of course, this approach raises immediate concerns about cost-effectiveness. Requiring a dentist to frequently stop treatment means delaying the completion of treatment. However, these studies have shown that offering children brief escape takes no more time away from restorative procedures than does the time and effort devoted to dealing with the disruptive behavior when the breaks are not used. Of more concern, however, is the demand the procedure places, not on the dentist's time, but on his or her concentration and attention. The approach requires the dentist to continuously notice cooperative behavior. This is not easily achieved. As with most adults, noticing and responding to problem behavior comes much easier than noticing and responding to appropriate behavior.

In an effort to reduce the demand on the dentist, Allen and colleagues modified the procedure to eliminate the requirement that the dentist monitor child behavior. Instead, they arranged for the brief breaks to be delivered based on time rather than based on child behavior. The pleasantness of the dental environment is enhanced by simply making frequent brief breaks a regular part of the procedure, independent of how the child behaves. In this way, the dentist is freed from the need to monitor child behavior. In this approach, the dentist wears an electronic prompter (MotiVator, Behavioral Dynamics, Inc.) that signals when a break is due. This approach has proven as effective as the contingent procedure in reducing disruptive behavior, again with very young children (O'Callaghan et al., 2005).

Conclusions and Recommendations

Good behavior management starts with recognizing that the key to success resides in the creation of a pleasant experience for the child. Although outside influences such as parenting and previous experiences may have some impact on some children, the most potent sources of influence lie directly within the dental operatory and are under the control of the dentist. Although much has been done and continues to be done to reduce the pain and discomfort associated with restorative dentistry, the dental operatory can still be experienced as unpleasant. Children's perceptions of unpleasantness are important sources of distress and must be acknowledged and addressed. Years of research and experience suggest that, to create a maximally pleasant experience for children and reduce the likelihood of disruptive behavior, the following approaches make sense:

- Use topical anesthetics and slow injection rates to reduce procedural discomfort.
- Allow parents of young children to accompany them in the operatory and ask them to remain silent or limit their discussions to nonprocedure-related topics.
- Offer pleasing distractions. The operatory itself should be equipped with either a TV/DVD combination unit or stereo unit for which children can select, in advance, DVDs or CDs of their choice. Children would be able to scan the DVDs or CDs throughout the visit, providing them with some control and choice. Headphones would be available to wear for either the TV or stereo to help attenuate operatory sounds and enhance listening ability.
- Communication should be kept relatively simple and positive, focusing praise on observed cooperative behavior. Efforts should be made to give three to four times more positive comments to each child than negative, directive, or controlling comments. Threats or promises about either negative or positive consequences to come at the end of the visit should be kept to a minimum, recognizing that, in this type of situation, children live for the moment not the future.
- Brief breaks should be offered frequently, regardless of how the child behaves, although additional breaks based on cooperative behavior can be effective too.

The emphasis here on nonpharmacological methods derives, in large part, from recent calls for greater promotion of these methods (Ng, 2004). Changing attitudes about the acceptability of some traditional management techniques have made the search for effective alternatives more salient and the need to establish training competencies more urgent. Fortunately, there do exist an assemblage of reasonable techniques that offer benign, low-risk, empirically supported approaches. Each of these approaches appears relatively easy to implement with minimal training or cost in terms of dollars or time. Perhaps more important, however, is that each has the potential of making the dental experience more pleasant for both the child and dentist alike.

Acknowledgments

Supported in part by Project #8188 from the Maternal and Child Bureau (Title V, Social Security Act), Health Resources and Services Administration, Department of Health and Human Services and by grant 90DD0533 from the Administration on Developmental Disabilities (ADD), Administration for Children and Families, Department of Health and Human Services.

References

Adair, S., Rockman, R., Schafer, T., & Waller, J. (2004). Survey of behavior management teaching in pediatric dentistry advanced education programs. *Pediatric Dentistry, 26(2)*, 151–58.

Adair, S., Schafer, T., Rockman, R., & Waller, J. (2004). Survey of behavior management teaching in predoctoral pediatric dentistry programs. *Pediatric Dentistry, 26(2)*, 143–50.

Adair, S., Waller, J., Schafer, T., & Rockman, R. (2004). A survey of members of the American Academy of Pediatric Dentistry on their use of behavior management techniques. *Pediatric Dentistry, 26(2)*, 159–66.

Addelston, H. (1959). Child patient training. *CDS Review, 38* (7), 27–29.

Allen, K. D., & Stokes, T. F. (1987). The use of escape and reward in the management of young children during dental treatment. *Journal of Applied Behavior Analysis, 20(4)*, 381–90.

——. (1989). Pediatric Behavioral Dentistry. In M. Hersen, R. Eisler, & P. Miller (eds.), *Progress in Behavior Modification*. Newbury Park, CA: Sage Publications, Inc.

Allen, K. D., Hutfless, S., & Larzelere, R. (2003). Evaluation of two predictors of child disruptive behavior during restorative dental treatment. *Journal of Dentistry for Children, 70(3)*, 1–5.

Allen, K. D., Kotil, D., Larzelere, B., Hutfless, S., & Beiraghi, S. (2002). Comparison of computerized anesthesia delivery with traditional syringe in preschool children. *Pediatric Dentistry, 24*, 315–20.

Allen, K. D., Loiben, T., Allen, S., & Stanley, R. (1992). Dentist-implemented contingent escape for the management of disruptive child behavior. *Journal of Applied Behavior Analysis, 25*, 629–36.

Allen, K. D., Stark, L. J., Rigney, B. A., Nash, D., & Stokes, T. F. (1988). Reinforced practice of children's cooperative behavior during restorative dental treatment. *Journal of Dentistry for Children, 55(4)*, 273–77.

American Academy of Pediatric Dentistry. (2003). Clinical guideline on behavior management. *Reference Manual 2003–2004. Pediatric Dentistry* http://www.aapd.org/members/referencemanual/pdfs/02-03/G_BehavMgmt.pdf

Asarch, T., Allen, K. D., Petersen, B. S., & Beiraghi, S. (1999). Efficacy of a computerized local anesthesia device in pediatric dentistry. *Pediatric Dentistry, 21(7)*, 421–24.

Barrios, B., & O'Dell, S. (1998). Fears and anxieties (pp. 249–337). In E. Mash & R. Barkley (eds), *Treatment of Childhood Disorders*. 2d ed. New York: Guilford Press.

Bo, C. (2004). Applying the social learning theory to children with dental anxiety. *Journal of Contemporary Dental Practice, 5(1)*, 1–8.

Brill, W. A. (2000). Child behavior in a private pediatric dental practice associated with types of visits, age, and socio-economic factors. *Journal of Clinical Pediatric Dentistry, 25(1)*, 1–7.

Bross, D. C. (2004). Managing pediatric dental patients: issues raised by the law and changing views of proper child care. Pediatric Dentistry, 26 (2), 125–30.

Carlson, A., Humphries, G. M., Lee, G., & Birch, R. (1993). The effect of pre-treatment enquiries on child dental patient's post-treatment ratings of pain and anxiety. *Psychology and Health, 8,* 165–174.

Casamassimo, P., Wilson, S., & Gross, L. (2002). Effects of changing US parenting styles on dental practice: perceptions of diplomates of the American Board of Pediatric Dentistry. *Pediatric Dentistry, 24,* 18–22.

Chan, H. (2001). Effects of injection duration on site-pain intensity and bruising associated with subcutaneous heparin. *Journal of Advances in Nursing, 35(6),* 882–92.

Coombs, J. A. (1980). Application of behavioral science research to the dental office setting. *International Dental Journal, 30,* 240–48.

Corah, N. L., Gale, E. N., & Illig, S. J. (1979). Psychological stress reduction during dental procedures. *Journal of Dental Research, 58,* 1347–51.

Cotton, K. T., Seale, N. S., Kanellis, M. J., Damiano, P. C., Bidaut-Russell, M., & McWhorter, A. G. (2001). Are general dentists' practice patterns and attitudes about treating Medicaid-enrolled preschool age children related to dental school training? *Pediatric Dentistry, 23(1),* 51–55.

Dunegan, K. M., Mourino, A. P., Farrington, F. H., & Gunsolley, J. C. (1994). Evaluation of the Eyberg Child Behavior Inventory as a predictor of disruptive behavior during an initial pediatric dental examination. *Journal of Clinical Pediatric Dentistry, 18,* 173–79.

Edelstein, B. L. (2000). Public and clinical policy considerations in maximizing children's oral health. *Pediatric Clinics of North America, 47(5),* 1177–89.

Filcheck, H., Allen, K. D., Ogren, H., Darby, B., Holstein, B., & Hupp, S. (2004). The use of choice-based distraction to decrease the distress of children at the dentist. *Child & Family Behavior Therapy, 26* (4), 59–68.

Frankl, S., Shiere, F., & Fogels, H. (1962). Should the parent remain with the child in the dental operatory. *ASDC Journal of Dentistry for Children, 29,* 150–63.

Gibson, R., Allen, K. D., Hutfless, S., & Beiraghi, S. (2000). The Wand vs. traditional injection: a comparison of pain related behaviors. *Pediatric Dentistry, 22(6),* 458–62.

Gonzalez, J., Routh, D., & Armstrong, D. (1993). Effects of maternal distraction versus reassurance on children's reactions to injections. *Journal of Pediatric Psychology, 18(5),* 593–604.

Greenbaum, P., Lumley, M., Turner, C., & Melamed, B. (1993). Dentist's reassuring touch: effects on children's behavior. *Pediatric Dentistry, 15(1),* 21–24.

Greenbaum, P., Turner, C., Cook, E., & Melamed, B. (1990). Dentists' voice control: effects on children's disruptive and affective behavior. *Health Psychology, 9(5),* 546–58.

Grembowski, D., & Milgrom, P. M. (2000). Increasing access to dental care for medicaid preschool children: the Access to Baby and Child Dentistry (ABCD) program. *Public Health Reports, 115(5),* 448–59.

Harper, D., & D'Alessandro, D. (2004). The child's voice: understanding the contexts of children and families today. *Pediatric Dentistry, 26(2),* 114–20.

Havener, L., Gentes, L., Thaler, B., Megel, M., Baun, M., Driscoll, F., Beiraghi, S., & Agrwal, S. (2000). The effects of a companion animal on distress in children undergoing dental procedures. *Issues in Comprehensive Pediatric Nursing, 24,* 137–52.

Houpt, M. I., Heins, P., Lamster, I., Stone, C., & Wolff, M. S. (1997). Evaluation of intraoral Lidocaine patches in reducing needle-insertion pain. *Compendium, 18,* 309–17.

Johnson, R., & Baldwin, D. C. (1969). Maternal anxiety and child behavior. *Journal of Dentistry for Children, 36,* 87–92.

Kamp, A. (1992). Parent child separation during dental care: a survey of parent's preference. *Pediatric Dentistry, 14,* 231–35.

Maragakis, G. M., & Musselman, R. J. (1996). The time used to administer local anesthesia to 5 and 6 year olds. *Pediatric Dentistry, 20,* 321–23.

Marcum, B. K., Turner, C., Courts, & F. J. (1995). Pediatric dentists' attitudes regarding parental presence during dental procedures. *Pediatric Dentistry, 17* (7), 432–36.

Matthews, R., Ball, R., Goodley, A., Lenton, J., Riley, C., Sanderson, S., & Singleton, E. (1997). The efficacy of local anaesthetics administered by general dental practitioners. *British Dental Journal, 182,* 175–78.

Ng, M. W. (2004). Behavior management conference panel IV report-educational issues. *Pediatric Dentistry, 26 (2),* 180–83.

O'Callaghan, P. M., Allen, K. D., Powell, S., Roberts, H., Kelley, M. L., & Salama, F. (2005). *The Efficacy of Noncontingent Escape for Decreasing Disruptive Behavior During Dental Treatment.* Presented at the 31st Annual Convention of the Association for Behavior Analysis, Chicago.

Peretz, B., & Zadik, D. (1998). Attitudes of parents towards their presence in the operatory during dental treatments to their children. *Journal of Clinical Pediatric Dentistry, 23(1),* 27–30.

Pfefferle, J., Machen, J., Fields, H., & Posnick, W. (1982). Child behavior in the dental setting relative to parental presence. *Pediatric Dentistry, 4,* 311–16.

Quinonez, R., Santos, R. G., Boyar, R., & Cross, H. (1997). Temperament and trait anxiety as predictors of child behavior prior to general anesthesia for dental surgery. *Pediatric Dentistry, 19,* 427–31.

Raadal, M., Milgrom, P., & Weinstein, P. (1995). The prevalence of dental anxiety in children from low income families and its relationship to personality traits. *Journal of Dental Research, 74(8),* 1439–43.

Radis, F. G., Wilson, S., Griffen, A. L., & Coury, D. L. (1994). Temperament as a predictor of behavior during initial dental examination in children. *Pediatric Dentistry, 16,* 121–27.

Sheller, B. (2004). Challenges of managing child behavior in the 21st century dental setting. *Pediatric Dentistry, 26(2),* 111–13.

Sokol, D. J., Sokol, S., & Sokol, C. K. (1985). A review of nonintrusive therapies used to deal with anxiety and pain in the dental office. *Journal of American Dental Association, 110* (2), 217–22.

Travell, J. (1955). Factors affecting pain of injection. *Journal of American Medical Association, 158,* 368–71.

Venham, L. L., Bengston, D., & Cripes, M. (1978). Parent's presence and the child's response to dental stress. *ASDC Journal of Dentistry for Children, 45* (3), 213–17.

Venham, L. L., Goldstein, Gaulin-Kremer, E., Minster F., Bengston-Audia, D., & Cohan, J. (1981). Effectiveness of a distraction technique in managing young dental patients. *Pediatric Dentistry, 3* (1), 7–11.

Waldman, H. B., & Perlman, S. P. (1999). Are we reaching very young children with needed dental services? *ASDC Journal of Dentistry for Children, 66(6),* 390–94.

Weikart, D. (2002). The origin and development of preschool intervention projects (pp. 245–64). In E. Phelps, F. Furstenburg, A. Colby (eds.), *Looking at Lives: American Longitudinal Studies of the 20th Century.* New York: Russell Sage Foundation.

Weinstein, P., Getz, T., Ratener, P., & Domoto, P. (1982). The effect of dentists behaviors on fear-related behaviors in children. *Journal of American Dental Association, 104,* 32–38.

——. (1982b). Dentists' responses to fear and non-fear related behaviors in children. *Journal of American Dental Association, 104,* 38–40.

Wright, G. Z. (2000). Psychological management of children's behaviors (pp. 34–51). In R. E. McDonald & D. R. Avery (eds.), *Dentistry for the Child and Adolescent* (7th ed.). St. Louis, MO: Harcourt.

Nonpharmacological Approaches to Managing Pain and Anxiety

Eugene Hittelman and Saul Bahn

Pain and dentistry are connected in the minds of many people, often resulting in treatment postponement, avoidance, and disruptive behaviors and discomfort during treatment. Anticipation and fear of pain, past pain experiences and pain behavior during treatment, and memory of responses to pain after treatment all pose significant problems for the dentist and the dental patient. Studies have suggested that one of the primary causes of dental anxiety is the anticipation and/or fear of dental pain resulting from an actual painful or "second hand" traumatic experience during dental treatment. The fear of dental pain is a major barrier for many individuals who need dental care. In a major epidemiologic study (Maggirias & Locker, 2002), fear of pain in dental treatment was reported as a concern by 42.5% of the respondents. The purpose of this chapter, therefore, is to provide dental health professionals with some techniques for management of the pain experience and related emotional and behavioral responses arising during dental treatment.

Receiving invasive dental treatment is usually associated with pain of moderate or severe intensity. Levels of reported pain are often closely correlated with the patients' level of dental anxiety and/or indications of negative attitudes toward dentists and the processes of dental care. Studies of the fears of injury from the needle and bleeding indicate a special challenge for the dentist because treatment often starts with the injection of a local anesthetic. These pain-procedure associations form quickly. They often generate disruptive behaviors, which delay treatment and elicit avoidance behaviors resulting in dental pathology. These problems often can be prevented or caught at an early stage rather than being allowed to reach a more serious level before care is provided (Meit et al., 2004).

Individuals who are to receive even routine dental treatment usually require some assistance with pain and anxiety to reduce their experience of discomfort associated with restorations, extractions, and even dental impressions. In addition, some patients may need extensive help coping with postoperative discomfort and distress. Attempts by the dental professional and the patient receiving dental care to respond to anticipated and/or actual painful experiences may range from denial to suggesting or requesting chemical and pharmacologic strategies, to minimizing sensation or awareness. In today's practice of dentistry, many dentists offer "painless dentistry" solutions, and some anxious patients may attempt self-medication in preparation for a dental visit. Although these strategies often may be helpful to the dentists and/or the patients, each additional pharmacological intervention increases the possibility of adverse physiologic or interpersonal reactions and may lead to problems of "overmedication."

A variety of approaches to pain management are available to the practicing dentist. These approaches range from pain blocking procedures involving various levels of anesthesia; pharmacologic intervention to reduce anxiety and arousal; and behavioral, physical, and cognitively based strategies (see table 15.1). These strategies, in combination, provide powerful resources for use by the general practitioner in responding to problematic physiologic, behavioral, evaluative, and emotional patient reactions to the sensations experienced during treatment and for eliciting and facilitating productive coping strategies by the patient during treatment process.

The dental patient's experience related to both the anticipation of a painful experience and the actual discomfort of treatment can pose significant interferences with optimal patient care. Any attempt to reduce the potential difficulties involved must include a clear understanding of the nature of the pain experience and the development of effective strategies for reducing patient discomfort, problematic behavioral responses prior to, during, and after the dental visit.

The dentist's attempts to modulate the patient's discomfort and anxiety, by using local anesthesia or sedation alone, may be experienced by the patient as mechanical, uncomfortable, and frightening. If the patient feels "it hurts," as far as the patient is concerned, it hurts. Attempts by the dentist to minimize the patient's experience of discomfort through the use of sedation may be felt as dismissive or an attempt to relieve the patient's responsibility for participating in the care provided. The pain experience involves sensory (nociperception), affective (suffering and anxiety), and evaluative or cognitive (sense of tissue damage) components. The patient is attempting to "make sense" of what is felt during treatment. If the patient reports feeling pain, the pain is real to the patient and should not be treated as just an expression of an overanxious patient. This response must involve interpersonal attention as well as chemomechanical intervention.

Pain management will differ depending upon whether the pain is self-limiting, short lasting (acute), or persistent (chronic). Chronic pain, which may involve neural changes, psychological and lifestyle adaptations, and associated neuropathies, usually requires a multidisciplinary team because of its complex etiology (Holdcroft & Power, 2003). However, during the dental visit, all pain requires some form of immediate palliative response. Behavioral, cognitive, physiological levels of arousal, and neurophysiological re-

Table 15.1   Management of Pain Experience (Strategies to Reduce Suffering and Anxiety)

Educational Strategies
- Tell–Show–Do
- Rehearsal
- Informed consent
- Description of the treatment process

Pharmacologic
- NSAIDS
- Opioids
- Conscious sedation
- Local anesthetics
- Membrane stabilizers
- Psychotropic medications
- Steroids

Behavioral-Interpersonal Strategies
- Cognitive strategies
  - Iatrosedation
  - Reframing
  - Thought stopping
- Strengthening sense of self-efficacy
- Building a therapeutic alliance—interpersonal support
- Increasing sense of control
  - Informational control
  - Physical control
  - Decision making
- Distraction

Biomechanical
- Surgical intervention
- Pressure
- Cold applications
- Physical therapy

sponses (see table 15.2) (including those caused by pharmacologic intervention) will influence the level of the pain response (Holdcroft & Power, 2003). If the stimulus is unpleasant, the patient is likely to interpret the sensation as pain and to express his/her discomfort, withdraw, and/or avoid the situation or activity. To the patient in the dental chair, all pain is acute. The fact that some of the pain is a result of a chronic condition or prior injury does not eliminate or make irrelevant the feeling of pain experienced during treatment. This chapter will focus upon the management of (acute) pain and pain behavior occurring during the dental visit.

Pain management studies have begun to evaluate the role of nerve cells, pain pathways, and gating mechanisms (influencing attention and activation) in the central nervous system and the neurochemical processes that occur during signal transmission. Included are studies of psychosocial and cognitive mechanisms that determine the sensory, motivational-affective,

Table 15.2 Pain Factors Affecting Experience

Quality of the Nociceptive Sensation
- Sharp, piercing
- Pressure
- Temperature (hot, burning, stinging)

Intensity of the Pain Experience
- Visual Analogue Scale (relation to the worst pain ever felt)

Onset of the Stimulus Experience
- Initial surprise
- Situational cues
- Relationship to other stimulus experiences

Time Factors
- Duration of the stimulus
- Frequency of the experience

Psychological Factors
- Personal meaning (attribution) of the sensation
- Level of anxiety, fear, and/or arousal
- Sense of control
- Motivation
- Neurohormonal responses
   Endogenous endorphin and enkephalin production
   Serotonin 1-6
   Dopamine
   GABA
   Glutamate
   Cortisol
   Epinephrine
   Norepinephrine

and cognitive-evaluative process that leads to the experience of discomfort and suffering. The patient's affective and evaluative responses to this pain and/or to the threat of pain begin with cognitions triggered by nociceptive related sensory impulses, and/or hormonal signals registered by cortical structures primarily within the limbic system.

Initial pain-stimulus awareness will activate the amygdala, which in turn will activate the hypothalamic-pituitary-adrenal axis resulting in immediate arousal of the sympathetic and parasympathetic systems. The brain areas activated during peripheral stimulation involve the anterior cingulate, the insular, prefrontal, and somatosensory cortices. Continued stimulation will involve the hippocampus, which in turn activates the prefrontal and temporal structures resulting in cognitive appraisal and interpretation (Ledoux, 2000) The translation of peripheral stimulus to cortical awareness is not automatic but is mediated by arousal level (including the amount of neurohormonal activity) and emotional state, interference from other stimuli, intensity and quality of the stimulus, and the patient's level of attention (vigilance).

Table 15.3   Approaches to Pain Control in Treatment

Block transmission of sensation to central nervous system
- Local anesthesia
- Cold
- Vibration
- Electrical stimulation
- Pressure
- Counterstimulation
- Anoxia

Block neuromodulation of stimulus
- NSAIDS
- Membrane stabilization
- Anxiolytic medications

Block perception
- Opioids
- Placebo and Hypnosis
- Distraction
- Exercise
- Counterstimulation

Block behavioral responses
- Muscle relaxants
- Condition incompatible response to stimulus
- Sedation
- Immobilization
- Threat of punishment or damage
- Relaxation training

Differential responses to the expectation of pain or the direct experience of pain, ranging from instinctive "fight-flight" physiologic activation to emotional and behavioral responses, are evoked by differences in the areas of the cortex activated (Ploghaus et al., 1999). These responses to a direct or anticipated threat serve to signal the need to engage in a defensive or protective response. Depending upon the individual's vigilance, emotional state, competing stimuli, and past experiences, the nociceptive or other sensory pathways may activate the cortical structures eliciting a cognitive appraisal of pain by the patient (Melzack, 2001). As such, these perceptual responses can be modulated or even prevented by pharmacologic, physical, and/or behavioral intervention (see table 15.3). Because these experiences are actually "perceptions" or "attributions" rather than a direct analog of the sensations traveling from the site of an injury, they can be influenced by the reactions of the dentist and/or dental staff. Whether the patient's experience of a physical stimulus is unpleasant and/or frightening, merely annoying, or even pleasurable is dependent not only on its physical intensity and quality but also upon the patient's present psychoemotional state and physiological arousal, the setting, the patient's perception of the "meaning" of the sensation, and the quality of the response from the dental staff.

Pain, fear, and anxiety responses are variations of a similar neurophysiologic event but differ primarily in their relationship to the temporal presentation of the stimulus and the patient's awareness of the threat. Pain is the sense of experiencing an actual or perceived tissue injury; fear is the anticipation of a specific, imminent threat of injury; and anxiety is a sense of dread or anticipation of an unknown potential loss or damage. Anxiety tends to be characterized by catastrophizing while fear tends to be characterized by avoidance (Sullivan et al., 2004). However, the level of discomfort experienced by the individual (also often what is measured as "pain" on most subjective scales) may be more intense when the patient is anticipating the "painful" event than when the actual event occurs. Pain behavior may be more problematic during the fear stage than during the actual stage of nociperceptive activity. Each of these reactions are elicited by a combination of retrieval of earlier learning and retrieved memories, physiological arousal, emotional state, and attribution processes. The dentist can modulate the patient's experience of discomfort and distress by employing a variety of interpersonal strategies such as cognitive restructuring, emotional support, instruction, relaxation techniques, distraction, and support for positive coping skills.

In addition to the emotional and cognitive reactions of the patient, the dentist must also manage the patient's behavioral response. Behavioral reactions are much less responsive to pharmacologic intervention than are emotional and cognitive reactions. The behavioral reaction may be voluntary (under the purposeful control of the patient) or involuntary (a momentary reaction that is instinctual or learned). Pain behaviors during treatment can slow or block treatment or, at times, expose the patient or dentist to actual injury. The patient may jump, pull away, attempt to escape, or even strike out when first feeling "pain." The patient may also begin to create a disturbance (by yelling or screaming, for example)—upsetting other patients in the office—or exhibit a physiological response such as hyperventilation, cardiac changes, or shock. In reaction to the discomfort, the patient may begin to exhibit fear behaviors, increased sensitivity, and possible avoidance of future treatment. Finally, as a result of the "pain experience," the patient may exhibit a lower threshold for experiencing pain during future treatment (Grau & Meagher, 1999). These hypersensitive patients may require more behavioral and pharmacologic intervention and increased use of local anesthetics. Any behavioral interventions for helping patients cope with their adverse dental experience must include strategies for minimizing disruptive patient behavior; responding to the patient's emotional, cognitive, or physiologic state; and responding to the patient's experience of discomfort.

Control of pain, decreasing fear, and reducing anxiety often involve more than trying to calm the patient, blocking the nociceptive pathway, or sedation. It is also usually necessary to focus on the cognitive experience. Although changes in the source of the physical insult, alterations of the neural transport processes, and blocking the release of specific neural products can modify the patient's discomfort, changes in the meaning of the sensations experienced will also impact upon the patient's emotional, cognitive, and behavioral responses. For example, local injections, to control pain, are not usually seen as painless by the patient, although most dentists tend to minimize the discomfort experienced. For many patients, the injection process is their most feared and "traumatizing" experience. The actual level of sensation caused by a local injection, the quality of the discomfort created by a dental procedure using modern equipment, or the suffering experienced during treatment by a well-anesthetized patient will usually be much less intense than the sensation experienced after stubbing a toe, banging a limb on a hard object, or sustaining a cut or burn while cooking. Also, the patient's response to a major traumatic injury occurring during active play will often go unnoticed while a low-level stimulation during a dental procedure might seem to be terribly painful. Since each pharmacological intervention involves some medical risk, it is important that the dentist utilize nonpharmacological, behavioral strategies in addition to appropriate pharmacological interventions to minimize the patient's adverse experience.

Painful stimuli evoke two successive and distinct sensations over dual pain fiber pathways. Initially, the thin myelinated fibers (Aδ) will signal a sharp localized sensation. The first impulse is more rapid and is related to the immediate activation of cortical activity. This results in a sense of danger and rapid activation of the fight-flight response, and initiates immediate withdrawal (often in the form of startle or quick movements). The cortical reception threshold for this impulse is somewhat dependent upon the patient's current level of arousal, anxiety, and vigilance. The second neural transmission is slower and is more long lasting, providing information on the location, quality, and intensity of the pain signal. This is a result of the activation of the unmyelinated, slower firing fibers (C-fibers). Continued activation of the C-fibers tends to modify the characteristics of the neural transmission making it intolerable. This activates behavioral and cognitive responses intended to limit further injury (Plon et al., 2002). Peripheral and central pain medications can minimize, to an extent, the intensity and quality of the sensation. Parallel to this physiologic process, perceptions of and cognitive reactions to acute pain can be divided into three thresholds governing the patient's response. Sensory detection theory makes a distinction between the actual quality, the intensity of the stimulation, the individual's personal criteria for judging and reporting the level of pain being experienced, and the patient's decision as to when to attempt to escape the sensation.

A pain threshold is the stimulus intensity at which a subject will report experiencing pain to be present with 50% of the stimuli presented at that level (Clark, 1974). Experimental and clinical pain research has identified three thresholds for pain (see table 15.4). Most of the initial work defining the pain thresholds was experimental. In 1958, pain thresholds were divided between "pain perception" and "pain reactions" using heat, pressure, and pricking (Wolff & Wolf, 1958). Subsequent studies using techniques such as the Cold Pressure Test, identified a third threshold, which involved tolerance. Clinical applications describing the pain experience have differentiated these three pain response thresholds as sensation or the awareness of nociceptive stimulus, suffering or cognitive appraisal of the stimulus as damaging, and suffering or inability to tolerate the stimulus (Perl & Kruger, 1996; Giddon, 1974). Although the subjects in experimental situations with carefully controlled nociceptive stimuli do have a different physical and cognitive experience—the experimental subjects are aware that the research design

Table 15.4   Pain Response Thresholds

Threshold 1: Awareness of a Sensation (Signal of Danger)
- Cognitive responses
    Orientation (Awareness)
    Danger (Alert)
- Emotional response
    Fear and apprehension
    Anger and defensiveness
    Tension
- Behavioral response
    Frozen flight
    Startle and quick movements
    Withdrawal

Threshold 2: Perception of Tissue Damage or Injury
- Cognitive response
    "I am being injured or damaged."
    "I am in danger."
    "This is very painful."
- Emotional response
    Discomfort and suffering
    Fear and anxiety
- Behavioral response
    Grimacing, flinching, teeth clenching, tightening muscles
    Moaning, groaning, crying out, and complaining
    Requests for more anesthesia or sedation
    Passivity and searching for comfort

Threshold 3: A Feeling That the "Pain" Is Unbearable
- Cognitive response
    "This is too much, I can't stand the pain."
    "The pain is going to go on forever."
    "I can't survive the pain."
- Emotional response
    Panic and a sense of loss of control
    Fear
    Suffering
    Anger

- Behavioral response
    Demands to stop procedure
    Attempts to escape
    Loud cries
    Striking out, aggression

has been developed in such a way that they will not experience harm, while clinical patients do not feel that assurance—the pain thresholds remain the same. Strategies for moderating the pain experience, which have been studied experimentally, can be applied clinically (Baron, Logan, & Hoppe, 1993). Different pain management strategies are suggested for each of the three pain thresholds.

Threshold 1 ("awareness"): involves the immediate detection or awareness of a stimulus. The patient "feels something" and reacts with startle, avoidance, and arousal. The intensity and the quality of the sensation are less important than the awareness. An individual is just as likely to become startled and pull back when touching a cold stove or brushing against a cobweb as when touching a hot iron or being stung by a bee. It is not the intensity or the quality of the stimulus (nociceptive characteristic) but the sudden awareness. This threshold is sensitive to levels of attention (vigilance), psychophysiological arousal (anticipatory anxiety), intensity and quality of the stimulus, and individual differences (Fernandez & Turk, 1992; Williams, 1999).

Threshold 2 (an experience of discomfort or pain): follows as the patient begins to assign meaning to the sensation. This affective response is the result of the attribution of danger or damage to the stimulus experience. The nociperceptive signal is evaluated against prior experience, the current situation, the perceived meaning of the sensation, and the patient's self-perception as to the ability to cope with and/or control his/her response (Williams, 1999). At this point, the hippocampus and related cortical structures have been activated (Price, 2000) and the stimulus is cognitively processed against prior memories and experiences as well as an appraisal of the present situation (Rainville et al., 1997). It involves the "interpretation" or "attribution" that the sensation is indicating tissue damage or insult to body integrity. Typically, the patient will allow the dentist to continue but will complain, become upset, and possibly develop a negative anticipatory response to future treatment. The patient experiences suffering and, perhaps, fear but manages to allow the activity to continue.

Threshold 3 (a sense of suffering, being unable to tolerate the sensation, and the desire to escape): is a continuation of the interpretive process and is the point at which the patient moves from pain to suffering to panic and possibly with ensuing escape behavior. The patient may actively try to interfere with treatment or begin to plead with the dentist to stop. It does not appear that the actual intensity or the quality of the stimulus is the governing factor related to when this threshold is crossed. The patient's motivation, sense of control over the termination of the stimulus, and sense of potential duration of the stimulus will all affect the patient's ability to tolerate the painful experience.

Many of the strategies for managing patient's experience of pain and their subsequent pain behavior are based on attempts to raise the response threshold at which the patient experiences the sensations as noxious and dangerous. Since the intensity and the quality of the nociceptive stimulus only contributes but does not determine the patient's awareness and interpretation of the sensation, many of these strategies involve behavioral interventions (see table 15.5)

Threshold 1, detection of a sensation, is affected by attention, arousal, and anxiety. Each of these can be modulated by behavioral interventions. The primary goal of these interventions is to prevent "startle reactions" and excessive physiological responses by decreasing the patient's level of anticipatory anxiety and tension. The greater the patient's apprehension and vigi-

Table 15.5 Behavioral Strategies to Raise Pain Response Thresholds

Threshold 1: Focus on Decreasing Amygdala Responsiveness
- *Lower level of vigilance and arousal* (Relaxation strategies: Jacobson Progressive Relaxation; Breathing strategies: diaphragmatic breathing; Exercise; Create a sense of safety and predictiveness, e.g., rehearsal)
- *Block awareness of the sensation* (Distraction: verbal, music, television, etc.; counterstimulus: palpation, pinching, rubbing; distraction activities: guided movements)
- *Decrease sense of surprise* (Increase continuity of the treatment process. Maintain finger rest—decrease sense of transitions of treatment process.)
- *Lower sense of threat* (Interpersonal strategies: positive relationship, safe environment, trust)

Threshold 2: Modify Cognitive Appraisal of Stimulus
- *Reframing: Change meaning of sensation* (Explain the sensation as pressure rather than as pain. Explain that local anesthetic will block "pain" but not feeling of vibration.)
- *Tell-Show-Do* (Clarify the treatment process and suggest appropriate responses.)
- *Iatrosedation* (Change the personal—associative—meaning of the treatment process.)
- *Hypnosis*

Threshold 3: Decrease Panic and Increase Sense of Control
- *Specify the time period the pain will last* (e.g., Count to five and the pain will stop.)
- *Allow the patient to signal dentist to stop* ("Raise your left hand.")
- *Have patient "monitor" the sensation* (Cognitive control)
- *Have patient "enter the pain"* (Accept the sensation as sensation.)
- *Change the motivation* (Redefine the value of "standing the pain.")

lance, the lower the detection threshold will be. Distraction, counterstimulation, and imagery can serve to redirect the patient's attention from the anticipated discomfort and will result in a higher pain detection threshold. Standard anxiety and arousal control strategies can be employed to help the patient. Relaxation techniques (e.g., progressive relaxation), breathing techniques (e.g., diaphragmatic breathing), iatrosedation, appropriate touch, preparing the patient for the experience (rehearsal), and increasing environmental cues (minimizing surprise) will often serve to lower the arousal and anticipatory responses. Attempts to decrease the patient's sense of danger with hypnosis, placebo, and suggestion have had some effect but, other than lowering arousal and providing distraction, tend not to greatly effect the startle response and awareness threshold (Katcher, Segal, & Beck, 1984).

Threshold 2, interpretation of the sensation as painful, is the result of the patient's attributing the cause of the sensation as tissue damage or threat to bodily integrity. In other words, the patient believes that the sensation is signaling a need to prevent further damage. In this situation, it is the patient's perception or attribution as to the meaning of the sensation that is creating the problem. Techniques such as "cognitive reframing" ("After the needle actually passes the skin, you will feel pressure from the fluid being released but the 'pain nerve' will have been anesthetized"), explaining the source of the sensation ("as we continue extracting your tooth, the 'cracking' that you hear/feel is the result of the periodontal tissues releasing the tooth"), and changing the meaning of the sensation ("the 'tingling' you feel is an indication the anesthesia is taking hold") will all decrease the likelihood that patient will experience the necessary sensations of treatment (pressure, vibration, and throbbing) as painful.

Many patients will benefit from the Tell-Show-Do procedure because they expect many of the sensations and have a sense of how to respond to these sensations. Hypnosis, suggestion, and placebo all have a place in helping the patient cope with his/her sense of danger. Although the patient may be aware of the sensation, under hypnosis and suggestion, the patient is unlikely to translate the sensation into pain but will cognitively process the experience in a different manner (Chaves & Dworkin, 1997). Brain-imaging studies have demonstrated that hypnosis can selectively alter the unpleasantness of noxious stimuli by modifying the cortical processes that encode the stimulus (Rainville et al., 1997). Helping patients interpret sensations is often a strategy for decreasing their distress and apprehension. To help patients cope with the sensations they feel during restorative procedures, the dentist may need to tell them that, although they have received a local anesthetic, they will still experience sensations such as vibration, noise, and pressure from the tissues but that this is not predictive of a strong and intense sensation, they usually experience as sharp pain.

Threshold 3 is the point at which the patient begins to experience the discomfort as unbearable suffering and to demand that the treatment be halted. To be helpful to the patient, the dentist must realize that pain, once started, feels like it has existed forever and will go on forever. The patient's reaction is essentially the result of feeling out of control and being unable to reestablish safety. For this reason, several behavioral interventions are possible. First, if the patient knows exactly when the pain is going to stop, it will be much easier to withstand the discomfort ("the anesthetic will stop the pain by the time you count to 6"). Second, if the patient is able to stop the procedure, then the threshold will be raised ("raise your hand when you feel you have to stop"). For this second strategy, it is essential that the patient believes the dentist will stop and that the patient is committed to the importance of completing the procedure (e.g., "hold your hand over this candle and I will give you a dollar for each second you can stand the discomfort without pulling back"). Finally, the more important or valuable the completion of the procedure is to the patient, the more discomfort the patient will feel is acceptable.

Interpersonal pain management attempts will be more effective when they are consistent with the patient's preferred coping strategies, sense of self, and locus of control (Bandura, 1997) relative to perception of the treatment situation. Depending on whether they perceive that they can control the situation, patients will vary in their desire or need to exert or be able to exert control over the dental process. This control may be cognitive (being able to understand and/or predict treatment events), physical (being able to stop a procedure), or physiological (being able to control gagging or arousal) (Law, Logan, & Baron, 1994). In addition, the patient's perception of "self-efficacy" (and later "health self-efficacy") will influence the patient's willingness to cooperate with the suggestions made by the dentist. For example, patients who evidence a strong need to be in control fare better with strategies such as monitoring the sensations experienced, using information provided by the dentist regarding the procedure and the meaning of the sensations experienced. In contrast, patients who are "other directed"—that is, who perceive that events are controlled by forces external to them (i.e., external locus of control)—may feel better by giving up control to the dentist and not monitoring the actual process or their sensations. Such patients usually will fare better with distraction strategies (Baron, Logan, & Hoppe, 1993).

Control of acute pain is an important aspect of dental treatment. Patients who experience trauma during treatment often are reluctant to return for regular maintenance and needed care. Although much of the discomfort experienced in a modern dental office, as compared to dental care of the past, has been decreased through the use of high-speed instrumentation, lasers, air and water for cooling, and local anesthetic techniques, patients still fear discomfort from dental care. Pharmacologic strategies developed to lower anxiety and the actual nociceptive experience will aid in the management of discomfort. However, even these biomedical strategies will not be enough to relieve all the distress produced during dental care and may increase the expense of the treatment, risk of side effects, and time necessary for treatment. The dentist, using current behavioral strategies, can reduce the level of biomedical intervention needed, increase the patient's sense of safety and self-efficacy, and decrease the interference with treatment that occurs when patients are apprehensive, uncomfortable, and feeling vulnerable.

References

Bandura, A. (1997). *Self-Efficacy: The Exercise of Control*. New York: W. H. Freeman and Company.

Baron, R. S., Logan, H., & Hoppe, S. (1993). Emotional and sensory focus as mediators of dental pain among patients differing in desired and felt dental control. *Health Psychology, 12(5)*, 381–89.

Chaves, J., & Dworkin, S. (1997). Hypnotic control of pain: historical perspectives and future prospects. *The International Journal of Clinical and Experimental Hypnosis, 45(4)*, 356–76.

Clark, W. C. (1974). Pain sensitivity and the report of pain. *Anesthesiology, 40(3)*, 272–87.

Fernandez, E., & Turk, D. (1992). Sensory and affective components of pain: separation and synthesis. *Psychological Bulletin, 112(2)*, 205–17.

Giddon, D. B. (1974). Psychophysiological factors in sensation, perception, and tolerance of pain in the teeth and periodontal tissues (abridged version). In A. I. Chasens & R. S. Kaslick (eds.), *Mechanisms of Pain and Sensitivity in the Teeth and Supporting Tissues* (pp. 6–11). Hackensack, NJ: Farleigh Dickinson University.

Grau, J., & Meagher, M. (1999). Pain modulation: it's a two-way street. *Psychological Science Agenda, 12*, 10–12.

Holdcroft, A., & Power, I. (2003). Recent developments: management of pain. *British Medical Journal, 326*, 635–39.

Katcher, A., Segal, H., & Beck, A. (1984). Comparison of contemplation and hypnosis for the reduction of anxiety and discomfort during dental surgery. *American Journal of Clinical Hypnosis, 27(1)*, 14–21.

Law, A., Logan, H., & Baron, R. (1994). Desire for control, felt control, and stress inoculation training during dental treatment. *Journal of Personality and Social Psychology, 67(5)*, 926–36.

Ledoux, J. (2000). Cognitive-emotional interactions: listen to the brain. In R. D. Lane & L. Nadel (eds.), *Cognitive Neuroscience of Emotion* (pp. 129–55). New York: Oxford University Press.

Maggirias, J., & Locker, D. (2002). Psychological factors and perceptions of pain associated with dental treatment. *Community Dentistry and Oral Epidemiology, 30(2)*, 151–59.

Meit, S., Yasek, V., Shannon, C. K., Hickman, D., & Williams, D. (2004). Techniques for reducing anesthetic injection pain: an interdisciplinary survey of knowledge and application. *Journal of the American Dental Association, 135(9)*, 1243–50.

Melzack, R. (2001). Pain and the neuromatrix in the brain. *Journal of Dental Education, 65(12)*, 1378–82.

Perl, E., & Kruger, L. (1996). Nociception and pain. In L. Kruger (ed.), *Pain and Touch* (pp. 180–202). New York: Academic Press.

Ploghaus, A., Tracey, I., Gati, J., Clare, S., Menon, R., & Rawlins, N. (1999). Dissociating pain from its anticipation in the human brain. *Science, 284(5422)*, 1979–81.

Ploner, M., Gross, J., Timmermann, L., & Schnitzler, A. (2002). Cortical representation of first and second pain sensations in humans. *Proceedings of the National Academy of Sciences, 99(19)*, 12444–48.

Price, D. (2000). Psychological and neural mechanisms of the affective dimensions of pain. *Science, 288*, 1769–72.

Rainville, P., Duncan, G. H., Price, D. D., Carrier, B., & Bushnell, M. C. (1997). Pain affect encoded in human anterior cingulate but not somatosensory cortex. *Science, 277(5328)*, 968–71.

Sullivan, M., Thorn, B., Rodgers, W., & Ward, C. L. (2004). Path model of psychological antecedents to pain experience: experimental and clinical findings. *Clinical Journal of Pain, 20(3)*, 164–73.

Williams, D. A. (1999). Acute pain (with special emphasis on painful medical procedures). In R. Gatchel & D. Turk (eds.), *Psychosocial Factors in Pain* (pp. 151–63). New York: Guilford Press.

Wolff, H., & Wolf, S. (1958). Anatomy and physiology: measurement of threshold for reaction to pain. In R. F. Pitts (ed.), *Pain: A Monograph in American Lectures in Physiology* (2d ed.). Springfield, IL: Charles C. Thomas.

Self-Efficacy Perceptions in Oral Health Behavior

Anna-Maija Syrjälä

Bandura (1977) proposed a theory of self-efficacy that serves as an important determinant of behavior. According to this theory, "efficacy expectation" is the conviction that the person is able to successfully accomplish a behavior that is needed to bring about certain outcomes. Expectation of self-efficacy determines the beginning of the coping behavior, the amount of effort used, and the time to sustain the behavior in the face of obstacles. In addition to expectation, component capabilities are also needed to produce the hoped-for behavior. These include suitable skills and relevant incentives. People are afraid of and avoid situations that they find unmanageable, whereas they undertake activities they evaluate themselves able to cope with. The theory also defines the term "outcome expectancy," which is an individual estimate that a specified action will lead to a certain outcome. Efficacy and outcome expectations affect behavior differently because one may believe that a certain action will lead to a certain outcome, but if the person feels unable to perform the action, this information will not affect his/her action.

Efficacy expectations have several variable dimensions, such as magnitude, generality, and strength. Magnitude implies that efficacy expectations may be restricted to easy tasks or include very demanding ones. Generality, on the other hand, means that some tasks create restricted self-efficacy expectations and some others a more generalized expectation of mastery. Strength also varies, meaning that weak self-efficacy expectations may be thwarted by undermining experiences, while persons with strong expectations will cope despite such experiences (Bandura, 1977).

The sources of self-efficacy include "performance accomplishment, vicarious experience, verbal persuasion, and physiological states" with performance accomplishment being the most powerful source because it consists of personal experiences of mastery (Bandura, 1977). Reliance on one's own experiences is not the only source of expectations. Vicarious experiences also affect self-efficacy expectations, for example, observing another person succeed in performance may increase the efficacy expectations of the observing person. Verbal persuasion can be used to convince people that they have capabilities that help them to attain their objectives, and while the power to induce long-term growth of self-efficacy may be limited, it may help a person to succeed in performance if the evaluation is realistic. People rely partly on their physiological state when they evaluate their capabilities so that when tasks demand perseverance and strength, they evaluate their pains, aches, and fatigue as signs of physical inefficacy (Bandura, 1982).

A person's belief in his/her ability to cope with stressing factors has an effect on the biological systems mediating disease and health. If one is exposed to stressors but does not perceive the efficacy to cope with them, the opioid, autonomic, and catecholamine systems are activated (reviewed by Bandura, 1992). Furthermore, a poor sense of social efficacy is related to depression (Holahan & Holahan, 1987), which reduces immunity (Herbert & Cohen, 1993).

Bandura's social cognitive theory includes self-efficacy as a determinant of health behavior with an effect on the control of health habits and the progression of biological aging. The person's self-efficacy beliefs about behavior and motivation affect the change of behavior, that is, the contemplation of changing health habits, the necessary perseverance and motivation, the maintenance of the achieved habit, and the sensitivity to relapse (Bandura, 2000). Self-efficacy has been found to relate to various health-related practices, such as diet (Robinson & Thomas 2004), smoking avoidance (Fagan et al., 2003), and health-promoting lifestyle (Gillis, 1993). Improvement of self-efficacy can be used in various health-related practices, such as reduction of dental phobia (Do, 2004) and the management of chronic disease (O'Leary et al., 1988). Self-efficacy is also a determinant of health behavior in the Theory of Planned Behavior and Theory of Protection Motivation (Bandura, 2000). Further, self-efficacy in health behavior has been found to correlate with locus of control beliefs, self-esteem, and intention to health behavior (Syrjälä et al., 2004).

Dental Self-Efficacy in Determining Oral Health Behavior and Oral Health Status

McCaul, Glasgow, & Gustafson (1985) analyzed self-efficacy and outcome expectations concerning brushing and flossing to predict these behaviors among 131 college students. Dental knowledge and brushing and flossing skills were also analyzed. Self-efficacy and outcome expectations predicted retrospectively reported brushing and flossing and also self-monitoring of these behaviors, but skills and dental knowledge did not predict these behaviors. Tedesco, Keffer, & Fleck-Kandath (1991) analyzed the theories of reasoned action and self-efficacy to describe the reported oral health behavior of 39 patients. The study included variables of the theory of reasoned action, such as items of intention to perform oral health behavior and dental attitude, subjective norms, behavioral beliefs, and evaluation of dental outcomes. It was found that variables of the theory of reasoned action were related to reported brushing and flossing. Addition of variables concerning self-efficacy into the theory of reasoned action increased the variance of the reports to brush and floss the teeth.

McCaul, O'Neill, & Glasgow (1988) analyzed brushing and flossing in the context of theories of reasoned action and self-efficacy in a sample of 131 students. The study included variables of the theory of reasoned action, such as behavioral beliefs, attitudes, normative beliefs, subjective norms, and intention to perform oral health behavior. The intentions to brush and floss were related to brushing and flossing frequency. Addition of self-efficacy variables into the model of the theory of reasoned action did not enhance the prediction of oral health habits. Wolfe, Stewart, & Hartz (1991) used the Dental Coping Belief Scale to analyze the correlations between health beliefs and oral hygiene among 99 male veterans. The scale included items of locus of control, self-efficacy, and oral health beliefs. Self-efficacy items were not related to the plaque index.

Stewart et al. (1997) developed questionnaires to measure self-efficacy beliefs in tooth brushing and flossing and the expected outcomes concerning dental beliefs. Questionnaires filled in by 103 employees were analyzed. Self-efficacy for brushing and flossing correlated significantly with the frequencies of brushing, flossing, and dental visits. The outcome expectations of dental disease correlated significantly with flossing and the willingness to spend money in order to save one's teeth. The outcome expectations of brushing and personal beliefs correlated with dental visits and the willingness to spend money to save one's teeth. The writers interpreted their results to suggest that questionnaires on outcome expectations and self-efficacy expectations differentiate between domains of oral hygiene beliefs.

Syrjälä, Kneckt, & Knuuttila (1999) proposed a self-efficacy scale for insulin-dependent diabetic patients, including items on tooth brushing self-efficacy, approximal cleaning self-efficacy, and dental visiting self-efficacy. They also studied the association between dental self-efficacy and oral health behavior and dental plaque among 149 insulin dependent diabetes mellitus (IDDM) patients. They found the correlations of tooth brushing self-efficacy with the reported frequency of tooth brushing, approximal cleaning self-efficacy with the reported frequency of approximal cleaning, and dental visiting self-efficacy with the reported frequency of dental visits. Dental plaque correlated inversely with tooth brushing self-efficacy and dental visiting self-efficacy.

Kneckt et al. (1999) reported other results from the same research project. They used the sum score of brushing and dental visiting self-efficacy as a combined dental self-efficacy scale. Dental self-efficacy was associated with the sum of decayed surfaces. Dental self-efficacy and diabetes self-efficacy were mutually correlated.

Syrjälä et al. (2004) reported a comparative analysis, which psychological characteristics such as self-efficacy, locus of control, intention, or self-esteem most comprehensively explained oral health habits, deepened periodontal pockets, dental caries, diabetes adherence, and HbA1$_c$. The sores for both dental and diabetes self-efficacy were found to be associated with oral health habits and diabetes adherence. Psychological characteristics explained the clinical variables with a minor proportion of variance. Only self-efficacy was associated with both oral health habits and diabetes adherence.

Sources of Dental Self-Efficacy in Oral Health Behavior

According to Bandura (1981), the formation of perceived self-efficacy begins in infancy, grows as a result of interaction with the family, and widens in interaction with peers. Self-efficacy is affected by transitional experiences in adolescence, and by the new demands encountered in adulthood, and reappraised along with advancing age. Many health-imperiling habits develop in childhood and adolescence (Bandura 2000). To improve the perception of dental self-efficacy in patient-centered interaction, it is important to understand the formation and role of dental self-efficacy. Syrjälä, Knjuuttila, & Syrjälä (2001) used the test scores of a quantitative questionnaire to select five persons with either a good or a poor orientation to dental matters. Focused interviews were conducted to obtain qualitative data. In the interview, there were questions about tooth brushing, dental visits, and the use of dental floss in various taxing situations. Perceptions of self-efficacy concerning dental self-care and the source of self-efficacy were also assessed. In the analysis of the qualitative data, participants' discussion was classified by means of thematic units varying from individual words to several sentences.

Cognitive Dimension

The primary dimension of poor self-efficacy seemed to be a lack of knowledge. Two persons spontaneously reported lack of knowledge as the source of their poor self-efficacy: "It is ignorance. . .you see, and you have to care more about it." "I just haven't been to any place where they would show you what you should do. I mean, the dentist has never shown me."

Experiential Dimension

Personal experiences of dental self-care as contributing to better oral health seemed to be related to better self-efficacy. The experience of one's insufficient oral health behavior as contributing to poor oral health seemed to be related to poor self-efficacy. Subjective experience as a source of dental self-efficacy is shown in the following comments: "I mean, when the gums stop bleeding you know you're beginning to get it right" (moderate self-efficacy). "Maybe it is that I have no decay nor any other problems" (fairly good self-efficacy). "Well, I dunno, it seems to me that it's a bit like, well things haven't gone the way I'd've wanted . . . you know . . . I still got cavities" (poor self-efficacy).

Supportive Dimension

The persons with better dental self-efficacy said that the dentist had given them support, whereas poor dental self-efficacy was related to a lack of supportive experiences. This can be seen in the following comments concerning the support received during dental visits:

"especially when I was younger, the way the dentist looked and behaved had an influence, I can remember how, 20 years ago, it was really nice to go to the dentist even when I had tooth decay because I got a little present" (fairly good self-efficacy). "Now that I've been visiting the dentist, I clean the spaces between my teeth more thoroughly, I used to have kind of overfilled teeth, but then I began to visit another dentist, and he fixed my teeth so well that I can now clean all the spaces with dental floss. We (the subject and her husband) have a good relationship with our dentist" (fairly good self-efficacy).

Negative Emotions

Two subjects with unpleasant experiences continued to show a phobia, which still prevented their regular dental care and also seemed to be related to their poor self-efficacy: "there were such difficulties in pulling it out . . . they were . . . beyond description, so that . . . the dentist just couldn't get it out . . . and they had to give me more anesthetic" (poor self-efficacy). Two other subjects had had negative experiences, but they had lived down these negative experiences, which had induced a desire to attempt to keep their teeth in a good condition and resulted in better self-efficacy: "yes, it was something in the first contact, I remember when I was in my first year at school we went to this dentist's surgery, and the room was absolutely awful, and then they pulled out loads of my teeth . . . so that somehow I got this horrible . . . , for ages I was scared of dentists" (fairly good self-efficacy).

Model in Childhood

Those who had had a distinct model of regular dental care in childhood had better self-efficacy, while those with no model or an unambiguous model had poorer self-efficacy. One subject gave the following account of the source of her fairly good perception of dental self-efficacy: "perhaps it is very much from home . . . from home and school."

Interventions in Self-Efficacy to Improve Oral Health Behavior

Hölund (1990) reported about an intervention among fourteen-year-old students, who learned about health matters by teaching younger students. Their knowledge about dental caries and sugar, nutrition and sugar, self-efficacy, and beliefs concerning susceptibility were evaluated before and after the intervention. In the *computer group*, dietary habits were analyzed among the fourth graders. The *culture group* analyzed local and national factors affecting the dietary habits. The *food and fashion group* dealt with commercials and body image. The *health group* compared caries prevalence between the fourth and eighth grades. The eighth graders had to present their results on posters to the fourth graders. The intervention had no effect on posttest self-efficacy, but self-efficacy was slightly improved at two-month follow-up.

Stewart et al. (1996) reported on an intervention among 123 veterans. Before the intervention, the subjects' self-efficacy concerning brushing and flossing was evaluated. The participants also completed the Dental Health Knowledge Questionnaire before the study and at five weeks. All participants received a demonstration of tooth brushing and dental flossing. The *educational intervention* included information sessions about periodontal disease and motivation to oral hygiene. The *psychological intervention* included four sessions based on the model of Prochaska and DiClemente (1983). It turned out that the flossing self-efficacy increased significantly in the intervention groups and in the control group. The *psychological intervention group* had significantly greater changes in flossing self-efficacy compared to the other groups.

Wolfe et al. (1996) used the Dental Coping Belief Scale (DCBS) to evaluate cognitive changes in dental intervention among one hundred male veterans. The subjects in the *educational intervention group* were given oral hygiene instruction by a dentist. In the *cognitive behavioral intervention*, the subjects were provided the same instruction as in the *educational intervention*, and they additionally received one session provided by a psychologist, where they were helped to develop plans to maintain good oral hygiene and to prevent relapse into routine oral hygiene. The *attention intention group* had a cognitive intervention followed by an educational intervention. After the intervention, the DCBS self-efficacy score increased in all intervention groups.

Self-Empowerment to Help Patients to Change Their Oral Health Behavior and to Improve Their Self-Efficacy

This approach is a modification of Anderson et al. (1996) about helping the patient to change diabetes health behavior and including principles of educational and counseling psychology. Three basic principles are proposed:

1. The patient accomplishes a large part of dental care, and the patient thus plays an essential role in controlling and making decisions on his/her own dental care.
2. The dental professional has the important task of providing knowledge and psychosocial support, so that the patient is able to make decisions concerning his/her daily oral health behavior.
3. Adults are more likely to change their behavior and to maintain the changes if these changes are freely chosen and personally reasonable.

There are various obstacles related to the dentist in the use of self-empowerment. The dentist may be reluctant to bring up the emotional content of dental problems. Adults rarely make considerable changes if they do not feel any demand for it. In order to succeed in changing the patient's behavior, the dentist must elicit the patient's feelings about the anticipated change. The dentist must create an atmosphere where patients can freely express their emotional experiences concerning dental diseases. The dentist may naturally solve the problems concerning the patients' oral health behavior instead of doing it together with them. The dentist should, however, help the patients to find their own competence to solve their problems, which will confirm their self-efficacy and individual responsibility.

The patients may also face obstacles in implementing the empowerment approach. They may be reluctant to consult the dentist about oral-health-related problems (e.g., eating disorders) as noted by Giddon and Anderson (2005). They may have been criticized and blamed for their dental care, which has made them unwilling to visit the dentist and to tell dental professionals about their dental care and their controversial opinions about it. If the dentist wants to successfully employ the empowerment approach, the patients should regard themselves as real partners in the caring process. The purpose of the self-empowerment approach is to help the patients to understand that they are liable for their daily oral health behavior, to prioritize their problems concerning dental care, to become psychologically and emotionally committed to change and maintain their oral health behavior, and to develop a plan for behavior change.

Self-Empowerment Model for Changing Behavior

The following questions help to change behavior. The questions should not be used in a rigid manner, but the order of the questions may vary depending on the situation: some questions may be deleted or new questions may be added. An important factor in the discussion is the patient's knowledge of dental issues. The questions are aimed to support a patient-centered process of decision making; yet, the interaction should be mainly guided by the dentist's evaluation concerning the patient's needs.

The dentist: *What do you think is most difficult in oral self-care?*
The patient answers: *The use of dental floss is so difficult* (The dentist: *Do you have definite examples?*)
The aim of this question is to concentrate on the patient's perception concerning dental care. The dentist and the patient may have different opinions about what is most important in dental care. The patients change their health behavior most probably in order to eliminate the problems they find significant and meaningful.

The dentist: *How do you feel about the (above) situation? (Do you feel confused, etc.?)*
The patient may answer: *On the other hand, I would have to floss and care for my teeth better (guilty), I am so frustrated about the use of dental floss, because I cannot do that. The use of dental floss is so hard, because the floss gets frayed between the back teeth.*
When the patients can speak about their unpleasant feelings and frustrations, they will most probably practice things on their own.

The dentist: *How could we change and improve the situation?* The dentist may ask: *How would do you feel if you began to use dental floss? If you don't do anything about that, how would you feel then?*

This question aims to make the patients think of the situation and the ways to improve it.

The dentist: *Would you like to do something yourself in order to improve the situation? Is it important to you that the situation would change? Do you want to change the situation?*

This question assists the patient to work out his/her commitment to change the situation. The patient should, however, choose freely whether or not to commit to the behavior. It is essential that the patient does not feel enforced to change his/her behavior in order to please the dentist, because if changes are made as a reaction to such imposition, they do not last.

The dentist: *Is there something you could do to proceed toward the optimal situation? What kind of difficulties or obstacles do you have in using dental floss?*

The patient: *What should the floss to be like, if I decided to buy it? The spaces between the teeth are so small that the floss gets frayed.*

The dentist explains: *The fillings must be filed down, so that the floss glides well into spaces between the teeth. A thin waxed floss would be good for you. We will test a flosser, which is an easier way to use dental floss than by your fingers.*

The dentist: *Is there something that you could do about this now?*

The dentist asks if there is something that the patient could do about this matter at home.

The patient answers: *I could floss in the evening.*

The change may be difficult for the patient and the dentist. However, when the alterations in the roles have taken place, both the dentist and the patient may feel satisfaction with the partnership, which results in enhanced self-efficacy and better oral health behavior.

Conclusions

From previous studies, dental self-efficacy seems to determine oral health habits quite well. Improvement of self-efficacy in one aspect of health behavior may have an effect on other aspects of health behavior. Thus, in order to improve oral health behavior in clinical practice, it is important to enhance dental self-efficacy in patient-centered interaction. Sources of dental self-efficacy have only been analyzed in one case study. That report showed that the important sources of better dental self-efficacy are subjective experience of success in dental care, and consequently, better oral health, support from the dentist, a family model internalized in childhood, and an ability to overcome negative dental experiences, such as fear. Poorer self-efficacy was related to not having acquired knowledge about dental matters, experience of insufficient oral health behavior contributing to poor oral health, lack of supportive experiences during dental visits, no or an unclear model about dental care in childhood, and inability to overcome negative experiences. Thus, the dentist can improve and shape the patient's perception of dental self-efficacy in the following ways:

1. Provide information concerning oral health
2. Encourage the patient, give support to the patient, and provide positive feedback to improve his/her successful experiences in oral home care

3. Provide models concerning oral health behavior
4. Create a safe, peaceful atmosphere to minimize dental fear and emotional arousal concerning dental visits
5. Use an empowering approach to help the patients to find their competence to solve their dental problems and to develop a plan for behavior change, which confirms their self-efficacy and individual responsibility. It is important to create an atmosphere where the patient can freely make a decision on whether or not to commit to good oral health behavior.

References

Anderson, R. M., Funnel, M. M., & Arnold, M. S. (1996). Using the empowerment approach to help patients change behavior (pp. 163–72). In B. Anderson & R. Rubin (eds.), *Practical Lessons from Psychology for Diabetes Clinicians*. Alexandria, VA: The American Diabetes Association.

Bandura, A. (1977). Self-efficacy: toward a unifying theory of behavioral change. *Psychological Review, 84*, 191–215.

——. (1981). Self-referent thought: a developmental analysis of self-efficacy. In J. H. Flavell & L. Ross (eds.), *Social Cognitive Development: Frontiers and Possible Futures* (pp. 200–239). Cambridge: Cambridge University Press.

——. (1982). Self-efficacy mechanism in human agency. *American Psychologist, 37*, 122–47.

——. (1992). Self-efficacy mechanism in psychobiologic functioning. In R. Schwarzer (ed.), *Self-Efficacy: Thought Control of Action* (pp. 355–94). Washington, DC: Hemisphere.

——. (2000). Health promotion from the perspective of social cognitive theory. In P. Norman, C. Abraham, & M. Conner (eds.). *Understanding and Changing Health Behavior: From Health Beliefs to Self-Regulation* (pp. 299–339). Amsterdam: Psychology Press.

Do, C. (2004). Applying the social learning theory to children with dental anxiety. *The Journal of Contemporary Dental Practice, 5*, 1–8.

Fagan, P., Eisenberg, M., Frazier, L., Stoddard, A. M., Avrunin, J. S., & Sorensen, G. (2003). Employed adolescents and beliefs about self-efficacy to avoid smoking. *Addictive Behaviors, 28*, 613–26.

Giddon, D. B., & Anderson, N. K. (2005). Attitudes toward expanded roles for paramedical personnel. *American Journal of Health Studies, 19* (4), 220–25.

Gillis, A. J. (1993). Determinants of a health-promoting lifestyle: an integrative review. *Journal of Advanced Nursing, 18*, 345–53.

Herbert, T. B., & Cohen, S. (1993). Depression and immunity: a meta-analytic review. *Psychological Bulletin, 113*, 472–86.

Holahan, C. K., & Holahan, C. J. (1987). Self-efficacy, social support, and depression in aging: a longitudinal analysis. *Journal of Gerontology, 42*, 65–68.

Hölund, U. (1990). Effect of a nutrition education program, "Learning by teaching," on adolescents' knowledge and beliefs. *Community Dentistry and Oral Epidemiology, 18*, 61–65.

Kneckt, M. C., Syrjälä, A.-M. H., Laukkanen, P., & Knuuttila, M. L. E. (1999). Self-efficacy as a common variable in oral health behavior and diabetes adherence. *European Journal of Oral Sciences, 107*, 89–96.

McCaul, K. D., Glasgow, R. E., & Gustafson, C. (1985). Predicting levels of preventive dental behaviors. *Journal of American Dental Association, 111*, 601–5.

McCaul, K. D., O'Neill, H. K., & Glasgow, R. E. (1988). Predicting the performance of dental hygiene behaviors: an examination of the Fishbein and Ajzen model and self-efficacy expectations. *Journal of Applied Social Psychology, 18,* 114–28.

O'Leary, A., Shoor, S., Lorig, K., & Holman, H. R. (1988). A cognitive-behavioral treatment for rheumatoid arthritis. *Health Psychology, 7,* 527–44.

Prochaska, J. O., & DiClemente, C. C. (1983). Stages and processes of self-change of smoking: toward an integrative model change. *Journal of Consulting Clinical Psychology, 51,* 390–95.

Robinson, C. H., & Thomas, S. P. (2004). The Interaction Model of Client Health Behavior as a conceptual guide in the explanation of children's health behaviors. *Public Health Nursing, 21,* 73–84.

Stewart, J. E., Strack, S., & Graves, P. (1997). Development of oral hygiene self-efficacy and outcome expectancy questionnaires. *Community Dentistry and Oral Epidemiology, 25,* 337–42.

Stewart, J. E., Wolfe, G. R., Maeder, L., & Hartz, G. W. (1996). Changes in dental knowledge and self-efficacy scores following interventions to change oral hygiene behavior. *Patient Education and Counseling, 27,* 269–77.

Syrjälä, A.-M. H., Kneckt, M. C., & Knuuttila, M. L. E. (1999). Dental self-efficacy as a determinant to oral health behavior, oral hygiene and HbA1$_c$ level among diabetic patients. *Journal of Clinical Periodontology, 26,* 616–21.

Syrjälä, A.-M. H., Knuuttila, M. L. E., & Syrjälä, L. K. (2001). Self-efficacy perceptions in oral health behavior. *Acta Odontologica Scandinavica, 59,* 1–6.

Syrjälä, A.-M. H., Ylöstalo, P., Kneckt, M. C., & Knuuttila, M. L. E. (2004). Relation of different measures of psychological characteristics to oral health habits, diabetes adherence and related clinical variables among diabetic patients. *European Journal of Oral Sciences, 112,* 109–14.

Tedesco, L. A., Keffer, M. A., & Fleck-Kandath, C. (1991). Self-efficacy, reasoned action and oral health behavior reports: a social cognitive approach to compliance. *Journal of Behavioral Medicine, 14,* 341–55.

Wolfe, G. R., Stewart, J. E., & Hartz, G. W. (1991). Relationship of dental coping beliefs and oral hygiene. *Community Dentistry and Oral Epidemiology, 19,* 112–15.

Wolfe, G. R., Stewart, J. M., Maeder, L. A., & Hartz, G. W. (1996). Use of dental coping beliefs scale to measure cognitive changes following oral hygiene interventions. *Community Dentistry and Oral Epidemiology, 24,* 37–41.

Behavioral Issues in Geriatric Dentistry

Joseph L. Riley III

During the past several decades, the percentage of older adults who have retained their natural teeth has increased steadily (Burt & Eklund, 1999). However, the surgeon general's report on oral health and other studies indicate the overall dental health status of older adults is less than optimal (*Oral Health in America*, 2000). This growing population poses special challenges to the dental practitioner from technical, physiological, social, and behavioral standpoints.

Practitioner-Related Issues

Ageism and Stereotypes

Ageism is the root of many myths and misunderstandings about older adults. Ageism is a concept that was introduced by Robert Butler (Butler, 1969), the first director of the National Institute on Aging, to describe discrimination that is based solely on age. Ageism exists among some health-care professionals, undoubtedly influenced by the fact that providers often see older persons who need help or are ill (Scharf et al., 1996). The influence these negative perceptions have on patient and caregiver has been largely ignored. Stereotypes are at the base of ageism and are ideas that set individuals apart based on supposed characteristic qualities. Although the elderly constitute the most diverse and individualized age group within the entire population, they continue to be stereotyped by the following misconceptions:

- Old people are sick and disabled.
- Senility comes with old age.
- People either get very tranquil or very cranky as they age.
- Old people have lower intelligence and are resistant to change.
- There are few satisfactions in old age.

For a majority of older persons, the above statements are not true. With improved diet, physical fitness, public health, and health care, more adults are reaching age 65 in better physical and mental health than in the past. Although normal aging is a gradual process that ushers in some physical decline, age alone is a poor marker of functioning (Scharf et al., 1996). These stereotypes are counterproductive in both the long and short term and maintain negative attitudes toward aging that may play a role in the inhibition of successful aging (Giles et al., 1992).

Attitudes of Dentists Toward Older Patients

Barriers to optimal oral health for older adults include dentists that incorporate many of these stereotypes into their perception of older adults. Understanding how these attitudes influence the treatment decisions made by oral-health-care providers is important. Unfortunately, there is little research in this area that goes beyond documenting these attitudes and beliefs.

Although dentists usually view older patients' behavior as positive, many indicate that the elderly are the least rewarding group to treat, and they hold inaccurate beliefs concerning the elderly. For example, Kiyak and Miller (1982) surveyed dentists to explore their attitudes toward older patients. Approximately two-thirds showed inaccurate perceptions of older adults that included "their health status shows a sharp decline upon retirement," "people are likely to become lonely and isolated as they grow older," and "most people eventually become a financial burden to their children." Despite these misconceptions, the dentists reported favorable feelings toward the elderly. They also found that dentists whose practices included older patients that paid for treatments themselves or had private dental insurance held fewer stereotypes and more favorable views of the elderly. Strayer, DiAngelis, & Loupe (1986) surveyed private-practice dentists about their perception of older patients' values and expectations. They were generally confident in their ability to treat them, but found older patients were less satisfying to treat than younger patients.

A study by Wilson, Holloway, & Sarll (1994) compared the views of dentists and older patients on barriers to treatment. The dentists assumed that these older patients would have more negative dental attitudes than their middle-aged patients. In reality, there were no differences between middle-aged and older patients' views on barriers to the receipt of dental care. This suggests that the value placed in dental care by older patients and their ability to pay may be underestimated. It is possible that similar misconceptions may cause providers to choose less-aggressive or lower standards of care for older patients (Kiyak, 1986). Although dentists may not be conscious of their ageist behavior, it is important to recognize these attitudes and recognize their potential effects.

Patient Death and Bereavement

With older patients retaining more dentition, dentists are encountering dying patients and patient deaths with increasing frequency. These events call upon dentists and their staffs to provide support for the terminally ill and for survivors of the deceased. Only two studies (Henry et al., 1995; Chiodo & Tolle, 1988) have surveyed dentists about these experiences. Henry et al. (1995) found that general dentists reported an average of seven patients who die each year, with those in specialty areas reporting an average of two such patients per year. The dentists indicated that patient deaths cause considerable stress, with the greatest personal stress occurring when talking with the patient's family. Chiodo and Tolle (2000) concluded that the basis for dealing effectively with a dying patient's need for open and honest discussion is mandated by ethical obligations associated with the doctor-patient relationship. These ethical requirements carry over to providing some level of bereavement support for the surviving family members of the deceased and addressing the professional duties of compassion and care. They also suggest that sending a card with a personal note, attending the patient's funeral, or making a telephone call to the patient's family are appropriate, beneficial, and appreciated.

Normal Aging

Understanding the process of aging is important to the practice of dentistry because cognition, sensory-perceptual processes, personality, and social relationships affect oral health and dental care. Therefore, it is important to distinguish between normal and pathological changes in these areas. When changes are observed, the dental team should question the older person and his or her family members, to determine the underlying cause for any changes that are observed.

Cognition

Research on cognition in aging has traditionally sought to develop generalizations about changes associated with age that hold regardless of the context within which a cognitive process operates. We review attention span, memory, and problem-solving abilities.

There are three aspects of attention that are important to understanding older adults: *selective attention, divided attention*, and *sustained attention*. Selective attention involves the focus on a specific aspect of an experience while ignoring others that are irrelevant. Generally, older adults are less adept at this than younger adults (Rogers & Fisk, 2001). However, on simple tasks involving limited stimuli and sufficient practice, age differences are minimal (Humphrey & Kramer, 1997). Divided attention involves concentrating on more than one activity at the same time. When the two competing tasks are reasonably easy, age differences among adults are minimal or nonexistent. However, as competing tasks become more difficult, older adults divide attention less effectively than younger adults (Stein-Morrow & Soederberg

Miller, 1999). Sustained attention is the state of readiness to detect and respond to changes occurring at random times in the environment. Researchers have found that older adults perform as well as middle-aged and younger adults on measures of sustained attention (Berardi, Parasuraman, & Haxby, 2001).

Memory is the process of sorting and retrieving information and includes a number of capacities that make up the system that allows us to remember. Immediate memory maintains a literal copy of the stimulus for up to two seconds. Immediate memory does not decline with aging (Santrock, 2004). Short-term memory requires attention and retention of information for periods up to fifteen minutes, and long-term memory stores and retains information for longer periods. Memory decline with age is likely to be affected by retrieval difficulty rather than any decrease in storage capacity of long-term memory (Santrock, 2004). The practicality of these distinctions in everyday life is that even though some older adults show decrements in processing information and attention tasks, the majority of functioning remains intact and sufficient.

Problem solving also can show some deterioration over time, however, the reasons are slower reaction time, susceptibility to interference and stimulus overload, short-term memory difficulty, and rigid abstract thinking (Hooyman & Kiyak, 1988). Although there are gradual declines, the rate varies considerably. Older adults adapt by relying on still intact systems (e.g., they stand closer, use nonverbal cues, etc.; Kiyak & Bennett, 1982). Other changes are attributable to secondary processes from disease, environmental conditions, and increased caution in responding.

It seems that cognitive decline is less in those who engage more frequently in cognitively stimulating activities—use it or lose it. For example, data from the Seattle Longitudinal Studies of adult intelligence suggested that the observed decline in many community-dwelling older people is probably a function of disuse and is often reversible. It was found that some two-thirds of participants in a cognitive training program showed significant improvement, and 40% of those who had declined significantly were returned to their earlier (predecline) level of cognitive functioning (Schaie, 1998).

Dementia

Although many older adults experience a decline in certain cognitive abilities, this decline is usually not pathological, but rather parallels a number of common decreases in physiological function that occur in conjunction with normal developmental processes. For some older persons, however, declines go beyond what may be considered "normal" and are progressive. Dementia is a variety of conditions that are caused by or associated with brain-tissue damage. They are characterized by a change in a person's ability to recall events in recent memory and problems with comprehension; attention span; judgment; and orientation to time, place, and person. Dementia is estimated to affect 1% of those older than sixty years of age and doubles every five years to reach 30% to 40% by the age of eighty-five (Hendrie, 1998).

Many dental patients with dementia may have never had a diagnostic evaluation and therefore will not identify themselves as having dementia. In addition, family members may incorrectly attribute signs of dementia to normal aging. For this reason, if a dental patient does not have a previously established diagnosis but shows some of the signs and symptoms, medical consultation should be recommended.

The chief problems of persons with dementia are behavioral (Henry, 1999). In the early stages, dental appointments and instructions are forgotten. There is an increasing dependence on the caregiver to provide oral hygiene, and the dentist has a significant role in ensuring that caregivers are able to take on these tasks. Families are reassured when the dentist understands the problems of dementia and the underlying nature of the disease (Moody, 1990). From a dental management perspective, major dental procedures should be performed in the early stages. If the treatment plan involves the fitting of new dentures, this should occur while the older patient can still adapt to changes and communicate any problems with fit. In more advanced cases, frequent recall and preventive measures should be continued with treatment plans designed with minimal changes to the oral cavity and should not involve complete rehabilitation (Kiyak, 1988).

Oral Physical Senses

Taste and olfaction are two senses that are associated with taste perception (Schiffman, 1997). Although older people frequently report to dentists that the taste of food is less intense than it once was (Hoffman, Ishii, & MacTurk, 1998), these complaints are equally attributable to factors such as disease, smoking, and medications (Winkler, 1999; Weiffenbach et al., 1990). This phenomenon is of importance to dentists because it can have a long-term negative effect on the efficiency of dental treatment through loss of appetite and related neglect of nutritional needs. In the past it was thought that age brought about a decrease in the number of taste buds on the tongue, however, more recent studies indicate that this may not be true (Miller, 1988). Rather, the perception of salty and bitter tastes declines with age, but sweet and sour perceptivity does not (Weiffenbach et al., 1982).

Also affecting the experience of taste is the gradual olfactory loss with age (Winkler et al., 1999). Older adults have increased olfactory thresholds, perceive odors as being weaker, and do not recognize and identify common odors (Cain & Stevens, 1989; Doty 1989). They are also more prone to olfactory habitation and are slower to recover threshold sensitivity (Schiffman, 1997). As with all physical senses, taste and smell are also affected by the cognitive and emotional context of the applied stimulus. As food can become tasteless and unappetizing as the result of declining taste and smell, geriatric patients should be encouraged to add seasonings to their food instead of relying on excessive consumption of salt and sugar to give their food flavor. Dental staff should incorporate systematic smoking cessation services into routine patient care (Warnakulasuriya, 2002) and should promote the use of proven cessation products by patients who are attempting to quit (Brothwell, 2001). Tongue cleaning can also be recommended for geriatric dental patients as it can have an enhancing effect on taste (Quirynen et al., 2004).

Other Sensory Deficits

A number of sensory changes occur with age as the result of the process of aging. Hearing impairments are the most common sensory deficit for older adults (Chavez & Ship, 2000). While hearing deficits do not directly affect oral health because of its close relationship to speech, it disrupts the process of communication between patients and dentists (Ship et al., 1996). Communication and comfort can be improved by simple measures such as asking patients to wear hearing aids when indicated.

Visual impairments are another common sensory problem for older adults (Chavez & Ship, 2000). Although some systemic diseases such as diabetes that may cause visual impairment also affect the oral cavity, visual disturbances themselves do not have direct effects on oral health (Ghezzi & Ship, 2000; Ship, 1992). However, the oral health of these patients may suffer indirectly through the decreased ability to assess their own oral hygiene or detect oral problems by sight.

Psychosocial Issues

Personality

Although personality is generally stabile, some changes in personality style occur that relate to how individuals cope with aging. An instance of where personality changes with age is the tendency for reduced sex-typed behavior for both males and females. For example, men acknowledge their need for affiliation and nurturance, while women are more accepting of their aggressive or egocentric needs. Older people may also display greater caution and even appear to become more introverted (Santrock, 2004). This is particularly apparent in the need for more time to make decisions about dental treatment, a desire to reject extensive and costly dental procedures, and in some cases a decision to avoid dental care altogether. Personality styles also influence how individuals cope with and adapt to the external and internal changes. The process of aging can involve numerous stressful life experiences. How well older persons respond to and manage these stressors can have a significant influence on their long-term well-being (Aldwin et al., 2001).

Most theories of personality have argued that personality traits are relatively stable beyond adolescence and have few implications for aging. Erik Erikson's approach focused on psychosocial development throughout the life cycle (Hooyman & Kiyak, 1988). According to his model, a person undergoes stages of development with the final stage occurring in late adulthood. Growth occurs through solving a major crisis or conflict that becomes the foundation of success in the later stages. An older person in the last stage of life is confronted with the crisis of ego integrity versus despair, which involves the acceptance of the inevitability of mortality, and achieves wisdom and perspective, or despairs because he or she has not come to grips with death and lacks ego integrity. A major task associated with this last stage is to integrate the experiences of earlier stages and to realize that one's life has had meaning.

The value of healthy teeth for maintaining self-concept and sense of attractiveness for younger adults is well accepted (Levinson, 1990). There is considerable evidence that aging itself does not result in a loss of this need for attractiveness (Levinson, 1990; Goldstein & Niessen, 1998). Davis et al. (2001) found that persons who experienced difficulties in accepting their tooth loss were more likely to feel less confident, restrict food choice, enjoy food less, avoid laughing in public, and avoid forming close relationships than those people who had no difficulties accepting tooth loss. It is important to help older patients maintain and even enhance their oral health status with restorations of existing teeth, fixed and removable prostheses if needed, and even cosmetic dentistry (Bryant & Zarb, 2002). Therefore, older adults should not be discouraged from consulting a dentist regarding cosmetic dentistry or surgery.

One measure of an older person's self-concept and self-esteem is the importance he or she places on oral health. For example, an older patient who views himself as near death just because he is seventy-five years old is likely to neglect his oral health altogether and reject any dental treatments beyond emergency care (Friedlander et al., 2003). This can be a challenge to the dental team and requires patience and the ability to convince the patient that old age does not preclude good oral health. Similarly, the patient with low self-esteem will be less motivated to maintain good oral health than one who has high self-esteem (Gardiner & Raigrodski, 2001; Chu & Craig, 1996). Indeed, if the dental team observes signs of declining oral hygiene in their older patients, these signs may point to a more severe loss of self-esteem as in depression or may indicate dementia (Ghezzi & Ship, 2000). These conditions and their impact on dental care are discussed below.

Finally, adjusting to new situations may require greater effort by older persons as noted earlier in this section. For this reason, an older person who is making his or her first visit to a dentist in a number of years may experience considerable apprehension. This feeling of stress may be displayed as anxiety about dental care, lack of compliance with treatment recommendations, and other problems in the dental chair, creating the appearance of an uncooperative patient. The dental team must therefore take the time to orient the patient to the operatory and explain the purpose of the equipment and the steps involved in providing dental care. Taking these extra few minutes of time will result in a worthwhile improvement in patient understanding and cooperation.

Depression

Psychiatric disorders are not inherent to normal aging, but they can have important implications for dental care. Depression is the mental health problem of greatest frequency and magnitude that affect the aged population. Although it is estimated that approximately 3% of the population over age sixty-five meet the DSM-IV criteria for a major depressive disorder (Alexopoulos, 1995), some fifteen million elders suffer from some degree of depression (Gallo and Lebowitz, 1999). Depression should be thought of as being on a continuum from mild, brief sadness, to intense reaction to loss or severe depression (Alexopoulos, 1995).

Certainly dentists do not have primary responsibility for the psychiatric care of older patients. However, dentists and the office staff should be aware of any signs and symptoms of depressed mood and thoughts of suicide among their older patients (Kiyak, 1983). This is best accomplished by the establishment of rapport so that older persons can trust the dental team. Consequently, patients will feel comfortable expressing grief and sadness over life stressors, including declines in their own health and that of their spouse, or grief over the death of a loved one. This is particularly true for older persons who are isolated and have few friends and family members remaining. For these reasons, it is imperative for the dental team to allow more time to obtain social and medical histories from their older patients. The dental team must avoid the potential complacency of assuming that older people's lives do not change much. Therefore, a quick question such as, "Any changes in your health or living situation since your last visit?" is suggested.

Studies have found that depressed patients are prone to neglect of oral hygiene, have diminished salivary flow, increased smoking, and altered immune function (Friedlander & Mahler, 2001; Friedlander et al., 2003), as well as decreased oral health quality of life (Kressin et al., 2002). In addition, medications taken for the treatment of depression have a range of adverse oral reactions that include xerostomia, altered taste sensation, and increased incidence of oral infection (Little, 2004). However, Anttila, Knuuttila, & Sakki (2001) did not find a direct association between depressive symptoms and dental caries, periodontal status, or number of teeth. They did find that dentate women with high rates of depressive symptoms had a more negative attitude toward preserving their natural teeth, used sugary products more frequently, reported a longer time since their last dental visit, and tended to have a higher percentage of unfilled tooth surfaces than the nondepressed dentate women.

Pain Response/Somatization

Pain is a personal experience that signals the possibility of injury and is one of the most common reasons to seek medical and dental treatment (Turk & Melzack, 2001). There are many myths about the experience of pain in the elderly. For clinical pain conditions in general, prevalence appears to peak in older individuals between fifty-five and seventy years of age. For oral pain conditions, prevalence decreases with age for toothache, oral sores, and jaw joint pain but increases with age for burning mouth (Lipton, Ship, & Larach-Robinson, 1993). Laboratory studies of the effects of aging on pain perception tend to yield somewhat mixed findings with older participants tending to report less sensitivity to noxious stimuli than their younger counterparts (Gagliese & Melzack, 1997; Gibson & Helme, 2001). One source of variability is the chosen method of pain induction. Edwards and Fillingim (2001) have speculated that the effects of age on pain responses may vary as a function of the stimulus because aging may differentially affect the various types of afferent fibers that transmit information concerning pain. A recent study did not find age differences in the perception of oral needle stick pain from the initial insertion of a needle puncturing the skin or from the subsequent injection of an analgesic agent (Carr, France, & Horton, 2002).

Changes occurring in the sensory, emotional, cognitive, and behavioral systems may influence pain perception and expression in old age. There is some evidence that older adults have greater expectations of pain and greater interference of pain with daily activities (Gibson et al., 1994). Because individuals interpret pain in the context of their lives, attitudes toward aging are likely to contribute to the response to pain (Leventhal & Prohaska, 1986). For example, the tendency to attribute physical symptoms to the aging process has been shown to be greater for older than younger medical patients and associated with reduced emotional response to these symptoms (Prohaska et al., 1987). The elderly may accept pain-related losses as an aging related natural reduction in overall health and experience less negative emotion related to their symptoms. It should not be concluded that older adults are less likely to experience pain during dental treatment, rather they may be less likely to complain of them.

If the elderly are really less willing to report low-intensity stimuli as painful, a possible alternative to convey the feelings of pain to the dentist may be through the nonverbal channel of facial expression. However, physical changes in the face that occur with age (wrinkling of skin, loss of subcutaneous fat, loss of elastic fibers, loss of hair, etc.), as well as psychiatric disorders that are more prevalent in the elderly, can influence the facial expression of pain by the elderly (LeResche & Dworkin, 1985). The failure of the dentist to decode (and relate to) such signs can lead to anxiety and frustration on the part of the patient.

Social/Family Support

There is considerable evidence that the social network of family and friends is an important determinant of general health status for older adults (Bowling & Browne, 1991). Social support provides not only emotional and/or financial support but also aids behavioral adaptation to disease such as disability or treatment (Gallo, 1982; Rise & Sogaard, 1991). Definitions of social support can vary from the presence of other family members at home, some contact with family or friends, to membership within organizations (Gottleib, 1991). Greater social support and social networks are known to be associated with reduced tooth loss (Drake, Hunt, & Koch, 1995; Hanson, Liedberg, & Owall, 1994), lower risk for periodontitis (Monteiro da Silva et al., 1996; Merchant et al., 2003), and reduced risk of being edentulous (McGrath & Bedi, 2002). The utilization of dental care by the elderly is also affected by various aspects of the social network. For example, perceived social support and marital status were more predictive of the time since last visit to a dentist than functional ability and general health (Osterberg et al., 1998; Tennstedt et al., 1994; McGrath & Bedi, 2002). A study by Rickardsson and Hanson (1989) also found that social participation was associational with regular dental care.

Issues of Dental Care

With increased attention to oral health earlier in their lives and greater number of natural teeth (Stoopler, Sollecito, & DeRoss, 2003), the current cohort of seniors may suffer with a relative increase in coronal and root caries, periodontal diseases, and preventive needs (Lamster, 2004; Fox & Eversole, 2002). Traditionally, older adults have been among the groups least likely to use dental services, despite the fact that the elderly usually use medical care to a much higher extent than younger populations (Kiyak, 1989). Several authors suggest that current older adults are better educated than previous generations and have higher expectations about maintaining and preserving their oral health (Gift & Newman, 1993; Schwab & Pavlatos, 1991). For example, Macek et al. (2004), reporting data from the 1999 National Health Interview Survey, found that 71% of dentate and 20% of edentulous older adults had made a dental visit in the previous year. The primary reason for the visit was preventive or diagnostic. Respondents without a dental visit in the past year typically did not report a need for one; however, dentate adults were more likely to identify a need than were edentulous adults.

As the number of older adults with dental needs increase, many aging Americans will be experiencing a diminished capacity to access oral health care because of retirement and the resultant loss of income and dental coverage (Manski et al., 2004; Jones et al., 1990). Consistent with this assertion, Macek et al. (2004) reported that for those who recognized a need but did not visit a dentist, cost was the most frequently reported barrier. Certainly there is a growing group of elders that are able to afford dental care, although this is less true for older minority adults (Lamster, 2004). Manski and Goldfarb (1996) reported that among older Americans aged fifty-five to seventy-five, being dentate, female, non-Hispanic White, higher income, and educated and having dental insurance coverage were each independently associated with an increased likelihood of a dental visit.

Dentate older adults need to be aware that restorative procedures completed in the past do not guarantee their oral health now or in the future. Current oral-hygiene measures, appropriately used and in conjunction with regular professional care, are capable of nearly preventing caries and most periodontal disease and maintaining oral health for all ages including older patients (Reynolds, 1997). Oral hygiene approaches should be tailored to lifestyles and abilities of the elderly in order to enable them to make decisions to improve personal oral hygiene and oral health (Choo, Delac, & Messer, 2001). Initial exams of older patients should include assessment of not only the patient's oral health but also his/her ability to perform oral hygiene (Reynolds, 1997). Kiyak (1984) summarized several principles in the administration of effective preventive oral care to the elderly. Since cognitive processing may occur more slowly in older adults, presenting information several times, using verbal and visual information is suggested (Ham et al., 2002). Written material in large-format print with contrasting figure-ground relations should be used. Frequent and brief sessions are preferred to a few long sessions. Motivation can be significantly enhanced with regular feedback to participants regarding their success in achieving predetermined oral health goals.

Summary

With the elderly retaining more of their natural teeth, they are becoming an increasingly larger and important part of dentists' practices due to increased life expectancy, declining edentulous rates, and improvements in dental specialties such as endodontics and periodontics. Older patients may present with more complex dental conditions due to many years of "wear and tear" as well as with numerous complex medical conditions. Dentists, accordingly, may be reluctant to treat them or offer rational care tailored to their unique needs. Misconceptions about the value of oral health to older adults and that current dental practitioners are coming from a cohort often very different than that of the older patient may influence dentists' views about the type and level of care these patients require. Reviews of education in geriatric dentistry indicate trends toward a focus on clinical techniques rather than a curriculum with an emphasis on adaptation to the aging process. Although all U.S. dental schools report teaching at least some aspects of geriatric dentistry, 67% of schools reported having a clinical component to geriatric dental teaching, and only 30% have a specific geriatric dentistry clinic within the school (Mohammad et al., 2003). A recent review of oral health disparities among the elderly urged for increased training emphases on geriatrics (Pyle & Stoller, 2003). Dentists must be educated in the roles required of them to improve the oral health of older adults. Training in geriatric dentistry must include the development of sensitivity to the medical, psychological, and financial issues of these patients.

References

Aldwin, C. M., Spiro, A., 3d, Levenson, M. R., & Cupertino, A. P. (2001). Longitudinal findings from the Normative Aging Study: III. Personality, individual health trajectories, and mortality. *Psychology of Aging, 16*, 450–65.

Alexopoulos, G. S. (1995). Mood disorders. In H. Kaplan & B. Sadock (eds.), *Comprehensive Textbook of Psychiatry*. 6th ed. Baltimore: Williams & Williams.

Anttila, S. S., Knuuttila, M. L., & Sakki, T. K. (2001). Relationship of depressive symptoms to edentulousness, dental health, and dental health behavior. *Acta Odontologica Scandinavia, 59*, 406–12.

Berardi, A., Parasuraman, R., & Haxby, J. V. (2001). Overall vigilance and sustained attention decrements in health aging. *Experimental Aging Research, 27*, 19–39.

Bowling, A., & Browne, P. D. (1991). Social networks, health, and emotional well-being among the oldest old in London. *Journal of Gerontolology, 46*, S20–32.

Brothwell, D. J. (2001). Should the use of smoking cessation products be promoted by dental offices? An evidence-based report. *Journal of the Canadian Dental Association, 67*, 149–55.

Bryant, S. R., & Zarb, G. A. (2002). Outcomes of implant prosthodontic treatment in older adults. *Journal of the Canadian Dental Association, 68*, 97–102.

Burt, B. A., & Eklund, S. A. (1999). *Dentistry, Dental Practice, and the Community*. 5th ed. Philadelphia: W. B. Saunders Co.

Butler, R. N. (1969). Ageism: another form of bigotry. *Gerontologist, 9*, 243–46.

Cain, W. S., & Stevens, J. C. (1989). Uniformity of olfactory loss in aging. *Annals of the New York Academy of Science, 561*, 29–38.

Carr, M. P., France, R. P., & Horton, J. E. (2002). A comparison of perceived injection pain with and without anesthetic between elderly and young female subjects. *Special Care Dentistry, 22*, 75–79.

Chavez, E. M., & Ship, J. A. (2000). Sensory and motor deficits in the elderly: impact on oral health. *Journal of Public Health Dentistry, 60*, 297–303.

Chiodo, G. T., & Tolle, S. W. (1988). Patient death and bereavement: what is the dentist's role? *Special Care Dentistry, 8,* 198–200.

———. (2000). The dentist's role in bereavement support. *General Dentistry, 8,* 500–505.

Choo, A., Delac, D. M., & Messer L. B. (2001). Oral hygiene measures and promotion: review and considerations. *Austrian Dental Journal, 46,* 166–73.

Chu, R., & Craig, B. (1996). Understanding the determinants of preventive oral health behaviors. *Probe, 30,* 12–18.

Davis, D. M., Fiske, J., Scott, B., & Radford, D. R. (2001). The emotional effects of tooth loss in a group of partially dentate people: a quantitative study. *European Journal of Prosthodontic Restorative Dentistry, 9,* 53–57.

Doty, R. L. (1989). Influence of age and age-related diseases on olfactory function. *Annals New York Academy of Science, 561,* 76–86.

Drake, C. W., Hunt, R. J, & Koch, G. G. (1995). Three-year tooth loss among black and white older adults in North Carolina. *Journal of Dental Research, 74,* 675–80.

Edwards, R. R., & Fillingim, R. B. (2001). Age-associated differences in responses to noxious stimuli. *Journal of Gerontology: Biological Science Medical Science, 56,* M180-5.

Fox, P. C., & Eversole, L. R. (2002). Diseases of the salivary glands. In S. Silverman, L. R. Eversole, & E. L. Truelove (eds.), *Essentials of Oral Medicine* (pp. 260–76). Ontario, Canada: BC Decker Inc.

Friedlander, A. H., & Mahler, M. E. (2001). Major depressive disorder: psychopathology, medical management and dental implications. *Journal of the American Dental Association, 132,* 629–38.

Friedlander, A. H., Friedlander, I. K., Gallas, M., & Velasco, E. (2003). Late-life depression: its oral health significance. *Intentional Dental Journal, 53,* 41–50.

Gagliese, L., & Melzack, R. (1997). Chronic pain in elderly people. *Pain, 70,* 3–14.

Gallo, F. (1982). The effects of social support networks on the health of the elderly. *Social Work and Health Care, 8,* 65.

Gallo, J. J., & Lebowitz, B. D. (1999). The epidemiology of common late-life mental disorders in the community: themes for the new century. *Psychiatric Service, 50,* 1158–66.

Gardiner, D. M. & Raigrodski, A. J. (2001). Psychosocial issues in women's oral health. *Dental Clinics of North America, 45,* 479–90.

Ghezzi, E., & Ship, J. A. (2000). Systemic diseases and their treatments in the elderly: impact on oral health. *Journal Public Health Dentistry, 60,* 289–96.

Gibson, S. J., & Helme, R. D. (2001). Age-related differences in pain perception and report. *Clinics in Geriatric Medicine, 17,* 433–56.

Gibson, S. J., Katz, B., Corran, T. M., Farrell, M. J., & Helme, R. D. (1994). Pain in older persons. *Disability Rehabilitation, 10,* 127–39.

Gift, H. C., & Newman, J. F. (1993). How older adults use oral health care services: results of a National Health Interview Survey. *Journal of the American Dental Association, 124,* 89–93.

Giles, H., Coupland, N., Coupland, J., Williams, A. & Nussbaum, J. (1992). Intergenerational talk and communication with older people. *International Journal of Aging and Human Development, 34,* 271–97.

Goldstein, R. E., & Niessen, L. C. (1998). Issues in esthetic dentistry for older adults. *Journal Esthetic Dentistry, 10,* 235–42.

Gottleib, B. H. (1981). *Social Networks and Social Support.* San Francisco, CA: Sage.

Ham, R. J., Sloane, P. D., & Warshaw, G. A. (2002). *Primary Care Geriatrics: A Case Based Approach.* 4th ed. St. Louis, MO: Mosby.

Hanson, B. S., Liedberg, B, & Owall, B. (1994). Social network, social support and dental status in elderly Swedish men. *Community Dentistry and Oral Epidemiology, 22,* 331–37.

Hendrie, H. C. (1998). Epidemiology of dementia and Alzheimer's disease. *American Journal of Geriatric Psychiatry, 6* (suppl 1), S3–S18.

Henry, R. G. (1999). Alzheimer's disease and cognitively impaired elderly: providing dental care. *Journal of the California Dental Association, 27,* 709–17.

Henry, R. G., Johnson, H. A., Holley, M. M., & Kaplan, A. L. (1995). Response to patients' death and bereavement in dental practice. *Special Care Dentistry, 15,* 20–25.

Hoffman, H. J., Ishii, E. K., & MacTurk, R. H. (1998). Age-related changes in the prevalence of smell/taste problems among the United States adult population. Results of the 1994 disability supplement to the National Health Interview Survey (NHIS). *Annals of the New York Academy of Science, 30,* 716–26.

Hooyman, N., & Kiyak, H. A. (1988.) *Social Gerontology: A Multidisciplinary Perspective.* Needham Heights, MA: Allyn & Bacon.

Humphrey, D. G., & Kramer, A. F. (1997). Age differences in visual search for feature conjunction and triple-conjunction targets. *Psychology and Aging, 12,* 704–17.

Jones, J. A., Adelson, R. A., Niessen, L. C., & Gilbert, G. H. (1990). Issues in financing dental care for the elderly. *Journal of Public Health Dentistry, 50,* 268–75.

Kiyak, H. A. (1983). Psychological and social factors in the dental care of the elderly. *International Dental Journal, 33,* 281–91.

——. (1984). Management of oral problems in the elderly. *Annual Review of Gerontological Geriatrics, 4,* 106–36.

——. (1986). Psychological changes associated with aging: implications for the dental practitioner. In A. F. Tryon (ed.), *Oral Health and Aging.* Littleton, MA: PSG Publishing.

——. (1988). Impact of patients' and dentists' attitudes on older persons' use of dental services. *Gerodontics, 4,* 331–35.

——. (1989). Reducing barriers to older persons' use of dental services. *International Dental Journal, 39,* 95–102.

Kiyak, H. A., & Bennett., J. (1982). Special problems of the geriatric patient. In B. D. Ingersoll (ed.), *Behavioral Aspects in Dentistry* (pp. 135–50). New York: Prentice Hall.

Kiyak, H. A., & Miller, R. R. (1982). Age differences in oral health attitudes and dental service utilization. *Journal of Public Health Dentistry, 42,* 29–41.

Kressin, N. R., Spiro, A., III, Atchison, K. A., Kazis, L., & Jones, J. A. (2002). Is depressive symptomatology associated with worse oral functioning and well-being among older adults? *Journal of Public Health Dentistry, 62,* 5–12.

Lamster, I. B. (2004). Oral health care services for older adults: a looming crisis. *American Journal of Public Health, 94,* 699–702.

LeResche, L., & Dworkin, S. F. (1985). Evaluating orofacial pain in the elderly. *Gerodontics, 1,* 81–87.

Leventhal, E. A., & Prohaska, T. R. (1986). Age, symptom interpretation, and health behavior. *Journal of American Geriatric Society, 34,* 185–91.

Levinson, N. A. (1990). Psychologic facets of esthetic dental health care: a developmental perspective. *Journal of Prosthetic Dentistry, 64,* 486–91.

Lipton, J. A., Ship, J. A., & Larach-Robinson, D. (1993). Estimated prevalence and distribution of reported orofacial pain in the United States. *Journal of the American Dental Association, 124,* 115–21

Little, J. W. (2004). Dental implications of mood disorders. *General Dentistry, 52,* 442–50.

Macek, M. D., Cohen, L. A., Reid, B. C., & Manski, R. J. (2004). Dental visits among older U.S. adults, 1999: the roles of dentition status and cost. *Journal of the American Dental Association, 135,* 1154–62.

Manski, R. J., & Goldfarb, M. M. (1996). Dental utilization for older Americans aged 55–75. *Gerodontology, 13,* 49–55.

Manski, R. J., Goodman, H. S., Reid, B. C., & Macek, M. D. (2004). Dental insurance visits and expenditures among older adults. *American Journal of Public Health, 94*, 759–64.

McGrath, C., & Bedi, R. (2002). Influences of social support on the oral health of older people in Britain. *Journal of Oral Rehabilitation, 29*, 918–22.

Merchant, A. T., Pitiphat, W., Ahmed, B., Kawachi, I., & Joshipura, K. (2003). A prospective study of social support, anger expression and risk of periodontitis. *Journal of the American Dental Association, 134*, 1591–96.

Miller, I. J., Jr. (1988). Human taste bud density across adult age groups. *Journal of Gerontology, 43*, B26–30.

Mohammad, A. R., Preshaw, P. M., & Ettinger, R. L. (2003). Current status of predoctoral geriatric education in U.S. dental schools. *Journal of Dental Education, 67*, 509–14.

Monteiro da Silva, A. M., Oakley, D. A., Newman, H. N., Nohl, F. S.,& Lloyd, H. M. (1996). Psychosocial factors and adult onset rapidly progressive periodontitis. *Journal of Clinical Periodontology, 23*, 789–94.

Moody, G. H. (1990). Alzheimer's disease. *British Dental Journal, 169*, 45–47.

Oral Health in America: A Report of the Surgeon General. (2000). Rockville, MD: National Institute of Dental and Craniofacial Research.

Osterberg, T., Lundgren, M., Emilson, C. G., Sundh, V., Birkhed, D., & Steen, B. (1998). Utilization of dental services in relation to socioeconomic and health factors in the middle-aged and elderly Swedish population. *Acta Odontologica Scandinavia, 56*, 41–47.

Prohaska, T. R., Keller, M. L., Leventhal, E. A., & Leventhal, H. (1987). Impact of symptoms and aging attribution on emotions and coping. *Health Psychology, 6*, 495–514.

Pyle, M. A., & Stoller, E. P. (2003). Oral health disparities among the elderly: interdisciplinary challenges for the future. *Journal of Dental Education, 67*, 1327–36.

Quirynen, M., Avontroodt, P., Soers, C., Zhao, H., Pauwels, M., & van Steenberghe, D. (2004). Impact of tongue cleansers on microbial load and taste. *Journal of Clinical Periodontology, 31*, 506–10.

Reynolds, M. W. (1997). Education for geriatric oral health promotion. *Special Care Dentistry, 17*, 33–36.

Rickardsson, B., & Hanson, B. S. (1989). Social network and regular dental care utilization in elderly men. Results from the population study "Men born in 1914," Malmo, Sweden. *Swedish Dental Journal, 13*, 151–61.

Rise, J., & Sogaard, A. J. (1991). Communication about dental health in Norwegian adults. *Community Dentistry Oral Epidemiology, 19*, 68–71.

Rogers, W. A., & Fisk, A. D. (1991). Are age differences in consistent-mapping visual search due to feature learning or attention training? *Psychological Aging, 6* (4), 542–50.

Santrock, J. W. (2004). *Life-Span Development*. 9th ed. New York: McGraw Hill.

Schaie, K. W. (1998). The Seattle Longitudinal Studies of adult intelligence. In M. P. Lawton & T. A. Salthouse (eds.), *Essential Papers on the Psychology of Aging* (pp. 263–71). New York: University Press.

Scharf, S., Flamer, H., & Christophidis, N. (1996). Age as a basis for healthcare rationing. Arguments against ageism. *Drugs and Aging, 9*, 399–402.

Schiffman, S. S. (1997). Taste and smell losses in normal aging and disease. *Journal of the American Medical Association, 278*, 1357–62.

Schwab, D., & Pavlatos, C. A. (1991). The geriatric population as a target market for dentists. In T. Papas, L. C. Niessen, & H. H. Chauncey (eds.), *Geriatric Dentistry: Aging and Oral Health* (pp. 331–34). St. Louis: Mosby.

Ship, J. A. (1992). Oral sequelae of common geriatric diseases, disorders, and impairments. *Clinical Geriatric Medicine, 8*, 483–97.

Ship, J. A., Duffy, V., Jones, J. A., & Langmore, S. (1996). Geriatric oral health and its impact on eating. *Journal of American Geriatric Society, 44,* 456–64.

Stein-Morrow, E. A. L., & Soederberg Miller, L. M. (1999). Basic cognitive processes. In J. C. Cavanaugh & S. K. Whitbourne (eds.), *Gerontology: An Interdisciplinary Perspective.* New York: Oxford University Press.

Stoopler, E. T., Sollecito, T. P., & De Ross, S. S. (2003). Desquamative gingivitis: early presenting system of mucocutaneous disease. *Quintessence International, 34,* 582–86.

Strayer, M. S., DiAngelis, A. J., & Loupe, M. J. (1986). Dentists' knowledge of aging in relation to perceived elderly patient behavior. *Gerodontics, 2,* 223–27.

Tennstedt, S. L., Brambilla, D. L., Jette, A. M., & McGuire, S. M. (1994). Understanding dental service use by older adults: sociobehavioral factors vs need. *Journal of Public Health Dentistry, 54,* 211–19.

Turk, D. C., & Melzack, R. (2001). *Handbook of Pain Assessment, vol. 2.* New York: Guilford Press.

Warnakulasuriya, S. (2002). Effectiveness of tobacco counseling in the dental office. *Journal of Dental Education, 66,* 1079–87.

Weiffenbach, J. M., Baum, B. J., & Burghauser, R. (1982). Taste thresholds: quality specific variation with human aging. *Journal of Gerontology, 37,* 372–77.

Weiffenbach, J. M., Tylenda, C. A., & Baum, B. J. (1990). Oral sensory changes in aging. *Journal of Gerontology, 45,* M121–5.

Wilson, M. C., Holloway, P. J., & Sarll, D. W. (1994). Barriers to the provision of complex dental treatment for dentate older people: a comparison of dentists' and patients' views. *British Dental Journal, 177,* 130–34.

Winkler, S., Garg, A. K., Mekayarajjananonth, T., Bakaeen, L. G., & Khan, E. (1999). Depressed taste and smell in geriatric patients. *Journal of the American Dental Association, 130,* 1759–65.

Professional Practice

IV

18

Oral Health Promotion with People with Special Needs

Paul Glassman

The changing demographics of our population along with advances in medical and social systems have resulted in the number of people with special needs who need oral health services rising dramatically (U.S. Department of Health and Human Services, 2000). In this context, people with special needs refers to those individuals who have barriers to achieving good oral health primarily because of a disability or medical condition. This includes people who are elderly; people who have disabilities; and those who may also have complex medical, physical, and psychological problems.

People with special needs have more dental disease, more missing teeth, and more difficulty obtaining dental care than other segments of the population (Oral Health America, 2000; Waldman et al., 2000). It is harder for people with special needs to find sources of dental care. Once a source of care is located, it can be more difficult to render dental treatment. Deciding on adequate treatment may require balancing complex medical and social factors and may sometimes require the use of sedative medications or even hospital treatment under general anesthesia. Many people with special needs are dependent on others to locate and arrange for dental treatment. Some caregivers are not themselves aware of the consequences of untreated dental disease and may not be aware of or use procedures known to prevent dental diseases. These factors can result in pain, suffering, and social stigma in these populations beyond that found in other segments of our society (Horowitz et al., 2000; Schriver, 2001).

It is clear that it is far better to prevent dental disease in people with special needs than attempt to treat disease that has already developed, as it is in all populations. However, the difficulty in providing treatment for people with special needs makes this focus on prevention even more imperative in this population.

Even with a focus on prevention, there are challenges with establishing effective preventive practices in people with special needs. As indicated above, many people in these groups are dependent on caregivers to perform preventive practices. Additional challenges may come from the presence of xerostomia, which is a side effect of many psychotropic and other medications used by people in this group. Some people and their caregivers may not understand how to prevent dental disease. Some people have physical problems that make it difficult for them to perform preventive procedures. Some people are resistant to performing these procedures. All these obstacles present challenges to maintaining dental health not experienced by most individuals in our society.

Overcoming Obstacles to Oral Health

Many people have developed techniques and programs to prevent dental disease in people with special needs (Glassman et al., 1994; Miller et al., 1998; CDC, 2001). The training package *Overcoming Obstacles to Dental Health* (Miller et al., 1998) is designed for caregivers of people with disabilities and is organized to address three primary barriers: informational barriers, physical barriers, and behavioral barriers. These materials, which include a videotape, workbook, and trainers manual, incorporate information about oral health and disease, oral hygiene practices, and behavioral interventions. There is an emphasis on developing an individual oral health plan for each individual. There is, in addition, information about the use of chemotherapeutic agents as part of an oral hygiene regimen.

The Pacific Center for Special Care at the University of the Pacific School of Dentistry held a conference in 2002 to examine the use of chemotherapeutic modalities in promoting oral health for people with special needs. This conference resulted in a set of protocols that were published in 2003 (Glassman et al., 2003; Glassman & Miller, 2003). These are described later in this chapter.

Overcoming Barriers

Barriers to prevention of dental disease for people with special needs can be classified into three types: informational, physical, and behavioral. As described in the training materials, *Overcoming Obstacles to Dental Health*, informational barriers include a lack of understanding among individuals and their caregivers about effective practices to prevent dental disease. Given the fact that people with special needs can be dependent upon a caregiver to carry out preventive practices, it is critical that the caregiver as well as the individual understand the causes of dental diseases and techniques for prevention. It is unlikely that caregivers will do more for the individuals they are caring for than they will do for themselves. Therefore caregivers must understand the importance and benefits of oral preventive practices as well as the techniques to accomplish them. Whatever the relationship between the caregiver and the individual being cared for, caregivers can be motivated by the knowledge that good oral health is a part of good general health, that good oral health can make an individual more independent in other areas of life, and that maintaining good oral health can make the life of the caregiver more pleasant as well as the life of the individual being cared for.

Caregivers can be direct-care staff members in a community residential care facility, an LVN in a nursing home, a parent of a child living at home, or many other people. Dental professionals can have an important role in educating these caregivers about the benefits of good oral health and the consequences of poor oral health. Dental professionals can also be important sources of information about techniques and practices that can lead to good oral health. The most effective preventive information education is that which is delivered in a "pyramid" training program where the dental professional trains a home health nurse or a residential facility manager or someone else who can then be responsible for training others in the techniques learned. Such a training program can greatly magnify the effectiveness of the dental professional. The *Overcoming Obstacles* training materials are designed to be used in this pyramid training approach.

Another barrier to prevention of dental disease is physical barriers. Some people understand what needs to be done, but lack the musculature, dexterity, or coordination to do it. For many people, the physical barrier is simply the inability to grasp a toothbrush or to manipulate dental floss. There are numerous adaptations and aids that can help overcome these physical barriers. Figure 18.1 shows toothbrushes that have been adapted with a larger handle using a tennis ball or bicycle handle grip. Figure 18.2 shows someone with limited dexterity using a large foam ball as a means of picking up a toothbrush. Similar adaptation can be made for floss holders. These adapted instruments can be much easier to grip than conventional implements.

People with special needs should be encouraged to do as much as possible for themselves. However, some people need help from caregivers in order to perform oral hygiene procedures. This situation in which the person does as much as possible and the caregiver does what the person cannot do is referred to as "partial participation." For some individuals, the caregiver

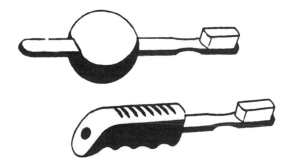

Fig. 18.1. Toothbrushes adapted for easier grip. (© 1998 University of the Pacific School of Dentistry, Department of Dental Practice and Community Services. Reprinted with permission.)

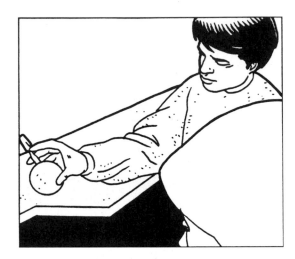

Fig. 18.2. Adapted toothbrush for someone with limited dexterity. (© 1998 University of the Pacific School of Dentistry Department of Dental Practice and Community Services. Reprinted with permission.)

needs to do much of the work. There are several positioning techniques that can make it easier for a caregiver to help someone complete oral hygiene procedures. Figure 18.3 is an illustration of a "tongue blade mouth prop." This type of mouth prop can be easily constructed by a caregiver from readily available materials and can be very useful in helping someone complete oral hygiene procedures. Figure 18.4 shows the use of a tongue blade mouth prop with someone who is sitting on the floor with head resting on the caregiver's shoulders. Note the use of the forefingers of the left and right hand in stabilizing the head. Figure 18.5 again shows the use of a tongue blade mouth prop. This time the individual may be less able to help and is positioned on a couch. Note the use of the right forearm and the tongue blade in stabilizing the head. These positions allow the caregiver to see and gain access to parts of the mouth that would be difficult in other positions. Again, dental professionals can play a pivotal role in educating caregivers about the use of physical adaptations and partial participation.

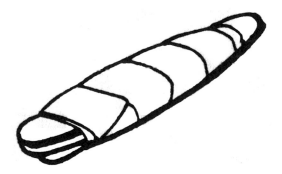

Fig. 18.3. A tongue blade mouth prop. (© 1998 University of the Pacific School of Dentistry Department of Dental Practice and Community Services. Reprinted with permission.)

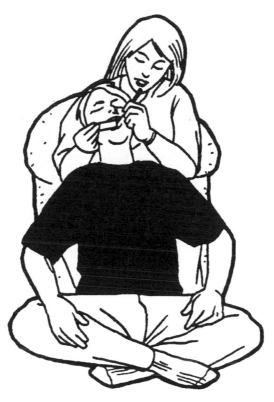

Fig. 18.4. Partial participation—using positioning and a tongue blade mouth prop. (© 1998 University of the Pacific School of Dentistry Department of Dental Practice and Community Services. Reprinted with permission.)

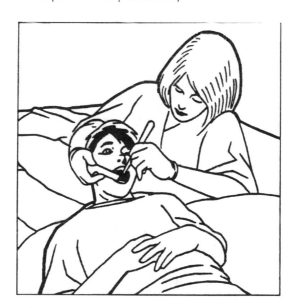

Fig. 18.5. Partial participation—using positioning and a tongue blade mouth prop. (© 1998 University of the Pacific School of Dentistry Department of Dental Practice and Community Services. Reprinted with permission.)

Some people or their caregivers may understand what needs to be done and possess the manual dexterity to do it, but the individual is resistant to participating in oral hygiene procedures or to letting the caregiver help. There are a number of techniques that can be used to overcome these behavioral barriers that are discussed in the *Overcoming Obstacles* training materials. Typically, the role of the dental professional is to work with the caregiver to educate the caregiver about the use of behavioral intervention strategies. Most dental professionals will not be able to be with the individual over the sometimes-extended time that a behavioral intervention program can take.

One technique is referred to as "structuring the environment." This refers to picking a place or time of day that is more conducive to gaining cooperation than other times or places. It may be a place or time where there are minimal distractions. It might include performing oral hygiene procedures in a setting that does not associate it with other unpleasant activities or people, or even better, makes oral hygiene procedures seem fun. In order to structure the environment for a given individual, it is necessary to get to know that individual and determine what type of environment would be conducive to a pleasant oral hygiene session. Caregivers may need to be trained to pay attention to how the individual responds in various environments or with various people present in order to make this determination.

Another technique is called "involving the individual." Many people with special needs, especially in group living or institutional living arrangements, may have very regimented lives. They may be told when to wake up, when to eat, when to use the bathroom, what to wear, and what they will do during the day. They can be most appreciative of anything that a caregiver can do to increase choices, and this in turn can aid cooperation. Increasing choices can be as simple as being able to choose when to brush ones teeth or what color a new toothbrush will be. It also involves counseling the caregiver to pay attention to how the person is doing and not to push him or her so far so that a pleasant oral hygiene session turns into an unpleasant one.

A basic behavioral intervention is the use of reinforcers or reward systems: determining and using reinforcers can be a critical component of a behavioral intervention plan for someone who is resistant to participating in oral health improvement procedures. A reinforcer is something that will result in having the individual want to continue or increase the activity that produced the reward. Caregivers can be educated to realize that carefully applied rewards can motivate people to become more and more independent in oral hygiene practices. As with the other behavioral interventions, it is critical that the caregiver pay attention to the individual and what she or he responds to in order to determine what reward may be reinforcing for them. It is important that the caregiver use things that are actually rewarding for that individual at that given time, monitor the effect of the reward over time, and change it if necessary. Caregivers can be educated to realize that social rewards like smiling and praise can be as powerful for people with special needs as they can for everyone else.

After mastering the idea of selecting and applying rewards, the caregiver can learn to use shaping procedures. Shaping is the reinforcement of an approximation of the task. For example, if the caregiver would like someone to brush for five minutes, she might use a reinforcer after thirty seconds at first. Later, the reinforcer might not be used until one or two minutes have passed. The caregivers must realize how critical it is to make sure that each session is a pleasant one and ends with individuals having a good feeling about themselves and their oral health. This can take coaching from the dental professional and practice on the part of the caregiver.

Caregivers can also learn about the idea of "generalization." For instance, they may be able to work with the individuals to teach them that its okay to have someone put a tongue blade in their mouths to look inside. Later, this may make it easier for the individual to accept help with toothbrushing.

The behavioral interventions described above can be critical for caregivers to master if they are to improve oral health for someone who is resistive to oral hygiene practices. Dental professionals can have an important role in educating caregivers about these behavioral interventions. More information about the techniques described above can be found in the *Overcoming Obstacles to Dental Health* training materials.

Using Chemotherapeutic Agents

The use of chemotherapeutic agents to prevent dental disease has been referred to as the medical model of dental prevention. As mentioned earlier in this chapter, the Pacific Center for Special Care at the University of the Pacific School of Dentistry developed a set of protocols for applying this medical model with people with special needs. An expert panel was convened that developed *Practical Preventive Protocols for Prevention of Dental Disease in People with Special Needs in Community Settings*. Although the use of the agents described in these protocols has been widely studied over many years, these studies typically excluded people with special needs in order to reduce the variables in the study. These agents may need to be used differently with people with special needs than with other individuals. These differences are the result of the need to have protocols that can be used with people who may have trouble fully following traditional oral health recommendations for control of plaque, who may not be able to rinse and spit out oral solutions, and who may need assistance from third parties in carrying out preventive recommendations. In addition, protocols for use with special needs populations must be applicable outside of the dental office in community settings since many people in these population groups have trouble finding dentists willing to see them or getting to dental offices for care. Also, these preventive practices must be applied on a frequent and in some cases a daily basis while visits to a dental office are occasional at best.

The protocols for the use of chemotherapeutic agents contain the following elements:

1. People with special needs should follow certain traditional and widely accepted preventive measures as much as possible for that individual. These fundamental practices include:

- Use of a fluoridated toothpaste accepted by the Council on Dental Therapeutics of the American Dental Association. (After the age of twelve, or when a dental professional finds that gingivitis is present in an individual under twelve years of age, use a fluoridated toothpaste accepted by the American Dental Association Council on Dental Therapeutics that contains an approved effective antigingivitis agent.)
- Effective removal of bacterial plaque using a soft manual or mechanical toothbrush and dental floss
- Daily use of fluoridated water for drinking and cooking (This may require the use of bottled fluoridated water where the community water supply is not optimally or adequately fluoridated.)
- Adopting a healthy diet with an emphasis on reduction of fermentable carbohydrates intake, especially between meals
- Regular professional oral health care including the use of professionally applied topical fluorides and pit and fissure sealants
- Controlling systemic factors that may affect oral health such as cessation and prevention of smoking and use of tobacco products and adequate treatment of systemic diseases that impact oral health such as diabetes

2. Use products containing xylitol (at least 50% by weight) as the predominant sugar with three exposures per day and five minutes per exposure. If xylitol-containing chewing gum can be used, it should be chewed for five minutes three times a day. Chewing may need to be supervised to ensure that the required exposure is achieved. For individuals who cannot chew gum, or where supervised gum chewing is not feasible, other xylitol-containing food products should be substituted. For infants, there are delivery systems that use pacifiers with a xylitol reservoir where a xylitol solution can be placed, or traditional baby bottles with xylitol-containing solutions. For other individuals, dissolving a xylitol-containing lozenge, mint, or lollipop can achieve the desired exposure.

3. Apply fluoride varnish using one of the following regimens. The panel recognizes that the use of fluoride varnish requires some removal of food debris by brushing or wiping off the teeth prior to application. There may be some individuals or circumstances where this is not possible. The selection of the regimen should be based on the feasibility of following that regimen for a given individual.
   - Apply fluoride varnish three times in one week (e.g., Monday, Wednesday, and Friday), once per year.
   - Or, apply fluoride varnish once every six months.

4. For individuals who are not able to fully use the primary preventive interventions described above or for those with persistent decay in spite of the above therapies, fluoride-containing rinses can be of benefit to prevent dental caries. Even if individuals are able to fully use the three primary preventive interventions described above, fluoride-containing rinses may provide an additional source of topical fluoride. Fluoride mouth rinse is currently an optional preventive choice for all people over the age of six who can safely rinse and expectorate without ingestion. The 0.05% NaF_2 fluoride has proven anticaries effects, and these effects are ad-

ditive to the use of fluoride-containing toothpaste. Use a fluoride rinse product that contains 230 ppm fluoride without alcohol. Rinse for one minute twice a day.

If an individual cannot rinse or spit out the solution, then apply the solution with a cotton swab or sponge applicator (Toothette) twice a day. Although the available evidence has not proven that there is an additive effect when 0.05% NaF_2 fluoride rinse is used with a fluoride varnish, such an effect has been demonstrated when used in conjunction with fluoridated toothpaste. A dental professional should be involved in the decision to add fluoride rinses as an intervention for a particular individual if the individual is under the age of six and/or is unable to rinse without ingestion.

5. The use of high-concentration fluoride toothpaste or gel should be considered for individuals where the previous recommendations are not working to adequately prevent dental caries or there is reason to believe that they will not work. One such circumstance could be an individual with xerostomia (dry mouth) resulting from medications, radiation treatment that involves the salivary glands, or other causes. The decision to use these products should also consider the ability of the individual or caregivers to supervise and control the application of these products since they contain concentrations of fluoride that could be toxic if sufficient quantities are ingested. Typically, these products contain 5000 ppm of fluoride, and the recommendation is to brush with the toothpaste or gel before going to sleep at night, spit out the excess, and leave the residual toothpaste or gel on the teeth while sleeping. Water should not be used to rinse out the excess, nor should water be consumed for one hour after use of the gel or toothpaste. Because of the considerations just listed, a dentist should be involved in the decision to add high-concentration fluoride toothpaste or gel as an intervention for a particular individual.

6. For individuals who are not able to fully use the primary preventive interventions described above or for those with persistent decay in spite of those therapies, using a chlorhexidine rinse can be of benefit to help prevent dental caries. Rinse with a half-ounce of chlorhexidine solution for one minute twice a day for two weeks. Repeat this four times a year.

If an individual cannot rinse or spit out the solution, then apply the solution with a cotton swab or sponge applicator (Toothette) twice a day. Because it is not clear that there is added benefit from this procedure for individuals who are able to use the primary protocols listed here, a dentist should be involved in the decision to add chlorhexidine rinses as an intervention for a particular individual.

Since chlorhexidine is more effective at reducing levels of caries producing microorganisms than is exposure to xylitol, for some individuals an initial course of chlorhexidine may be indicated prior to instituting a long-term regimen of xylitol exposure. It should be remembered that chlorhexidine has several side effects including diminution of taste and staining of oral tissues that make it less desirable than some of the other agents described above, especially for individuals who may need long-term therapy.

The Oral Health Care Plan

It is important to have a plan for applying the various techniques and agents described in this chapter. In many circumstances, this plan will need to be communicated among a variety of people. Some people with special needs, particularly those in group and institutional living situations, have numerous caregivers who may be helping them maintain oral health. It is critical that these caregivers understand the strategy being employed for that individual and coordinate their efforts. It is also helpful, even when the caregiver is a parent of an individual living in a family home, to have a specific plan for maintaining oral health. Figure 18.6 is an example of such a plan. This oral health care plan is a part of the *Overcoming Obstacles to Dental Health* training package.

There are several advantages to using a planning and communication document such as the one in figure 18.6. First, it serves to help caregivers organize their thinking about the treatment and preventive measures that are to be used for a particular individual. It helps them to think about specific interventions and measures that address the specific needs of that individual. Second, it acts as a communication vehicle so multiple caregivers can be kept up to date about the current strategies being used. Finally, it acts as a record of progress. If it is periodically updated, then caregivers can look back at old plans to review progress and use the sections of the current plan that act as reminders of future appointments or interventions.

Conclusions

People with special needs have the most dental disease and the least access to treatment services of any segment of our population. Therefore, it is critical that everything possible be done to prevent the occurrence of dental disease in these individuals. This chapter has reviewed strategies for overcoming informational, physical, and behavioral barriers to maintaining oral health. In addition, a summary has been provided of the results of a conference entitled *Practical Preventive Protocols for Prevention of Dental Disease in People with Special Needs in Community Settings*. These strategies and protocols are designed to compliment a system of supported community-based oral health care. The goal of this system is to help people with special needs enjoy a lifetime of oral health the same as other members of our society. Finally, a planning process using an oral health care plan has been described as a means of planning, communicating, and tracking strategies to improve oral health for people with special needs.

ORAL HEALTH CARE PLAN

Name _____ Caregiver Name _____ Date _____

Assessment
    a. Physical problems with oral hygiene: _____
    b. Behavioral problems with oral hygiene: _____

Physical Skills and Aids
    a. Skills being learned: _____
    b. Special aids: ❐ adapted toothbrush ❐ adapted floss holder ❐ electric toothbrush
    c. Schedule for using disclosing tablets: _____

Plan for **Partial Participation** (❐ not needed - person is independent)
    a. Best position for assisting with oral hygiene: ❐ couch, ❐ bean-bag chair, ❐ other: _____
    b. Techniques and/or aids used by caregivers: ❐ mouth prop, ❐ floss holder
    c. What part does caregiver perform: _____

Plan for **Structuring the Environment**
    a. Oral hygiene time and place: _____
    b. Are infection control procedures being used: _____
    c. Who will work with the individual: AM _____ PM _____

Plan for **Engaging the Client**
    a. Choices being offered: _____
    b. Limits the client can set: _____

Plan for **Reinforcers**
    a. What reinforcers are being used currently (e.g. music, book, TV): _____
    _____

Plan for **Shaping**
    a. What steps are being taught: _____
    _____
    b. What level of prompts is currently being used?
       ❐ Physical (hand-over-hand), ❐ Physical (touch), ❐ Pointing, ❐ Verbal

Other Prevention Actions
    a. Xylitol: ❐ 5 minute exposure 3 x / day. Form being used _____
    b. Fluoride varnish: ❐ Applied 2 x/ year. Next time: _____ ❐ Applied 3 times in one week 1 x/ year. Next time: _____
    c. Fluoride rinses: ❐ Person rinses and empties mouth, ❐ Caregiver uses swab technique
    d. High concentration fluoride toothpaste or gel: ❐ How and when to apply _____
    e. Chlorhexidine: ❐ Person rinses and empties mouth, ❐ Caregiver uses swab technique
    f. Diet: ❐ Decrease exposure to sugar and starches: ❐ How _____

Professional visits and recommendations
    a. Last dental cleaning appointment: Date _____ Next appointment date: _____
    b. Next dental check up or treatment appointment: _____

Fig. 18.6. The Oral Health Care Plan. (Pacific Center for Special Care at the University of the Pacific School of Dentistry, 2155 Webster Street, San Francisco, CA 94115; 415-749-3384 © 2002.)

References

CDC. (Nov 30, 2001). *Promoting Oral Health: Interventions for Preventing Dental Caries, Oral and Pharyngeal Cancers, and Sports-Related Craniofacial Injuries: A Report on Recommendations of the Task Force on Community Preventive Services.* CDC, MMWR 50(RR21), 1–13.

Glassman, P., & Miller, C. (2003). Preventing dental disease for people with special needs: the need for practical preventive protocols for use in community settings. *Journal of Special Care in Dentistry, 23(5),* 165–67.

Glassman, P., et al. (2003). Practical protocols for the prevention of dental disease in community settings for people with special needs: the protocols. *Journal of Special Care in Dentistry, 23(5),* 160–64.

Glassman, P., Miller, C., Wozniak, T., & Jones, C. (1994). A preventive dentistry training program for persons with disabilities residing in community residential facilities. *Journal of Special Care in Dentistry, 14(4),* 137–43.

Horwitz, S., Kerker, B., Owens, P., & Zigler, E. (2000). *The Health Status and Needs of Individuals with Mental Retardation.* Special Olympics. Available online at http://www.specialolympics.org/Special+Olympics+Public+Website/English/Initiatives/Research/Health+Status+report.htm

Miller, C., Glassman, P., Wozniak, T., & Gillien, N. (1998). *Overcoming Obstacles to Dental Health—A Training Program for Caregivers of People with Disabilities.* 4th ed. San Francisco, CA: Pacific Center for Special Care.

Oral Health America. (May 2000). *The Disparity Cavity: Filling America's Oral Health Gap.* Available online at http://www.oralhealthamerica.org/pdf/Disparitycavity.pdf

Schriver, T. (March 5, 2001). Testimony before a Special Hearing of a Subcommittee of the Committee on Appropriations of the United States Senate, One Hundred Seventh Congress, First Session. Anchorage, Alaska.

U.S. Department of Health and Human Services. (2000). *Oral Health in America: A Report of the Surgeon General.* Rockville, MD: U.S. Department of Health and Human Services, National Institute of Dental and Craniofacial Research, National Institutes of Health. Available online at http://www.surgeongeneral.gov/library/oralhealth/

Waldman, H. B., Perlman, S. P., & Swerdloff, M. (2000). Use of pediatric dental services in the 1990s: some continuing difficulties. *J Dent Child, 67,* 59–63.

Health Behavior and Dental Care of Diabetics

Mirka C. Niskanen and Matti L. E. Knuuttila

Introduction

There are about 150 million people with diabetes mellitus. The number is expected to rise to 300 million by the year 2025. Especially the prevalence of type 2 diabetes is rapidly increasing, and it also involves young patients. Diabetes mellitus and related complications in the eyes, kidneys, heart, blood vessels, and nerves affect the patients' quality of life, demand considerable medical resources, and cause morbidity. Thus, the effects of diabetes on both a personal level and in the economy as a whole will grow significantly in the future.

It has been shown that oral diseases are associated with diabetes mellitus. Diabetic patients have a two to four times greater risk of suffering from periodontal disease than nondiabetics (Taylor, 2001), and it has been found that diabetics are about five times more likely to be partially edentulous than controls (Moore et al., 1998). Diabetics also have a higher risk of xerostomia and oral mucosal lesions, and they may have impaired wound healing. On the other hand, the relationship is postulated to be two way: periodontitis as a chronic infection might impair metabolic control.

Several plausible biological mechanisms have been presented to explain the observed connection between diabetes and oral health. These are nonenzymatic formation of advanced glycation end products, changes in collagen metabolism, and altered host response. In addition to a causal link brought about by biological mechanisms, it is possible that part of the association is coincidental, which means there might be risk factors in common, such as smoking and other lifestyle factors. Similarly, common psychological factors that affect health behavior in dental and diabetes self-care can give a significant insight into the relationship between diabetes and oral health.

243

Good self-care is essential to maintain a good state of health, and therefore every effort must be made to remove obstacles to optimal self-care. Knowledge about oral diseases among diabetic patients is poor (Sandberg, Sundberg, & Wikblad, 2001), and diabetic patients require regular checkups and special attention by the dental profession. In order to have an impact on the behavioral aspects of diabetic patients' self-care practices, the whole dental appointment situation should be made safe and confidential. This means that dentists must be able to assess and prevent medical risks for diabetics as dental patients. To ensure good health-care results, dental professionals need to be conscious of the special needs of diabetics as dental patients. On the whole, close collaboration between diabetics, dental practitioners, and other health-care professionals is called for. This would allow them to share the responsibility for good health behavior in oral care and diabetes, making it possible to understand that oral health is an integral part of general health.

Diabetes Mellitus and Oral Diseases

There is epidemiological and clinical evidence that diabetes mellitus is a risk factor for periodontal diseases. More gingival bleeding, depth periodontal pockets, and extensive alveolar bone loss have been found in diabetic patients than in nondiabetics. However, diabetics are a very heterogenic group, and it is important to recognize those diabetic features that, as risk indicators, determine the association between diabetes and oral health (Taylor, 2001).

Research has shown that poor metabolic control (Tsai, Hayes, & Taylor, 2002), long duration of disease (Hugoson et al., 1989), and diabetic organ complications (Tervonen & Karjalainen, 1997) seems to be significant in making the periodontal disease worse. It has been proposed that a number of diabetes-related biologic changes can also increase the risk of periodontitis. These are impaired polymorphonuclear leukocyte function, decreased collagen synthesis, increased collagenase activity, glycosylating of proteins, and induced synthesis of cytokines, for example (Soskolne, 1998; Lalla et al., 2000).

Whether diabetics have an increased risk of dental caries is not clear. Some studies have found a higher occurrence of caries among diabetics than nondiabetics (Pohjamo et al., 1991; Jones et al., 1992; Karjalainen, Knuuttila, & Kaar, 1997; Twetman et al., 1992), while others showed no difference between the two (Swanljung et al., 1992; Moore et al., 2001). Some studies have even found less caries among diabetics than nondiabetics (Kirk & Kinirons, 1991). Furthermore, it is not clear whether there is an association between metabolic control and dental caries. Despite conflicting studies, the possibility cannot be excluded that poor metabolic control, salivary gland hypofunction, and high crevicular fluid glucose concentrations may increase the risk of dental caries in diabetics.

Other oral diseases related to diabetes are xerostomia and fungal infections. An increased risk of oral mucosal lesions, such as fissured tongue, irritation fibromas, traumatic ulcers, oral leukoplakia, and lichen planus, has been observed among diabetics. A link between diabetes and taste impairment and burning mouth syndrome has also been suggested.

Health Behavior

Oral Health Behavior

The main etiologic factor for periodontal diseases is microbial dental plaque with a biofilm structure. It has been demonstrated that good plaque control by the patients themselves is effective in preventing periodontal disease. However, supragingival plaque control alone is not sufficient. Professional mechanical subgingival biofilm and dental calculus removal is also necessary. Thus, controlling the plaque level and regular dental maintenance are essential for the prevention and treatment of periodontal diseases. As far as dental caries are concerned, microbial plaque and sugar in the diet are two major etiologic factors. Therefore, tooth brushing twice a day with fluoride toothpaste and avoiding sugar are effective ways of preventing dental caries.

Diabetes may lead to greater periodontal tissue destruction. Controlling causal etiological factors, such as plaque and calculus, is therefore significant. Whether diabetes predisposes to dental caries is not clear, but what is clear is that diet factors are of great importance to both of these diseases. Another reason for dental professionals to ensure that diabetic patients acquire proper knowledge and skills to perform oral hygiene practices is because a higher incidence of plaque has been detected among diabetics than nondiabetics (Bridges et al., 1996; Sandberg et al., 2000).

A number of studies have compared oral health behaviors between diabetic and nondiabetic patients, but only a few have included all self-care practices. Some of the oral health behavior studies include only diabetic patients, and moreover, the criteria for good oral health behavior vary. Comparisons between different studies is therefore difficult, but the results presented in table 19.1 give a general idea of oral health behavior among diabetics.

In the case of dental visits, Pohjamo et al. (1995) found that diabetics tend to miss more dental appointments than do nondiabetics. Diabetics require more emergency dental care than do nondiabetics (Thorstensson et al., 1989), and insulin dependent diabetes mellitus (IDDM) patients with poor metabolic control or diabetes-related complications visit the dentist less regularly than other diabetics (Karjalainen, Knuuttila, & von Dickhoff, 1994). It is observed that while diabetics were regular about their visits to the diabetes clinic, there were problems with the recommended dental treatment (Karikoski, Ilanne-Parikka, & Murtomaa, 2003). All in all, according to most of the studies, there are no major differences in oral self-care practices between diabetics and nondiabetics. Diabetics brush their teeth slightly less frequently than do nondiabetics, while interdental cleaning seems to be irregular in both groups. Instead, there were differences in how regular dental visits are, with diabetics showing more problems with attendance.

In conclusion, improved oral-health behavior is needed among all diabetics, and it should be focused particularly on patients with poor metabolic balance and complications. The aim is that health behavior of diabetics be-

Table 19.1 Oral Health Behaviors Among Diabetes Mellitus Patients and Possible Controls

	DM	Control	Brushing (%) DM	Brushing (%) Control	Interdental cleaning (%) DM	Interdental cleaning (%) Control	Dental visits (%) DM	Dental visits (%) Control
Thorstensson et al., 1989	152	77	88/75 (t) s/l	89	46/31 (d) s/l	30	11/17 (irreg)	3
Jones et al., 1992	202/107	706	94 (≥d)	83	—	—	61	45
Spangler & Konen, 1994	81/309	—	74/4 (t)	—	34/30 (d)	—	81/59 (a)	—
Collin et al., 1998	25	40	80 (d)	90	—	—	28% (a)	43
Syrjälä et al., 1999	149	—	50 (t)	—	15 (d)	—	54% (a)	—
Moore et al., 2000	390	202	72 (t)	80	33 (w)	30	69 (a)	76
Sandberg et al., 2001	102	102	91 (d)	94	52 (d)	60	15 (irreg)	5
Karikoski et al., 2002	258	—	38 (t)	—	27 (d)	—	66 (≤a)	—

Note: s = short-term diabetes mellitus; l = long-term diabetes mellitus; d = daily; t = twice a day; w = weekly; a = annually; irreg = irregularly.

come even better than that of others because diabetes itself is a predisposing risk factor for periodontal infections.

Diabetes Health Behavior

The purpose of daily self-care is to keep the level of blood glucose as close to normoglycemia as possible. Patients' self-care practices are indeed a crucial part of maintaining good metabolic control. Poor self-care causes poor long-term metabolic control, and this may lead to the development of diabetic complications. These consist of microangiopathic complications, such as retinopathy and nephropathy, neuropathy and a variety of macrovascular changes because of arteriosclerosis. This, in turn, increases the risk of stroke, myocardial infarction, and gangrene. Periodontal disease has also been regarded as one of the complications of diabetes.

The Diabetes Control and Complications Trial Research Group (1993) has shown that optimal blood glucose control delays and prevents diabetic complications. Indeed, any improvement in glycemic control among type 2 diabetics reduces the risk of diabetic complications. Numerous other studies have found that good self-care practices and proper adherence to the recommendations are associated with good HbA1$_c$ levels, but there is also evidence that appropriate self-care does not always guarantee a good metabolic balance. This is because various factors affect blood glucose levels: differences in insulin absorption, insulin sensitivity, exercise, stress, food absorption, hormonal changes, illnesses, and travelling (American Diabetes Association, 1998a, 1998b).

There are various terms to describe patients' own treatment practices. The term "self-management" emphasizes the responsibility of the patient, while "adherence" is defined as the level at which patients follow the regimens established by patient and health-care professionals. It has been suggested that adherence is a suitable term to describe optimal diabetes care (McNabb, 1997). Compliance, in turn, means only strict observance of instructions. Self-care can be either strict adherence to regimens or active self-care. Active self-care means self-monitoring, dietary and insulin adjustments for daily purposes, and regular exercise.

Diabetes self-care practices consist of:

- Insulin injections and adjustment of dosage—physiologically based injections
- Self-monitoring by blood glucose measurements—at least three to four times a day
- Dietary instructions—optimal serum lipid levels and calorie intake
- Regular exercise—improve cardiovascular fitness and lipoprotein profile, reduce blood pressure
- Regular foot care assessments—prevention and care of changes
- Smoking avoidance
- Good oral health—brushing teeth twice a day, daily interdental cleaning, regular dental attendance

Regular visits to diabetes care units are recommended to monitor metabolic control and intervene in the progression of complications. It has been

Table 19.2   Good Adherence to Diabetes Self-Care Practices

	Insulin (%)	Glucose testing (%)	Diet (%)	Exercise (%)	Not smoking (%)	Weight regulation (%)
Glasgow et al., 1987	92	70	—	—	—	—
Hanestad & Albrektsen, 1991	90	—	51	46	32	42
Hentinen & Kyngäs, 1992	84 adult 72 adolescent	28	11	—	—	—
Toljamo, 1999	—	—	23	35	65	—
Kneckt et al., 2000	64	47	39	41	—	—
Lerman, 2004	78	—	58	44	—	—
Chang, 2005	9	—	64	40	—	22

shown that infrequent attenders have more complications and poorer metabolic balance than regularly visiting patients (Griffin, 1998). The occurrence of missed diabetes control appointments varies considerably between studies, from 4% to 40%. The results of some recent studies on diabetes self-care practices are shown in table 19.2.

There are many reasons for inadequate diabetes self-care. Self-care is complex and requires commitment and specific lifestyle changes. Factors affecting diabetes self-care involve beliefs about benefits, reliability of regimens, stress, lack of time and support, being away from home, living alone, and fear of hypoglycemia. It has been observed that knowledge, social demands, and personal preferences and barriers at home or while shopping affect diet adherence in particular. Factors associated with diabetics' nonattendance consist of the patients' health beliefs and attitudes, the organization of the clinic, the costs of attendance, and the degree of patient participation. All in all, health-care professionals should be aware of the possible psychological barriers when setting treatment goals and developing plans to reach them.

Health Behavior Models

Health behavior is complex and affected by various psychological features, which have been explained by various complementary theoretical models. Since it might be possible to impact the significant psychological features, it is important to identify them. It is also important to recognize whether health behaviors are unidimensional or multidimensional. Unidimensionality implies that an individual who adheres to good health practice in one health behavior will probably act similarly toward other health behaviors, too. By contrast, the concept of multidimensionality means that some health behaviors occur together, while others are independent (Patterson, Haines, & Popkin, 1994).

Some studies have found a behavioral relationship between oral health and diabetes self-care by analyzing them by means of different psychological theories. It has been found that the perception of self-efficacy (Bandura,

1977) is a significant psychological feature affecting both oral and diabetes health behaviors, also showing overlapping relations between them (Kneckt et al., 1999b; Syrjälä, Kneckt, & Knuuttila, 1999). Self-efficacy in other self-care practices have been found to relate to health status of other areas too (Kneckt et al., 1999b). Self-esteem (Rosenberg, 1965) seems to be a psychological feature that influences certain specific practices of dental and diabetes care, namely tooth brushing and physical exercise (Kneckt et al., 2001). High self-esteem is seen to be important for good motivation and self-confidence. In Weiner's attribution theory (Weiner, 1985), relationships and similarities between attributions for success and failure in oral health and the status of diabetes were observed (Kneckt, Syrjälä, & Knuuttila, 2000). Using locus of control to explain health behavior or health status is not convincing (Kneckt, Syrjälä, & Knuuttila, 1999a).

The results can give insight into possible unidimensionality between oral and diabetes health behaviors. A similarity between the two health behaviors can be seen among some individuals, but they can also be distinct behaviors. On the whole, health education should be based on identifying and enhancing the psychological features affecting patients' health behavior. Knowledge about common psychological features should be applied in practice by health professionals.

Diabetics as Dental Patients

In order to be able to have an impact on the behavioral aspects of diabetics' self-care practices, the whole dental appointment situation should be made safe and confidential. Doctor-patient relationships require continuity. This section provides tools to assess and prevent medical risks for diabetics dental patients.

Emergency Situations

Diabetes-related emergencies are hypo- and hyperglycemia. Hypoglycemia is an acute, rapidly progressive life-threatening condition mainly among insulin-dependent diabetics. It results from insulin overdosage or lack of food intake. A variety of symptoms exist: problems with conversation, incoherence, lethargy, uncooperativeness, mood changes, hunger, nausea, sweating, tachycardia, stomach symptoms, and cold and wet skin. Without treatment, the patient loses consciousness and experiences seizures. Hyperglycemia, instead, is not acutely life threatening. It is caused by neglect of insulin therapy or by increased need for insulin. Symptoms include thirst, hunger, and urination with significant weight loss a couple of days before a hyperglycemic emergency. Other symptoms are itching, fatigue, headache, abdominal pain, nausea, vomiting, and mental stupor. After a long period of hyperglycemia, physical weakness; acetone breath; hot, dry skin; and bright red face can develop. Respiration becomes deep and rapid, the patient has tachycardia and hypotension. Eventually, hyperglycemia can lead to diabetic coma (Nunn, 2000).

The main difference is that a hypoglycemic person has cold and wet skin and manifests bizarre behavior, while a hyperglycemic patient has a hot and dry appearance and acetone breath. Until an exact diagnosis is been made, the patient should be treated as a hypoglycemic patient, because hypoglycemia can rapidly cause unconsciousness. Oral carbohydrates (sugared drink, honey, etc.) are given to cooperating patients. If the patient has an insulin pump and the diagnosis is not clear, the pump should be turned to suspend mode. Emergency services should be summoned if the patient loses consciousness or recovery does not take place. A subcutaneous glucagons injection and/or parental carbohydrate is administered to unconscious hypoglycemic patients. Above all, where diabetic patients are treated, there should also be proper tools for emergency situations, in other words, at least glucometers and oral carbohydrates. Moreover, general information on further emergency organization should be available.

Special Features of Treatment

The American Society of Anesthesiology (ASA) has developed a physical status classification system that also deals with diabetics (Malamed, 2000). Patients with well-controlled diabetes have minimal risk during treatment, whereas patients with uncontrolled diabetes are subject to significant medical risk during treatment. These patients should not be given dental treatment until their diabetes is under control. Each patient must be evaluated by type of medication and level of metabolic control.

Diabetic hypoglycemia can be prevented by discussing insulin intake before dental treatment. The best time for a dental appointment depends on the type of insulin (administration method, onset, peak time, duration of action). The best way is to adhere to the patient's individual life routines when scheduling dental appointments. Diabetes patients should bring their own glucometers with them and take blood glucose before treatment.

Diet control, blood sugar control, antibiotics, and stress reduction have to be addressed separately with each patient. Dental treatment can be a stressful situation and thus can increase the need for insulin. Stress reduction by pain control, premedication, and analgesia is essential. In every case, appointments should be as efficient as possible. Among well- and moderately well-controlled diabetes patients, prophylactic antibiotic is prescribed only when it would be prescribed to a nondiabetic patient. By contrast, antibiotic coverage should be considered among uncontrolled diabetes patients. Poorly controlled patients are advised to improve their control of blood glucose before surgery if it is possible to wait. After stressful dental treatment, the blood glucose level should be checked at least four times a day for several days (Malamad, 2000).

Recommendations to Dental Professionals

The following seven points summarize our recommendations to dental professionals:

- Be aware of the two-way relationship between dental health and diabetes: periodontitis as a chronic infection might have a negative impact on metabolic control and poorly controlled diabetes, and diabetic complications increase the risk of periodontal infections.

- Dentists might be able to detect undiagnosed diabetes while treating periodontal patients with abnormal responses to plaque, delayed wound healing, and lack of resolution of disease after conventional treatment. Dentists play an important role in counseling of patients on dietary factors and in motivating patients to stop smoking.
- Frequent dental visits are highly recommended for diabetic patients. For patients with poor metabolic control, diabetic complications, or reduced salivary gland function, dental visits about every three months may be advisable.
- Improved oral hygiene is significant for all diabetics but should be stressed particularly to patients with poor metabolic balance and complications. Other special groups are children and adolescents.
- When treating a diabetic as dental patient, determine the medical risks relating to the dental appointment and ensure that there are proper tools for emergency situations, in other words that there are at least glucometers and oral carbohydrates available. Find out about emergency organization in advance.
- Be aware of sensitiveness to infections especially among poorly controlled diabetics. Hence, be careful to provide a sterile and antitraumatic dental treatment and use prophylactic antibiotics.
- As a dental practitioner, make an effort to create collaboration between diabetic patients and other health-care professionals. Informing and educating nurses who deal with diabetes of dental issues benefits the patients. Medical professionals should share the responsibility for good health behavior in oral and diabetes care.

References

American Diabetes Association. (1998a). Nutrition recommendations and principles for people with diabetes mellitus. Position Statement. *Diabetes Care, 21,* S32–S35.

——. (1998b). Tests of glycemia in diabetes. Position Statement. *Diabetes Care, 21,* S69–S71.

Bandura, A. (1977). Self-efficacy: toward a unifying theory of behavioral change. *Psychological Review, 84,* 191–215.

Bridges, R. B., Anderson, J. W., Saxe, S. R., Gregory, K., & Bridges, S. R. (1996). Periodontal status of diabetic and non-diabetic men: effects of smoking, glycemic control, and socioeconomic factors. *Journal of Periodontology, 67,* 1185–92.

Chang, H. Y., Chiou, C. J., Lin, M. C., & Tai, T. Y. (2005). A population study of the self-care behaviours and their associated factors of diabetes in Taiwan: results from the 2001 National Health Interview Survey in Taiwan. *Preventive Medicine, 40,* 344–48.

Diabetes Control and Complications Trial Research Group. (1993). The effect of intensive treatment of diabetes on the development and progression of long-term complications in insulin-dependent diabetes mellitus. *New England Journal of Medicine, 329,* 977–86.

Glasgow, R. E., McCaul, K. D., & Schafer, L. C. (1987). Self-care behaviours and glycemic control in type 1 diabetes. *Journal of Chronic Disease, 40,* 399–412.

Griffin, S. J. (1998). Lost to follow-up: the problem of defaulters from diabetes clinics. *Diabetes Medicine, 15,* S14–S24.

Hanestad, B. R., & Albrektsen, G. (1991). Quality of life, perceived difficulties in adherence to a diabetes regimen, and blood glucose control. *Diabetes Medicine, 8,* 759–64.

Hentinen, M., & Kyngäs, H. (1992). Compliance of young diabetics with health regimens. *Journal of Advanced Nursing, 17,* 530–36.

Jones, R. B., McCallum, R. M., Kay, E. J., Kirkin, V., & McDonald, P. (1992). Oral health and oral health behaviour in a population of diabetic outpatient clinic attenders. *Community Dentistry and Oral Epidemiology, 20,* 204–7.

Karikoski, A., Ilanne-Parikka, P., & Murtomaa, H. (2002). Oral self-care among adults with diabetes in Finland. *Community Dentistry and Oral Epidemiology, 30,* 216–23.

——. (2003). Oral health promotion among adults with diabetes in Finland. *Community Dentistry Oral Epidemiology, 31,* 447–53.

Karjalainen, K. M., Knuuttila, M. L., & Kaar, M. L. (1997). Relationship between caries and level of metabolic balance in children and adolescent with insulin-dependent diabetes mellitus. *Caries Research, 31,* 13–18.

Karjalainen, K. M., Knuuttila, M. L. E., & von Dickhoff, K. J. (1994). Association of the severity of periodontal disease with organ complications in type 1 diabetic patients. *Journal of Periodontology 65,* 1067–72.

Kirk, J. M., & Kinirons, M. J. (1991). Dental health of young insulin dependent diabetic subjects in Northern Ireland. *Community Dental Health, 8,* 335–41.

Kneckt, M. C., Syrjälä, A-M. H., & Knuuttila, M. L. E. (1999a). Locus of control beliefs predicting oral and diabetes health behavior and health status. *Acta Odontologica Scandinavica, 57,* 127–31.

——. (2000). Attributions to dental and diabetes health outcomes. *Journal of Clinical Periodontology, 27,* 205–11.

Kneckt, M. C., Syrjälä, A-M. H., Laukkanen, P., & Knuuttila, M. L. E. (1999b). Self-efficacy as a common variable in oral health behavior and diabetes adherence. *European Journal of Oral Sciences, 107,* 89–96.

Kneckt, M. C., Keinänen-Kiukaanniemi, S. M., Knuuttila, M. L. E., & Syrjälä, A-M. H. (2001). Self-esteem as a characteristic of adherence with diabetes and dental self-care regimens. *Journal of Clinical Periodontology, 28,* 175–80.

Lalla, E., Lamster, I. B., Drury, S., Fu, C., & Schmidt, A. M. (2000). Hyperglycemia, glycoxidation and receptor for advanced glycation endproducts: potential mechanisms underlying diabetic complications, including diabetes-associated periodontitis. *Periodontology 2000, 23,* 50–62.

Lerman, I., Lozano, L., Villa, A. R., Hernández-Jiménez, S., Weinger, K., Caballero, A. E., Salinas, C. A., Velasco, M. L., Gómez-Pérez, F. J., & Rull, J. A. (2004). Psychological factors associated with poor diabetes self-care management in a specialized center in Mexico City. *Biomedicine & Pharmacotherapy, 58,* 566–70.

Malamed, S. F. (2000). *Medical Emergencies in the Dental Office.* 5th ed. St. Louis: Mosby.

McNabb, W. L. (1997). Adherence in diabetes: can we define it and can we measure it? *Diabetes Care, 20,* 215–18.

Moore, P. A., Orchard, T., Guggenheimer, J., & Weyant, R. J. (2000). Diabetes and oral health promotion. A survey of disease prevention behaviours. *Journal of the American Dental Association, 131,* 1333–41.

Moore, P. A., Weyant, R. J., Etzel, K. R., Guggenheimer, J., Mongelluzzo, M. B., Myers, D. E., Rossie, K., Hubar, H., Block, H. M., & Orchard, T. (2001). Type 1 diabetes mellitus and oral health: assessment of coronal and root caries. *Community Dentistry and Oral Epidemiology, 29,* 183–94.

Moore, P. A., Weyant, R. J., Mongelluzzo, M. B., Myers, D. E., Rossie, K., Guggenheimer, J., Hubar, H., Block, H. M., & Orchard T. (1998). Type 1 diabetes mellitus and oral health: assessment of tooth loss and edentulism. *Journal of Public Health Dentistry, 58,* 135–42.

Nunn, P. (2000). Medical emergencies in the oral health care setting. *Journal of Dental Hygiene, 74,* 136–55.

Patterson, R. E., Haines, P. S., & Popkin, B. M. (1994). Health lifestyle patterns of U.S. adults. *Preventive Medicine, 23,* 453–60.

Pohjamo, L., Tervonen, T., Knuuttila, M., & Nurkkala, H. (1991). Adult diabetic and nondiabetic subjects as users of dental services. A longitudinal study. *Acta Odontologica Scandinavica, 53,* 112–14.

Rosenberg, M. (1965). *Society and the Adolescent Self-Image.* Princeton, NJ: Princeton University Press.

Sandberg, G. E., Sundberg, H. E., & Wikblad, K. F. (2001). A controlled study of oral self-care and self-perceived oral health in type 2 diabetic patients. *Acta Odontologica Scandinavica, 59,* 28–33.

Sandberg, G. E., Sundberg, H. E., Fjellstom, C. A., & Wikblad, K. F. (2000). Type 2 diabetes and oral health: a comparison between diabetic and non-diabetic subjects. *Diabetes Research and Clinical Practice, 50,* 27–34.

Soskolne, W. A. (1998). Epidemiological and clinical aspects of periodontal disease in diabetics. *Annals of Periodontology, 3,* 3–12.

Spangler, J. G., & Konen, J. C. (1994). Oral health behaviors in medical patients with diabetes mellitus. *Journal of Dental Hygiene, 68,* 287–93.

Syrjälä, A. M., Kneckt, M. C., & Knuuttila, M. L. E. (1999). Dental self-efficacy as a determinant to oral health behaviour, oral hygiene and HbA1c level among diabetic patients. *Journal of Clinical Periodontology, 26,* 616–21.

Taylor, G. W. (2001). Bidirectional interrelationships between diabetes and periodontal diseases: an epidemiologic perspective. *Annals of Periodontology, 6,* 99–112.

Tervonen, T., & Karjalainen, K. (1997). Periodontal disease related to diabetic status: a pilot study of the response to periodontal therapy in type 1 diabetes. *Journal of Clinical Periodontology, 24,* 505–10.

Thorstensson, H., Falk, H., Hugoson, A., & Kuylenstierna, J. (1989). Dental care habits and knowledge of oral health in insulin-dependent diabetics. *Scandinavian Journal of Dental Research, 97,* 207–15.

Toljamo, M. (1999). Insuliinihoitoisten diabeetikkojen omahoito. *Acta University Ouluensis. D,* 504.

Tsai, C., Hayes, C., & Taylor G. W. (2002). Glycemic control of type 2 diabetes and severe periodontal disease in the US adult population. *Community Dentistry and Oral Epidemiology, 30,* 182–92.

Twetman, S., Nederfors, T., Stahl, B., & Aronson, S. (1992). Two-year longitudinal observations of salivary status and dental caries in children with insulin-dependent diabetes mellitus. *Pediatric Dentistry, 14,* 184–88.

Weiner, B. (1985). An attributional theory of achievement motivation and emotion. *Psychological Review, 92,* 548–73.

Interpersonal Communication Training in Dental Education

Toshiko Yoshida and Kazuhiko Fujisaki

Good communication is a window for understanding patients and a basis for providing better patient care. When patients are interviewed in a way that that makes them feel understood, their problems and concerns are well expressed. If dental health professionals comprehend precisely the patient's problems and concerns, they become more capable of responding to the patient's needs. As a result, an accurate diagnosis and an appropriate treatment plan will be achieved. It is therefore important for dental health professionals to learn and acquire effective interpersonal communication skills. In this chapter, we will refer to development, implementation, and evaluation of a successful training program focusing on utilizing simulated patients.

Effective interpersonal communication plays an important role in dental care, and has positive effects on outcomes. Existing literature suggests that effective dentist-patient communication increases patient satisfaction and compliance, and reduces patient anxiety and the risk of malpractice claims. Patient satisfaction appears to relate to the dentist's communication style. Street (1989) found that patients with higher satisfaction perceived their dentists as more attentive, responsive, and perceptive. Corah, et al. (1988) reported that dentists' empathy and communicativeness were important correlates of patient satisfaction.

Effective communication tends to make patients more cooperative and compliant. Klages, Sergl, and Burucker (1992) found that the dentist's encouraging behavior induced the patient to participate in a discussion. Sandell, Camner, and Sarhed (1994) indicated that establishing sympathy and informal relationships between the dentist and the patient contribute to attendance at follow-up sessions. *How* to communicate with patients is also related to reduction of dental anxiety. Explaining the procedures prior to treatment reduces the patient's level of fear (Soh, 1992) and the dentist's calm manner and reassurance for less pain helps to reduce patient anxiety (Corah et al., 1988).

Malpractice complaints seem to be associated with interpersonal communication with patients. Mellor and Milgrom (1995) explored dentists' dissatisfaction with the patients, and found a relationship between the dentists who experienced malpractice complaints and the lack of communication with their patients. Frustrating encounters with patients were more likely to lead to malpractice claims (Milgrom et al., 1996).

Compared to other doctor-patient encounters, dental consultations allow practitioners a better chance to observe and palpate directly the disease sites, often followed by surgical treatment. As a result, dental practitioners tend to rely less on the patient's subjective complaints, and verbal communication with the patient is too often restricted during dental treatment. Because of the nature of dental treatment services, more effective communication skills are needed for dental health professionals.

Interpersonal Communication Training in Education

Teaching patient-doctor (dentist) communication has been traditionally incorporated in clinical rounds both in medicine and dentistry where an excellent opportunity exists for the students to learn communication skills and clinical skills at the same time. Nevertheless, it appears that the students are less likely to have their patient interview monitored and to receive the benefit of feedback from the busy faculty. Mere repetition of skills without appropriate feedback cannot be expected to predictably lead to improvement. A survey conducted by the Association of American Medical Colleges (1999) indicated that in the current system there is a lack of structured framework that allows students to focus on communication. A recent survey revealed that in dentistry, the communication curriculum still lacks a system of exposing students to communication skills in a step-by-step fashion (Yoshida, Milgrom, & Coldwell, 2002).

The situation in Japan is much worse. It is assumed that the ability of interpersonal communication is an inborn trait, so that less attention is paid to learning and teaching communication skills. This has led to a poor theoretical background in communication education. The tendency to make much of manual techniques has also brought with it a neglect of effective communication in dental care. Students simply observe the way their superiors communicate with patients without receiving any formal teaching or guidance.

In recent years, more educators and practitioners have begun to realize the importance of interpersonal communicative competence among healthcare providers. A section on communication skills assessment was included rather abruptly in the Objective Structured Clinical Examination (OSCE), which is going to be required of medical and dental students. The sudden change in the exam format has made educators aware of the importance of providing communication training to their students and, as a consequence, the need to start searching for effective educational methods.

Factors Influencing the Design of Interpersonal Communication Training

A number of factors influence the development of communication training:

1. The learner's need and readiness and the level of the learner (from novice to expert) affect the design of a training program that can range from basic to advanced.

2. Goal setting that includes desirable interpersonal communication training to improve the trainee's knowledge, attitudes, and skills to be effective in clinical situations is critical. Successful training should help the trainee not only to expand the amount of knowledge but also to integrate the knowledge into problem solving to perform an appropriate task. The training design will be affected by any of the three components (knowledge, attitudes, and skills) that are emphasized. For these reasons, the goals need to be determined and adjusted for the student's level of training and proficiency.

3. An appropriate teaching method must be guided by the specific goal of a given training session. Passive instruction, such as a lecture, is suitable for information transmission, while performance-based methods should be included if the goal is to improve attitudes and personal behavior. Performance-based methods, such as role-playing and live-patient simulations, were recently introduced and have been increasingly employed in teaching, in place of passive instructions.

4. Resources including computer technology and audiovisual aids such as computer-based simulation and videotapes can be powerful training tools for problem-based learning. A small room with a one-way mirror may help the participants decrease the tension of being observed, and facilitates concentrating on being part of the simulation. Manuscripts for case studies and books/handouts for a lecture are also one of the invaluable factors for communication training. For appropriate staffing, it is recommended to have cooperation from facilitators with behavioral science/communication background and specific health professionals (Dickson, Hargie, & Morrow, 1997). While a sufficient number of staff is desirable, for live-patient simulations, the availability of simulated patients is critical.

5. Evaluation of performance, as Dickson et al. (1997) noted, is essential. *What* needs to be measured as well as *how* to undertake the measurement should be taken into consideration. What needs to be measured is tied to learning objectives. If the trainees are expected to improve mainly their cognitive aspects, any pencil-and-paper type of evaluation, such as quizzes, essays, and questionnaires, is applicable. The trainees' problem-solving ability can be assessed by an examination that requires written responses to a specific videotaped interview or printed dialogue. However, what the trainees *think* they should do is not necessarily the same as how they actually behave, supporting the preference for performance-based examinations when the goal is to acquire skills and to improve interpersonal behaviors.

Performance-Based Methodologies: Role-Playing and Live-Patient Simulation

Some trainees find role-playing a simulation difficult. Sometimes they are embarrassed because they consider it artificial and are afraid of exposing their incompetence to others. However, a compensatory benefit of this method is that it encourages the learners to be critical of their own performance, and permits them to be exposed to such experiences in a safe environment. A role-playing exercise allows the performers to understand the patient's perspective by putting themselves in the patient's position. If feedback from another person is available, the performers will realize and identify their own shortcomings so they can adjust their behavior to meet the needs. These experiences prove to be more appealing to students than a simple lecture.

Communication education and training programs using non-computer-simulated/standardized patients (SP) have been reported both in the United States and Japan (Johnson and Kopp, 1996; Yoshida, Itadani, & Shimono, 1999) as were evaluation studies of such programs (Logan et al., 1999; Yoshida et al., 2001). Ever since the SP was selected for use at some locations for the OSCE, the SP simulation methodology has attracted unexpected and considerable attention. The SP appears to be one of the most influential educational tools, and its use has gradually spread in Japan.

Background History of the SP as a Tool in Medical and Dental Education

The simulated/standardized patient (SP) is a layperson who is trained to portray the medical history as well as the psychological and social background of an actual patient case. The standardized patient is often distinguished from the simulated patient. The difference between them is whether the acting is standardized. The standardized patient is mainly used for assessment, and is expected to give consistent responses to the examinee's reactions. Both verbal and behavioral responses are strictly controlled. On the other hand, the *manner* in which the simulated patient provides information depends on the encounter situation between the patient and the health provider.

First reported by Barrows and Abrahamson (1964), the simulated patient was popular throughout the 70s in the United States. However, it was mainly for demonstration purposes, and few institutions used SP for assessment purposes. In the 1980s, the promise for assessing clinical competence of doctors and medical students by the SP methodology became widely recognized, along with objective assessment methods such as the OSCE (Harden, & Gleeson, 1979) with its primary focus on assessment (Coggan, Knight, & Davis, 1980; Stillman et al., 1986). As of 2004, the OSCE was established as the United States Medical Licensing Examination, and the SP became an essential part of medical education. The first utilization of the SP in dentistry, however, was not until 1990 (Johnson, Kopp, & Williams) and it was later introduced in teaching (Stilwell & Reisine, 1992). Although a gradual increase of interest in this type of method was noted, it was less popular to teach communication skills by the SP method in dental education than in medical education.

In Japan, the SP first appeared in dental education to teach interview and communication skills about ten years later than in the United States (Mataki et al., 1998). The growing patient demand for dentist's communication competence and an increasing risk of malpractice forced dental professionals to apply a new educational methodology. Because of the introduction of OSCE, the SP is currently used more in assessment than in training.

What Is the Benefit of SP Methodology?

Barrows proposed nine educational advantages of the SP (Uemura, 1984):

1. It can be used at any place and any time.
2. It can be used repeatedly.
3. The same patient settings can always be used.
4. The situations and conditions for a simulation can be adjusted.
5. Discussion concerning the patient is possible immediately after the simulation.
6. There is no harm to real patients.
7. Students can practice without anxiety.
8. Feedback from the SP is provided.
9. There are no time constraints.

An essential feature of SP is that it can be adapted for repeated presentations in training, where there is a high risk of mistakes to occur. Discussion immediately following the simulation helps to identify the troubling problem. Feedback from the SP as a recipient of medical services is a very important part of this practice, unlike role-playing that occurs only with medical peers.

There are several significant aspects that are helpful in understanding the dynamic of the laypersons' participation in the role of SP (Fujisaki, 2002). Above all, the participation of nonprofessionals greatly improves the student's attitude toward studying, since unlike lecturers with familiar faces, SPs are ordinary people who rarely come into a classroom. This fosters greater attentiveness and challenges students to behave politely to members of society who would not compromise easily, leading to effective learning. In addition, the voluntary participation of citizens in a medical education setting allows students to appreciate the expectations from society toward them, and to realize the social responsibilities to meet the expectations. Such expectations are hardly stressful, and rather serve as a strong motivation for studying. Furthermore, feedback from nonprofessional volunteer SPs are heard as voices of real patients. It is feedback to the entire medical world.

Some Essential Factors to Achieve a Successful Training Program

Many of the SPs in the United States are recruited from actor/actress trainees, while most of the SPs in Japan are nonactors and recruited from local communities. Some volunteers are listed in hospitals, and a recent survey revealed that about forty such groups make available some four hundred simulated patients in Japan (Fujisaki, 2002). However, there is no standard for SP qualification and each group (sometimes affiliated with hospitals and universities) has its own training standards. In her report, Adamo (2003) pointed out a similar situation with SP utilization in medical education in the United States.

The qualifications for volunteering as an SP are to be willing to help and to bear no enmity against health providers. The SP has two main roles: one is playing a role, and the other is giving verbal or written feedback. Playing a role is in itself not necessarily difficult even for nonactors, although an acting ability or experience may be helpful, since SPs are often expected to be able to give impromptu reactions during the training sessions. The demonstration of specific physical symptoms in a role does require prior training, if only by observing real patients and receiving guidance from health professionals. SPs should be well informed to be able to respond to medical questions from trainees on specific symptoms, in order to preserve the realism of the simulation. Since the interview can take different turns, preparation for any unexpected questions is necessary. Particularly when SPs are used for an evaluation purpose such as in the OSCE, more elaborated guidance and training are required to assure that SPs can give repeatable and consistent answers to the examiner's questions. When providing feedback, SPs must step out of their acting mode and recall how they felt during the encounter and what gave rise to their feelings, for example, "I was willing to share my feelings because you didn't criticize me" or "I couldn't fully understand what you explained to me, because you talked too fast." By mentioning the specific behavior or attitude that caused such feelings (e.g., the content of conversation, gestures, facial expressions, and other nonverbal signs), the trainees can learn to revise or retain their own behavior for similar encounters in the future. Feedback must always be concise and without excessive detail, and be sensitive to the trainee's readiness. If trainees suspect that the expectations are much higher than their current level of proficiency allows, they will easily give up trying to modify their behavior. Moreover, SPs should give constructive and objective feedback. If SPs persist in remaining in the acting role and give unrestrained negative emotions in the guise of a patient, it may offend the trainees' feelings, and contribute resistance to any behavior change.

The important point is that the feedback from the SP should be voiced from the patient's perspective. To be sure, when SPs become very familiar with clinical skills, they might then play a preceptor's role (Adamo, 2003). It is most important for the SP to identify with the patient's predicament since one of the training objectives is for the student to understand the patient's concerns, which is rarely available in actual clinical settings.

Case Development

A case scenario should embody the objectives that the trainees are expected to learn. The objectives should be matched with a particular case role. If an objective is for the trainees to learn how to listen to and deal with the patient's concerns, the SP's behavior should reflect a certain concern or problem. For example, the SP might voice fear of anesthesia because of a previous bad experience and is concerned about infection. For this type of objective, the training should focus on acquiring active listening skills such as responding to the patient's feeling. Unless a case scenario has clear objectives, the trainee's learning experience may become incoherent, and the effectiveness of the training suffers. In addition, the background information of the SP including lifestyle, occupation, family members, and attitude/habits toward dental/medical health should be described. Such information could be adjusted depending on the actual characteristics of the SP, so that the SP will have an easier role to play, which is especially important for nonactor SPs.

Faculty (Facilitator) Development and Quality Assurance

The facilitator is expected to establish the climate where all participants including SPs, trainees, and observers can discuss the training session in a free and open fashion. The facilitator might indicate some important aspects that the SP failed to mention in the feedback, as well as reinforce the SP's feedback by emphasizing its virtues. If there are some points to be learned that did not arise in the simulation, the facilitator must review them. It is also important to note whether the feedback is applicable to dentist-patient communication in general as opposed to a personal view of a certain type of patient. Trainees sometimes regard the feedback from the SP as applicable to any patient and may easily conclude that "all patients feel this way" or "this will work with any patients." Appropriate behavior depends on differentiating among the patients' characteristics, background, and needs. The facilitator should also point out discrepancies between the trainee's intention of executing a certain behavior and the SP's perception of what was delivered.

Since a case scenario is closely linked to learning objectives, the facilitator is often involved in designing the curriculum including case development. The facilitator is sometimes expected not only to train and monitor the SP performance, but also to coordinate the SP rotations when a shortage exists. Nevertheless, since faculty development in Japan is still evolving, some SPs may be asked to take the facilitator's place in the training, and this poses a question of defining the SP's role in the training. More serious perhaps is that the faculty often depend totally on the SP in implementing training, including case development, because of their own poor competence to serve as a facilitator.

One of the current challenges in conducting SP simulations in training is that there is a need to train not only SPs but also facilitators. To cope with this serious problem, a workshop on the training implementation for the medical and dental faculty was held in Japan, however, a shortage of skilled facilitators as well as SPs in Japan still remains. Faculty development in the educational institution is an immediate priority.

Evaluation of Interpersonal Communication Training with the SP

To assess the trainees' cognitive changes, it is useful to obtain feedback from the trainees about the impact of the training, such as what was useful and learned. A good example of evaluating behavioral changes is the medical interview situation that utilizes standardized patients in the OSCE. The OSCE can control the conditions, that is, the level of difficulty and the responses of patients, but it can evaluate only some of the trainee's skills. On the other hand, direct observation trainee communication with real patients in a clinical setting is a superb method to evaluate the trainee's overall competence. The disadvantage of this method rests in the difficulty in standardizing the conditions, which is not the case with the OSCE. It is therefore desirable to use both methods complementarily. A more appealing solution is to measure health outcomes such as patient satisfaction and adherence to health services and practice as proof of training effectiveness.

References

Adamo, G. (2003). Simulated and standardized patients in OSCEs: achievements and challenges 1992–2003. *Medical Teacher*, 25, 262–70.

Association of American Medical Colleges. (1999). *Contemporary Issues in Medicine: Communication In Medicine*. Medical Schools Objectives Project, Report. Washington, DC: Association of American Medical Colleges.

Barrows, H. S., & Abrahamson, S. (1964). The programmed patient: a technique for appraising student performance in clinical neurology. *Journal of Medical Education*, 39, 802–5.

Coggan, P. G., Knight, P., & Davis, P. (1980). Evaluating students in family medicine using simulated patients. *The Journal of Family Practice*, 10, 259–65.

Corah, N. L., O'Shea, R. M., Bissell, G. D., Thines, T. J., & Mendola, P. (1988). The dentist-patient relationship: perceived dentist behaviors that reduce patient anxiety and increase satisfaction. *Journal of American Dental Association*, 116, 73–76.

Dickson, D., Hargie, O., & Morrow N. (1997). *Communication Skills Training For Health Professionals*. London: Chapman and Hall.

Fujisaki, K. (2002). Simulated patient/standardized patient and the education of communication skills in Japan. In Japan Society for Medical Education (Ed.), *Igaku kyoiku hakusho 2002* (pp. 48–52). Tokyo: Shinoharashinsha. (Article in Japanese).

Harden, R. M., & Gleeson, F. A. (1979). Assessment of clinical competence using an Objective Structured Clinical Examination (OSCE). *Medical Education*, 13, 41–54.

Johnson, J. A., & Kopp, K. C. (1996). Effectiveness of standardized patient instruction. *Journal of Dental Education*, 60, 262–66.

Johnson, J. A., Kopp, K. C., & Williams R. G. (1990). Standardized patients for the assessment of dental students' clinical skills. *Journal of Dental Education*, 54, 331–33.

Klages, U., Sergl, H. G., & Burucker, I. (1992). Relations between verbal behavior of the orthodontist and communicative cooperation of the patient in regular orthodontic visits. *American Journal of Orthodontics and Dentofacial Orthopedics*, 102, 265–69.

Logan, H. L., Muller, P. J., Edwards Y., & Jakobsen, J. R. (1999). Using standardized patients to assess presentation of a dental treatment plan. *Journal of Dental Education*, 63, 729–37.

Mataki, S., Kawaguchi, Y., Teraoka, K., Shimura, N., Shimizu C., & Kurosaki, N. (1998). Medical interview with simulated patients at behavioral science in dentistry. *Kokubyo Gakkai Zasshi*, 65, 334–38. (Article in Japanese)

Mellor, A. C., & Milgrom, P. (1995). Dentists' attitudes toward frustrating patient visits: relationship to satisfaction and malpractice complaints. *Community Dentistry and Oral Epidemiology*, 23, 15–19.

Milgrom, P., Cullen, T., Whitney, C., Fiset, L., Conrad, D., & Getz, T. (1996). Frustrating patient visits. *Journal of Public Health Dentistry, 56*, 6–11.

Sandell, R., Camner L. G., & Sarhed G. (1994). The dentist's attitudes and their interaction with patient involvement in oral hygiene compliance. *British Journal of Clinical Psychology, 33*, 549–58.

Soh, G. (1992). Effects of explanation of treatment procedures on dental fear. *Clinical Preventive Dentistry, 14*, 10–13.

Stillman, P. L., Swanson, D. B., Smee, S., Stillman, A. E., Ebert, T. H., Emmel, V. S., Caslowitz, J., Greene, H. L., Hamolsky, M., Hatem, C., Levenson, D. J., Levin, R., Levinson, G., Ley, B., Morgan, G. J., Parrino, T., Robinson, S., & Willms, J. (1986). Assessing clinical skills of residents with standardized patients. *Annals of Internal Medicine, 105*, 762–71.

Stilwell, N. A., & Reisine, S. (1992). Using patient-instructors to teach and evaluate interviewing skills. *Journal of Dental Education, 56*, 118–22.

Street, R. L., Jr. (1989). Patients' satisfaction with dentists' communicative style. *Health Communication, 1*, 137–54.

Uemura, K. (1984). Simulated patient. In Japan Society for Medical Education (ed.), *Igaku kyouiku manual 5; simulation no ouyo, Igaku kyouiku niokeru simulation no syurui to tokucho.* (pp. 34–62). Tokyo: Shinohara syuppan Kabushikigaisha. (Article in Japanese)

Yoshida, T., Itadani, C., & Shimono, T. (1999). Adaptation of communication training in dental education using role playing and simulated patients. *Medical Education (Japan), 30*, 433–40. (Article in Japanese)

Yoshida, T., Itadani, C., Tsubouchi, J., Matsumura, S., Miyagi, J., Okamoto, Y., & Shimono, T. (2001). Effects of training with simulated patient for dental school students in clinical interviewing. *Medical Education (Japan), 32*, 153–58.

Yoshida, T., Milgrom, P., & Coldwell, S. (2002). How do U.S. and Canadian dental schools teach interpersonal communication skills? *Journal of Dental Education, 66*, 1281–88.

Community Health Promotion

Ray Croucher, Wagner Marcenes, and Allan Pau

Communities are specific groups living in a defined geographical area with common beliefs, values, and norms. Community membership may be based around factors such as occupation and social and leisure interests (Nutbeam, 1998). This chapter outlines how ideas of community have been incorporated into current concepts about health and health promotion, describes the epidemiology of oral diseases prevalent in communities, indicates how these approaches can be implemented within community settings, and proposes preventive approaches within these settings.

Health and Community

Health is a multidimensional idea, a "state of complete physical, mental and social well-being, and not merely the absence of disease" (World Health Organization, 1946). This positive, but abstract, concept emphasizes social and personal capabilities, in addition to physical capacity.

The place of community within health definitions is diverse. Durkheim (1897) demonstrated that healthiness is a population characteristic and that social environment determines individual behavior. Antonovsky (1979) proposed the importance of a sense of coherence, a psychological objective that is related to creating an awareness of community. Tarlov (1996) noted that health includes being able "to effectively negotiate the demands of the social environment." These ideas are reflected in the social capital construct (Putnam, 1993) and the argument that more egalitarian societies have better health because of greater community cohesion (Wilkinson, 1996; Pattussi et al., 2001).

Clinical and pharmaceutical interventions are not solely responsible for improving individual and community health (Lalonde, 1974). *Human biology, lifestyle, environment,* and *health care organization* are interdependently responsible. Diet (*lifestyle*) can alter the tooth structure resulting in caries (*biology*) that may lead to dietary changes. Lifestyle also interacts with the individual's *social* (family, friends, colleagues) and *physical environments* (exposure to irritants, infections, and physical hazards in settings as well as clean, safe places). *Policies and interventions* target factors such as immunizations, automobile seatbelt use, and *access to quality health care.* Health care may be received through community resources such as traditional healers, alternative therapies, or the mass media. Policy making may combine legislative, taxation, and organizational change. Finally, support for personal and social development is offered through providing information and enhancing skills.

These complex, multileveled links require integration, incorporating communities within general health activity to generate living and working conditions that are safe, stimulating, satisfying, and enjoyable. This is usually provided through health promotion activities, enabling people to increase control over the determinants of their health and thereby improve their health.

Health promotion is not owned by the health sector alone. It moves beyond clinical and curative services to communicate with the other sectors influencing health (World Health Organization, 1986). This "whole population"-based approach aims to reduce a risk factor's prevalence for everyone (Rose, 2001). Alternatively, a directed population strategy may be adopted, which focuses efforts on a targeted community identified as more vulnerable to disease. This approach addresses health disparities while saving resources.

Optimal community-based strategic interventions for oral diseases are not universally available or affordable because of escalating costs, limited resources, and lack of evidence of effectiveness. Oral health disparities related to socioeconomic status, ethnicity, gender, or general health, together with an insufficient emphasis on primary prevention, pose a considerable challenge for developing countries and countries with economies and health systems in transition. In many countries, oral health care is not fully integrated into national or community primary health care programs (Petersen, 2003b).

The evidence for effective community-based interventions to prevent and control dental caries supports community water fluoridation and school- or community-based pit and fissure sealant programs (Marinho et al., 2003). No recommendation either for or against use of interventions for the early detection of precancers and cancers or interventions to encourage use of helmets, face masks, and mouth guards to reduce oral-facial trauma in contact sports is available.

Evidence can be generated for effective health promotion strategies through cluster randomized trials, in which individuals are randomized in groups (i.e., the group is the unit of randomization, not the individual; Donner & Klar, 2000). For example, in a rural area with an oral condition, we might randomize whole villages to an intervention, or general practices, hospitals, families, or schools. In addition to convenience and cost-effectiveness, this recognizes that some interventions can only be administered to the group, such as adding fluoride to the water supply or a public oral health education campaign.

Are Oral Diseases Community Health Problems?

Oral diseases are characterized as community health problems. They are widespread, with costly impacts on the individual and community that result in pain and suffering, impairment of function, and reduced quality of life. Although all are potentially preventable (Centers for Disease Control, 2001), they are the fourth most expensive diseases to treat in most industrialized countries. In low-income countries, assuming treatment availability, the costs of treating dental caries alone in children would exceed the total health-care budget for children (Petersen, 2003b). The United States' estimated dental budget, at $60 billion per annum, involves approximately five hundred million dental visits. This does not include indirect expenses such as school and work hours lost each year and the cost of services by other health-care providers.

The social impact of pediatric oral diseases, such as pain and suffering, and problems with eating, speaking, and attending school (U.S. Department of Health and Human Services, 2003), is substantial and inequitable with more than fifty-one million school hours are lost each year. Poor children suffer nearly twelve times more activity-restricted days than rich children.

Another social outcome is work absence. A quarter of workers interviewed in one study reported at least one dentally related episode of work loss, averaging 1.7 hours, in the past twelve months. These data suggest a low social impact individually, but at the community level the impact from dental visits and oral conditions, especially among disadvantaged communities, is substantial (Reisine, 1984; Reisine & Miller, 1985; Gift, Reisine, & Larach, 1992). The impacts associated with oral conditions support the need for equitable health promotion interventions that prevent disease for everyone, whatever their life stage.

The Epidemiology of Community Oral Disease

Dental Caries

Dental caries affect 60–90% of schoolchildren and the vast majority of adults in most industrialized countries. Currently, the disease level is high in the Americas but relatively low in Africa. Changing living conditions indicate that dental caries incidence will increase in many parts of Africa, because of growing sugar consumption and inadequate fluoride exposure.

In the United States, the prevalence of dental caries among children aged twelve to seventeen years has declined from 90% during 1971–1974 to 67% during 1988–1991. Severity (i.e., the mean number of decayed, missing, or filled teeth) has also declined from 6.2 to 2.8 during this period. People with at least one decayed, missing, or filled permanent tooth increases with age, from 26% among five to eleven-years-olds to 67% among twelve-to-seventeen-years-olds, and 94% for dentate adults (with at least one natural tooth). Approximately 90% of caries in permanent teeth of children occur in tooth surfaces with pits and fissures, while two-thirds are on the chewing surfaces alone. Dental caries remains the most common U.S. chronic childhood disease, five and seven times more common than asthma and hay fever, respectively (Centers for Disease Control, 2001).

Although many countries have achieved the World Health Organization (WHO) Year 2000 goal of a mean DMF-T of three or less, the gains have been unequal. Some countries have large proportions of disease within a small percentage of the population. Eighty percent of dental caries in permanent teeth of children aged five to seventeen years in the United States occurs in 25% of children. Lower-income, Mexican-American, and African-American children and adults have more untreated caries than their higher-income or non-Hispanic white counterparts. Among low-income children, approximately one-third have untreated caries in primary teeth that could impact on pain, eating, and weight loss (Beltran-Aguilar, Estupinan-Day, & Baez, 1999).

Periodontal Disease

Most adults exhibit some periodontal disease without loss of a functional dentition. Nearly thirty-six million U.S. adults have periodontitis. Approximately 56.2 and 67.6 million persons who, on average, have about a third of their remaining teeth affected by at least three millimeters attachment loss and probing depth, respectively. Severe periodontal disease (measured as six millimeters of periodontal attachment loss) affects about 14% of U.S. adults aged forty-five to fifty-four years and 23% of sixty-five to seventy-four-year-olds. At all ages, men and people at the lowest socioeconomic levels are more likely to have more severe disease (U.S. Department of Health and Human Services, 2003; Albandar, Brunelle, & Kingman, 1999).

Dental Trauma

Reliable dental trauma data are lacking, particularly in developing countries. Worldwide, boys sustain more dental injuries than girls. Some Latin American countries report dental trauma for about 15% of schoolchildren, and prevalence rates of 5–12% are found in Middle Eastern children aged six to twelve years. One UK cross-sectional study assessed trauma in upper and lower permanent incisors of fourteen-year-olds, reporting a virtual doubling of the prevalence of traumatic injuries from 24% in 1995–96 to 44% in 1998–99. A community-derived index of deprivation and an overcrowded household were both significant predictors at both times, explaining a higher prevalence than that found elsewhere in the United Kingdom (Marcenes & Murray, 2002). Little is known about the U.S. prevalence of tooth or dental trauma, although the data suggest no significant change in prevalence over time. Data from a sample of 7,707 subjects aged six to fifty years showed a higher prevalence of trauma in both maxillary and mandibular incisors in males rather than females, and in both the younger and older age groups. Half of the individuals had only one incisor tooth classified as traumatized (Kaste et al., 1996).

The increasing prevalence of traumatic dental injuries relates to sports, unsafe playgrounds or schools, road accidents, or violence. In industrialized countries, the costs of care for dental-trauma patients are high (Petersen, 2003b).

Erosion

Dental erosion is defined as irreversible loss of dental hard tissue by a chemical process that does not involve bacteria. In a UK study of 17,061 children, over half of the five- and six-year-olds had erosion, 25% with dentinal involvement of the primary dentition. In the eleven-years-and-over group, almost 25% had erosion, with 2% with dentinal involvement in the mixed dentition. Dental erosion is now proposed as a developing UK public health problem, with high consumption of acidic beverages as the major etiologic factor (Gandara & Truelove, 1999). Deery et al. (2000) compared erosion in upper incisors between two UK and U.S. samples of eleven- and thirteen-year-old children and concluded that prevalence is similar.

Oral Cancer

Oral cancer is the eighth most common cancer in the world, with a life-threatening prevalence particularly high among men. In South Central Asia, oral cancer ranks among the three most common cancers. Sharp increases in its incidence rates have been reported in Northern, Central, and Eastern Europe and, to a lesser extent, Japan, Australasia, and the United States.

Oral cancers are preventable. The high incidence rates relate to smoking, the chewing of tobacco (either by itself or as a constituent of paan) and excessive alcohol consumption. The traditional practice of chewing tobacco in paan (betel quid) is popular in many parts of Asia and in Asian-migrant communities. Combining tobacco with alcohol use represents substantially greater risks than when either is consumed alone. Other causes of these cancers include viral infections, immunodeficiencies, poor nutrition, and, for lip cancers, exposure to ultraviolet light (Petersen, 2003b).

In the United States, thirty thousand mouth and throat cancers are diagnosed annually. Often diagnosed at late stages and treated by costly methods such as surgery, radiation, and chemotherapy, the outcomes may be disfiguring. Only half the persons diagnosed with oral cancer are alive five years after diagnosis. Mortality is nearly twice as high among minorities, especially African-American men, as among whites (Centers for Disease Control, 2001).

Malocclusion, Fluorosis, and Edentulism

Malocclusion is a set of dental deviations that may make a person less acceptable socially. Proffit, Fields, and Moray (1998) report that around 57–59% of each U.S. ethnic group has some degree of orthodontic treatment need, with severe malocclusion observed more frequently among blacks. Although evidence that orthodontic treatment enhances clinical dental health is limited (Petersen, 2003b), treatment is often justified by its potential for enhanced social and psychological well-being.

A survey in school children in 1986–1987 remains the only U.S. source of national data about enamel fluorosis prevalence. The prevalence of enamel fluorosis (ranging from very mild to severe) was 38 percent among children in communities with natural fluoride (0.7 to 4.0 parts per million (ppm) fluoride ions), 25.8 percent in the optimal fluoride group (0.7 to 1.2 ppm) and 15.5 percent in the suboptimal fluoride group (less than 0.7 ppm). Multiple exposures may explain an increase in enamel fluorosis. Exposure to fluoride from dietary supplements has decreased because of reductions in the recommended dosage. The simultaneous use of systemic fluorides with dietary supplements indicates the need to reinforce appropriate usage guidelines (Beltran-Aguilar, Griffin, & Lockwood, 2002) if an additional potential oral health challenge for communities is to be avoided.

Following improvements in oral health, the overall prevalence of tooth loss and edentulism has been declining in the United States. The most current estimates of the prevalence and distribution of tooth retention show that in 1988–91, 89.5% of the population was dentate, and 30.5% had retained all twenty-eight teeth. The partially edentate were most commonly missing the first and second molars. Age and ethnicity were strongly related to tooth retention and tooth loss after adjustment for other factors. Mexican-Americans had the lowest and black non-Hispanics the highest rates of tooth loss (Marcus et al., 1996).

The Common Risk Factor Approach to Prevention of Chronic Diseases

Noncommunicable chronic diseases, such as cancer and cardiovascular disease, are the largest cause of death in the world. Currently dominant in lower-middle and upper income countries, they are becoming increasingly prevalent in many of the poorest developing countries. This creates a polarized and protracted double burden, adding to the infectious diseases that still prevail in developing countries (Yach et al., 2004).

The common risk factor approach provides a cost-effective basis for appropriate oral health promotion. Common risk factors are the leading causes of morbidity and mortality—tobacco, excessive consumption of alcohol, nutrition and diet, exercise, environment, and hygiene. Controlling diet and nutrition reduces risk factors for dental caries, oral cancer, and craniofacial development diseases, while tobacco use (smoked and chewed) is a risk factor for conditions such as oral cancer, oral mucosal lesions, and periodontal disease. These interrelated behaviors are initiated during youth and fostered by sociopolitical policies and environmental conditions.

Community Settings for the Common Risk Factor Approach

Cities, workplaces, and schools offer local community settings for achieving global goals by translating concepts of health promotion into action. Action to promote health in settings can take many forms. All settings will aim to achieve their health-promoting potential through the interaction of the physical and social environmental with organizational and personal factors (Nutbeam, 1998).

Healthy Cities

The best example of a settings approach is provided by Healthy Cities, with several hundred cities currently participating worldwide. The Healthy Cities project was developed to put into practice the principles of the Ottawa Charter (WHO, 1986). The charter's authors argued that health is created within the various settings of everyday life where healthy public policy can be built by implementing the principles of strengthening community action, developing personal skills, creating supportive environments, and reorienting health services. This process provides a practical example of developing effective partnerships between different local government departments, health-care services, residents, NGOs, the private sector, community organizations, and academics. No standard formula builds effective partnerships. Leadership and managerial skills affect outcomes. Social pressure stimulates partnership development with organizations and individuals to enhance community-health promotion.

Health-Promoting Schools

One-fifth of the world's population is adolescent, aged ten to nineteen years. Young people with high self-esteem, good social skills, clear values, and access to relevant information have every chance to make positive health decisions. Significant mediating factors within a community include adolescent peer pressure, mass media messages, and industrial activity. A healthy school setting will provide a supportive environment for oral health through access to safe water, allowing general and oral hygiene programs. A safe physical environment reduces accident risk and dental trauma (WHO, 2003).

Health-Promoting Workplaces

A healthy workforce sustains social and economic development at national and community levels. Work settings promote the health of workers, their families, friends, and the community. Commonly, investments for health of working populations have been made in large-scale enterprises. Informal work settings and small-scale and micro enterprises are important new venues (Eakin & Weir, 1995). Workplace approaches should integrate physical, emotional, psychosocial, organizational, and economic factors. Links to existing setting programs should be established. Health benefits are gained by integrating health, environment, and safety issues in the overall management of the workplace. Outcomes can be evaluated at the community level, using the rate of work-related injuries and diseases and relevant WHO public health indicators.

Action Plans for Community Practice

The focus is on modifying risk factors within a favorable physical and social environment created by public policy.

Tobacco

Tobacco use has declined in some high-income countries, but continues to increase in low- and middle-income countries, especially among young people and women. The increasing number of smokers and smokeless-tobacco users among young people will affect the general and oral health of future generations. The prevalence of tobacco use in most countries is highest among people of low educational background, the poor, and the marginalized. The oral consequences of tobacco use impair quality of life, from halitosis and periodontal disease to oral birth defects and complications during wound healing (Petersen, 2003a).

Oral-health professionals should strengthen their contributions to tobacco-cessation activity. As effective as other clinicians in helping tobacco users, they can demonstrate the oral impacts of tobacco use. Regularly meeting children, youths, and their caregivers offers opportunities to influence individuals to entirely avoid, postpone initiation, or stop using tobacco. They may have more time with patients than many other clinicians. In addition, they treat women of childbearing age and can inform them about the potential harm to babies from tobacco use.

Diet

There are two kinds of malnutrition: associated with hunger (underweight) and dietary excess (overweight). Urbanization and economic development result in rapid diet and lifestyle changes, leading to chronic diseases such as obesity, diabetes, cardiovascular diseases, cancer, osteoporosis, and oral diseases (Moynihan & Petersen, 2004). This nutrition transition demonstrates how common risks impact on different aspects of the public's health.

Oral-health opportunities include:

1. *Implementing nutritional counseling, which covers general and oral health.* The posteruptive effect of sugar consumption is a key etiologic factor for dental caries.
2. *Promoting breastfeeding.* Breast milk prevents early childhood caries' occurring, caused by a child going to bed with a bottle of sweetened drink or drinking at will from a bottle during the day.
3. *Decreasing the consumption of acidic, sugary soft drinks, a major risk factor in dental caries and erosion.* Added sugars should remain below 10% of energy intake and the consumption of foods/drinks containing free sugars should be limited to a maximum of four a day.
4. *Advocating a healthy diet that includes fresh yellow-green fruits and vegetables, which can help prevent oral cancer.* Government ministries should implement intersectoral collaboration through taxation, pricing, and food labeling (Moynihan & Petersen, 2004; Yach et al., 2004).

Dental status impacts upon diet and nutrition. In a study of U.S. adults, the intake of carrots and tossed salads among denture-wearers was 2.1 and 1.5 times less than for the fully dentate, and dietary fiber intake was 1.2 times less (Nowjack-Raymer & Sheiham, 2003).

Fluoride

Fluoride is most effective when a low level is constantly maintained in the mouth. Community-based programs should implement the most appropriate means of maintaining this constant low level in as many mouths as possible. Long-term exposure to an optimal level of fluoride results in diminishing caries levels in both children and adults. Fluoride is globally available, usually as fluoridated toothpaste. This is particularly important because of the changing diet and nutrition status in developing countries. Achieving effective fluoride-based caries prevention without some degree of dental fluorosis may not be possible. A balance should be achieved between maximizing caries reduction and minimizing dental fluorosis (Petersen & Lennon, 2004).

Violence

Violence has a complex causation, indicating that multisectoral community activity can contribute to the successful implementation of violence-prevention programs. These approaches should implement and monitor a community violence-prevention plan; enhance capacity for collecting data on violence; define priorities for research on the causes, costs, and prevention of violence; and promote the primary prevention of violence (Krug et al., 2002).

Dilemmas for Community Practice

Reorienting oral-health activity toward community-based disease prevention and health promotion is recommended. Global goals for oral health by the year 2020 specify the need to develop high-quality oral health systems by applying evidence-based strategies in oral-health promotion, disease prevention, the treatment of oral diseases, and health systems research and development (Hobdell et al., 2003). Common dilemmas have to be faced. These include identifying sustainable levels of funding to develop an integrated approach to defined community issues and adopting guidelines for appropriate evaluation designs for community programs. The role of health professionals with clinical expertise alone should be developed toward promoting community health in their future professional lives. Community health-promotion efforts demand an integrated approach linking the individual and the social and physical environment with public-policy intervention.

Acknowledgment

We thank Ana Beatriz Gamboa for her help in researching the background to this chapter.

References

Albandar, J. M., Brunelle, J. A., & Kingman, A. (1999). Destructive periodontal disease in adults 30 years of age and older in the United States, 1988–1994. *Journal of Periodontology, 70,* 13–29.

Antonovsky, A. (1979). *Health, Stress, and Coping.* San Francisco: Jossey-Bass.

Beltran-Aguilar, E. D., Estupinan-Day, S., & Baez, R. (1999). Analysis of prevalence and trends of dental caries in the Americas between the 1970s and 1990s. *International Dental Journal, 49,* 322–29.

Beltran-Aguilar, E. D., Griffin, S. O., & Lockwood, S. A. (2002). Prevalence and trends in enamel fluorosis in the United States from the 1930s to the 1980s. *Journal of American Dental Association, 133,* 157–65.

Centers for Disease Control. (2001). *Promoting Oral Health: Interventions for Preventing Dental Caries, Oral and Pharyngeal Cancers, and Sports-Related Craniofacial Injuries: A Report on Recommendations of the Task Force on Community Preventive Forces. MMWR, 50,* 1–13.

Deery, C., & Wagner, M. L., Longbottom, C., Simon, R., & Nugent, Z. J. (2000). The prevalence of dental erosion in a United States and a United Kingdom sample of adolescents. *Pediatric Dentistry, 22(6),* 505–10.

Donner, A., & Klar, N. (2000). *Design and Analysis of Cluster Randomization Trials in Health Research.* London, England: Arnold.

Durkheim, E. (1897). *Le suicide.* Paris: F. Alcan. English translation by J. A. Spalding (1951). Toronto, Canada: Free Press, Collier-Macmillan.

Eakin, J. M., & Weir, N. (1995). Canadian approaches to the promotion of health in small workplaces. *Canadian Journal of Public Health, 86,* 109–13.

Gandara, B. K., & Truelove, E. L. (1999). Diagnosis and management of dental erosion. *Journal of Contemporary Dental Practice, 1,* 16–23.

Gift, H. C., Reisine, S. T., & Larach, D. C. (1992). The social impact of dental problems and visits. *American Journal of Public Health, 82,* 1663–68.

Hobdell, M., Petersen, P. E., Clarkson, J., Johnson, N. (2003). Global goals for oral health 2020. *International Dental Journal, 53 (3),* 285–88.

Kaste, L. M., Gift, H. C., Bhat, M., & Swango, P. A. (1996). Prevalence of incisor trauma in persons 6–50 years of age: United States, 1988–1991. *Journal of Dental Research, 75,* 696–705.

Krug, E. G., Mercy, J. A., Dahlberg, L. L., & Zwi, A. B. (2002). The world report on violence and health. *The Lancet, 360,* 1083–88.

Lalonde, M. (1974). *A New Perspective on the Health of Canadians: A Working Document.* Canada: Minister of Supply and Services.

Marcenes, W., & Murray, S. (2002). Changes in prevalence and treatment need for traumatic dental injuries among 14-year-old children in Newham, London: a deprived area. *Community Dental Health, 19,* 104–8.

Marcus, S. E., Drury, T. F., Brown, L. J., & Zion, G. R. (1996). Tooth retention and tooth loss in the permanent dentition of adults: United States, 1988–1991. *Journal of Dental Research, 75,* 684–95.

Marinho, V. C., Higgins, J. P., Logan, S., & Sheiham, A. (2003). Systematic review of controlled trial on the effectiveness of fluoride gels for the prevention of dental caries in children. *Journal of Dental Education, 67 (4),* 448–58.

Moynihan, P., & Petersen, P. E. (2004). Diet, nutrition and prevention of dental diseases. *Public Health Nutrition, 7,* Special Issue 1, 201–26.

Nowjack-Raymer, R. E., & Sheiham, A. (2003). Association of edentulism and diet and nutrition in US adults. *Journal of Dental Research, 82,* 123–26.

Nutbeam, D. (1998). *Health Promotion Glossary.* Geneva: World Health Organization.

Pattussi, M. P., Marcenes, W., Croucher, R., & Sheiham, A. (2001). Social deprivation, income inequality, social cohesion and dental caries in Brazilian school children. *Social Science and Medicine, 53(7)*, 915–25.

Petersen, P. E. (2003a). Global framework convention on tobacco control: the implications for oral health. *Community Dental Health, 20(3)*, 137–38.

———. (2003b). The World Oral Health Report 2003: continuous improvement of oral health in the 21st century—the approach of the WHO Global Oral Health Programme. *Community Dental Oral Epidemiology, 31*, 3–24.

Petersen, P. E., & Lennon, M. A. (2004). Effective use of fluorides for the prevention of dental caries in the 21st century: the WHO approach. *Community Dentistry and Oral Epidemiology, 32*, 319–21.

Proffit, W. R., Fields, H. W., Jr., Moray, L. J. (1998). Prevalence of malocclusion and orthodontic treatment need in the United States: estimates from the NHANES III survey. *International Journal of Adult Orthodontic Orthognathic Surgery, 13(2)*, 97–106.

Putnam, R. D. (Spring, 1993). The prosperous community: social capital and economic growth. *The American Prospect*, 35–44.

Reisine, S., & Miller, J. (1985). A longitudinal study of work loss related to dental diseases. *Social Science and Medicine, 21*, 1309–14.

Reisine, S. T. (1984). Dental disease and work loss. *Journal of Dental Research, 63*, 1158–61.

Rose, G. (2001). Sick individuals and sick populations. *International Journal of Epidemiology, 30*, 427–32.

Tarlov, A. R. (1996). An introduction to three studies assessing the impact of specific restrains on the delivery of pharmaceutical benefits. *Pharmacoeconomics, 10*, 48–49.

U.S. Department of Health and Human Services. (2003). *A National Call to Action to Promote Oral Health*. Rockville, MD: National Institute of Dental and Craniofacial Research.

Wilkinson, R. G. (1996). *Unhealthy Societies: The Afflictions of Inequality*. London and New York: Routledge.

World Health Organization. (1946). *Constitution*. New York: World Health Organization.

———. (1986). *Ottawa Charter for Health Promotion*. Geneva: World Health Organization.

———. (2003). *Oral Health Promotion Through Schools*. WHO Information Series on School Health. Document 11. Geneva: World Health Organization.

Yach, D., Hawkes, C., Gould, C., Linn, & Hofman, K. J. (2004). The global burden of chronic diseases. *Journal of the American Medical Association, 291*, 2616–22.

Index

Italic page numbers refer to figures.

Abrahamson, S., 258
Access, to quality health care, 266
Accidents, dental trauma and, 269
ACE. *See* Angiotensin-converting enzyme
Acetylcholine, 31
Acinar cells, primary saliva production and, 38
ACTH. *See* Adrenocorticotropic hormone
Action stage, in *Trans-Theoretical Model of Behavior Change*, 153, *153*
Active distraction activities, for children in dental settings, 181
Active electrodes, 59
Acupressure, dental fear management and, 116
Acute pain, control of, 200
Acute-phase protein, 32
Acute-phase response, 32
Adamo, G., 260
Adaptive toothbrushes, 233, *233, 234*
Adherence, optimal diabetes care and, 247
Adolescents
  health promotion for, 271
  orthodontics, oral-health-related quality of life, and, 25
  tobacco use by, 272
Adrenocorticotropic hormone, 31
Advice, role of, in facilitation of change, 154
AED. *See* Awareness enhancement device
Affordability of dental care, older minority adults and, 222
Africa, dental caries and, 267
African Americans. *See also* Minorities; Race
  dental caries in children, 268
  malocclusion and, 269
  oral cancer among men, 269
  tooth loss and, 270
Ageism, stereotypes and, 213–214
Aging
  cognition and, 215–216, 222
  dementia and, 216–217
  dental care issues and, 221–222
  dental pain and, 92, 93
  depression and, 219–220
  oral physical senses and, 217
  pain response/somatization and, 220–221
  personality and, 218–219
  sensory deficits and, 218

Aging (*continued*)
  social/family support and, 221
  tooth loss, edentulism, and, 270
Ajzen, I., 150
Albino, J. E., 8
Alcohol abuse
  chronic orofacial pain and, 108
  Motivational Interviewing and treat-
    ment of, 157–158
  periodontal disease and, 145, 146
Alcohol Use Disorders Identification
    Test, 108
Allen, K. D., 178, 183
Allergic rhinitis, 34
Alpha melanocyte-stimulating hormone
    (α-MSH), 31
Alveolar bone loss, in diabetic patients,
    244
Alzheimer's disease, salivary gland
    hypofunction and, 42
American Academy of Orofacial Pain,
    orofacial pain defined by, 80
American Dental Association, Council
    on Dental Therapeutics of, 238
American Medical Association, 66
American Society of Anesthesiology, 250
American Society of Clinical Hypnosis,
    74
Amitriptyline, bruxism and, 133
Amygdala
  pain response thresholds and decrease
    in responsiveness of, 198t
  pain-stimulus awareness and, 192
Analog information feedback, 54
Anderson, N. K., 209
Anderson, R. M., 208
Andrasik, F., 52, 56
Anesthesia
  dental fear and, 118
  general, 178
  "painless dentistry" solutions and,
    190
  surgical stress and, 33
  topical, 178, 184
Anger, facial expression and recognition
    of, 10
Angiotensin-converting enzyme, 31
Angiotensin II, 31
Animal magnetism, 66

Antecedent interventions, for thumb
    sucking, 165–166
Antibiotics, prophylactic, diabetic
    patients and, 251
Antigingivitis agents, people with
    special needs and, 238
Antitraumatic dental treatment, diabetic
    patients and, 251
Antonovsky, A., 265
Anxiety. *See also* Dental anxiety; Fear
  in children during dental treatment,
    177
  chronic orofacial pain and assessment
    of, 105, 106
  dental pain and, 92
  dry mouth and, 40
  models of, in dentistry, 82–83
  nonpharmacological approaches to
    management of, 189–200
  pain, fear, and, 194
  pain affected by, 79
  predictability and, 88
Anxiety sensitivity, expectancy model of
    fear and, 85
APP. *See* Acute-phase protein
Appointment attendance, communication/
    relationship with dental providers
    and, 86
Appraisal, chronic pain and, 102
APR. *See* Acute-phase response
Arteriosclerosis, diabetes and, 247
ASA. *See* American Society of
    Anesthesiology
Asmundson, G. J. G., 85
Assessment
  of chronic orofacial pain patients, 99
  of dental fear, 117
  of oral-health-related quality of life,
    22–23
  of thumb sucking, 164–165, 170
  of TMD pain patients, 111
Association of American Medical
    Colleges, 256
Asthma, 34
Atchison, K. A., 21, 24
Atherosclerosis, 32
Atopic dermatitis, 34
Attention, types of, in older adults,
    215

Attractiveness, judgments of, 7–8
Atypical odontalgia, 80, 100
Audiovisual aids, in communication training, 257
AUDIT-C. *See* Alcohol Use Disorders Identification Test
Auditory signals, from craniofacial area, 10
Auerbach, S. M., 88
Australasia, oral cancer in, 269
Authoritiarian style, in hypnotic communication, 72
Autogenic phrasing, 57
Autoimmune diseases
inflammation, stress response, and, 31
NEI network and, 34
Autonomic nervous system, low arousal states and avenues of entry to, 52
AVDR model, 109
Aversive interventions, thumb sucking and, 167–168, 170
Avoidance. *See* Fear-avoidance model
Awareness, pain response thresholds and, 196*t*, 197
Awareness enhancement device, thumb sucking and, 166, 168, 170

Bagramian, R. A., 21
Bandpass, 62
Bandura, A., 203, 204, 206
Barrows, H. S., 258, 259
Basmajian, J. V., 52, 56, 60
Beauty, cross-cultural studies on, 7–8
Behavior, chronic pain and, *102*, 103
Behavioral barriers, people with special needs and, 232, 236–237
Behavioral interventions, major problems with, 123
Behavioral reactions, pain management and, 194
Behavioral research, role of oral-health-related quality of life in, 23
Behavioral scientists, oral-health-related quality of life and, 26
Behavioral strategies
pain management and, 191*t*
raising patient's pain response thresholds with, 197–199, 198*t*

Behavior change
importance of, to oral health and dentistry, 149–150
linking to patient's values, 155–156
self-empowerment model for, 209–210
Behavior management, positive approaches to, with children, 177–178, 184
Behavior modification, dental fear management and, 116
Beliefs/attitudes/values, health behavior and, 150, *150*
Bernheim, 66
Bicarbonate buffer system, in saliva, 38
Biobehavioral assessment data, guidelines for obtaining/using, 109–111
Biobehavioral clinicians, dentists as, 109–111
Biofeedback
avenues of entry to nervous system and, 52, *53*
in clinical practice, 56–57
dental fear management and, 116
description of, 51–52
meta-analysis and, 54–56
selecting muscles for training and, 62
somatic anxiety and, 121
Biofeedback loop, schematic of, *52*
Biomaterials, 23
Biomechanical strategies, pain management and, 191*t*
Biomimetics, 23
Biopsychosocial model, 9
assessment of psychological and psychosocial factors, 104–105
of chronic pain/illness, *102*
discussion about, 101–109
dual-axis approach to assessment of dental and orofacial pain, 103–104
other measures of psychosocial functioning, 107–108
pain and treatment history, 105
parafunctional jaw behaviors, 105
physical and sexual abuse, 109
post-traumatic stress disorder, 108–109
psychological status, 105–106
psychosocial status, 106–107
sleep disturbance, 108
substance abuse, 108

Birbaumer, N., 55
Biting, 4
Blacks. *See* African Americans
Blood glucose levels, diabetic patients
    and, 247
Bochner, S., 82
Body dysmorphia, 13
Boersma, H., 9
Botulinum toxin (Botox) injections,
    bruxism and, 133
Boys, dental trauma in, 268
Braid, James, 66
Breast cancer, salivary biomarkers for,
    47
Breastfeeding, promoting, 272
Breathing, 57
  paced, dental fear management and,
    116, 119
  relaxation and, 52, *53*
Bromocriptine, bruxism and, 133
Broughton, R. J., 129
Brushing. *See* Tooth brushing
Bruxcore monitoring device, bruxism
    and, 131
Bruxism, 12, 103, 105, 127–134
  definition of, 127–128
  diagnosis of, 131–132
  effects of, 128–129
  etiological theories of, 129–131
  prevalence of, 128
  treatment of, 132–133
  uncovering and, 74
Budgets, dental, 267
Budyznski, T. H., 54
Bulimia nervosa, saliva function and, 41
Burke, B. L., 158
Burning mouth syndrome, 92, 220
Burucker, I., 255
Butler, Robert, 213

CAL. *See* Clinical attachment loss
Calcium hydroxyapatite, in saliva, 39
Calculus
  diabetic patients and removal of, 245
  low saliva flow rate and, 43
Camner, L. G., 255
Cancer, 270, 272
  oral, 269
  treatments for, 21

Candida albicans, 43
  salivary levels of, 47
Cannistraci, A. J., 54
CAPS. *See* Clinician Administered PTSD
    Scale
Cardiovascular disease, 270, 272
Caregivers, people with special needs,
    oral health, and, 232, 233, 234,
    236, 237, 240
Caries. *See* Dental caries
Carlsson, S. G., 54, 55
Case development, in successful training
    programs, 260–261
Cash, T. F., 6, 13
Catastrophizing, dental pain and, 86
Catecholamines, 32
CBST. *See* Cognitive behavioral skills
    training
CBT. *See* Cognitive-behavioral therapy
Central nervous system, 29
  low arousal states and avenues of
    entry to, 52
Cephalometric measures, independence
    of, from self-perceptions of face, 9
Cerebral lateralization, facial perception
    and, 7
Cevimeline hydrochloride, 46
CFAs. *See* Craniofacial anomalies
C-fibers, pain stimuli and, 195
"Chairside" manner, 79
Change
  initiating in people, 152–154
  readiness to, 153–154
  role of advice and education in facili-
    tation of, 154
  statements linked to facilitation of,
    155*t*
Channel, sEMG instruments and, 60
Charcot, Jean-Martin, 66
Chelions, importance of, in perception of
    facial expression, *11*
Chemomechanical caries removal, in
    children, 24
Chemotherapeutic agents, people with
    special needs and use of, 232,
    237–239
Chemotherapy, 21
  salivary gland hypofunction and, 41
Chewing gum, xylitol-containing, 238

Childhood, self-efficacy and dental care in, 207

Children
bruxism in, 128, 129
chemomechanical caries removal in, 24
dental caries in, 267–268
dental erosion in, 269
dental trauma in, 268
distraction of, 180–181, 184
enamel fluorosis in, 270
management of disruptive behavior by, 175–185
oral-health-related quality of life measurements for, 22, 23
orthodontic indices and self-esteem in, 8
parent presence in operatory with, 179, 184
positive approaches to behavior management with, 177–178, 184
prevalence of thumb sucking in, 163
reasons for disruptive behavior in, during dental treatment, 176–177
reduction of discomfort for, 178–179, 184
reinforcement of good behavior in, 181–182, 184
scheduled breaks for, 182–183, 184
surgical reconstruction and self-concept of, 9
urinary catecholamines and bruxism in, 130
Chiodo, G. T., 115
Chlorhexidine rinses, for people with special needs, 239
Christensen, A. P., 169
Chronic disease, common risk factor approach to, 270–271
Chronic orofacial pain
biobehavioral perspectives on, 99–111
toward a biopsychosocial model for, 100–101
"Chronic pain behavior," 103
Cigarette smoking, Motivational Interviewing and, 158
Cleft lip, 9
Cleft palate, 9
Clenching, 105, 127, 133
diagnosis of, 131–132

Clinical attachment loss, 141, 142, 143
Clinical hypnosis
brief history of, 65–66
map of, 68t
Clinical practice
biofeedback in, 56–57
oral-health-related quality of life and, 24–25
Clinical research, role of oral-health-related quality of life in, 23–24
Clinician Administered PTSD Scale, 109
CLP. See Combined cleft lip and palate
Cognition, aging and, 215, 222
Cognitive anxiety, 121
Cognitive behavioral skills training, 55
Cognitive-behavioral therapy, 110
Cognitive behavior modification, dental fear management and, 116
Cognitive behavior therapy, relaxation and, 52
Cognitive experience, pain management and, 194
Cognitive reframing, raising pain response thresholds and, 198t
Cognitive restructuring, dental fear management and, 116
Cohen, L. K., 21
Cold Pressure Test, 195
Combined cleft lip and palate, 9
Common risk factor approach
community settings for, 270–271
to preventing chronic disease, 270–271
Communication
with children in dental setting, 179–180, 184
craniofacially deformed individuals and, 10
dental fear management and, 116–118
dental pain and, 92
with dental providers, 86–87
effective, 255–256
Communication training, factors influencing development of, 257
Communities, defined, 265
Community, health and, 265
Community health problems, oral diseases as, 267
Community oral disease
epidemiology of, 267–270

Community oral disease (*continued*)
 dental caries, 267–268
 dental trauma, 268–269
 erosion, 269
 malocclusion, fluorosis, and edentulism, 269–270
 oral cancer, 269
 periodontal disease, 268
Community practice
 action plans for, 272–273
 dilemmas for, 273
Compliance, diabetic patients and, 247
Computer-based simulation, in communication training, 257
Computer-based surface EMG instruments, 60
Computerized local anesthetic delivery
 system, 178
Conditioned response, 83
Conditioned stimuli, 83
Confidentiality, diabetic patients and, 244
Cons, N. C., 8
Consequent interventions, thumb suck-
 ing and, 167–168
Contemplation stage, in *Trans-Theoretical
 Model of Behavior Change,* 153, *153*
"Contingent escape" approach, chil-
 dren's control over dental routine
 and, 183
Control
 of acute pain, 200
 pain response thresholds and increase
 in, 198*t*
Controllability
 defined, 88
 dental pain and, 88–91, 92
Corah, N. L., 255
Corah's Dental Anxiety Scale, 116
Cortical reception threshold, pain stimuli
 and, 195
Corticosteroid releasing factor, 32
Corticosteroids, 32
Corticotropin-releasing factor, 31
Corticotropin-releasing hormone, 29, 30
Cortisol, in saliva, 39, 40–41
Cosmetic dentistry, older patients and,
 219
Cosmetic surgery, depressed patients
 and, 13

Costen's Syndrome, 12
Council on Dental Therapeutics of the
 American Dental Association, 238
Counterstimulation, raising pain
 response thresholds and, 198
CR. *See* Conditioned response
Cram, J. R., 60
Craniofacial anomalies, 9
C-reactive protein, 32
CRF. *See* Corticotropin-releasing factor
CRH. *See* Corticotropin-releasing
 hormone
Crider, A. B., 54
CRP. *See* C-reactive protein
CS. *See* Conditioned stimuli
Culture, dental pain and, 91–92
Cunningham, M. R., 7
Curby cup, 46
Cytokines, 29, 31, 34

Dahlstrom, L., 55
DAI. *See* Dental Aesthetic Index
Darwin, Charles, 10
Davey, G., model for dental phobias by,
 83–84
Davidson, R. J., 121
Davis, D. M., 219
DCBS. *See* Dental Coping Belief Scale
Death and bereavement, dentists and,
 215
Deep bit, bruxism and, 130
Defensive coping style, *144*
 periodontal disease and, 141, 142, 143
DeLuca, C. J., 60
Dementia, 216–217
Dental Aesthetic Index, 8
Dental aesthetics, impact of, on social
 appearance concern, 8
Dental anxiety. *See also* Anxiety; Dental
 fear; Fear
 causes of, 189
 effective communication and reduc-
 tion in, 255
Dental appointments, dementia and, 217
Dental budgets, community health prob-
 lems and, 267
Dental care, social support and, 221
Dental caries
 in children, 267

African American and Hispanic, 268
community oral disease and, 267–68
in diabetic patients, 244
Dental Coping Belief Scale, 205, 208
Dental/dental hygiene education
background history of
simulated/standardized patient
in, 258–259
interpersonal communication training
in, 256–259
oral-health-related quality of life and,
25–26
Dental Education at the Crossroads, 149
Dental-facial attractiveness rating, 8
Dental fear. *See also* Anxiety; Dental
anxiety; Fear
assessing in patient, 117
nonrelaxation-based techniques,
116–119
communication, 116–118
distraction, 118–119
prevalence of, 115
quasi-relaxation based techniques for,
119–120
guided imagery, 120
reducing, chairside techniques for,
115–124
relaxation-based procedures for,
120–124
Dental health
oral-health-related quality of life and,
20
two-way relationship between diabetes
and, 250
Dental Health Knowledge
Questionnaire, 208
Dental health professionals, effective
communication and, 255–256
Dental impressions, pain management
and, 190
Dental insurance, older adults, dental
visits, and, 222
Dental pain. *See also* Pain
catastrophizing and, 86
conceptual issues in understanding of,
81–82
distraction and, 87–88, 92
dual-axis approach to assessment of,
103–104, *104*

emotional and environmental determinants of, 79–93
emotional determinants of, 82–85
anxiety and fear of pain models in
dentistry, 82–83
Davey's model, 83–84
expectancy model of fear, 85
fear-avoidance model, 84–85
Mowrer's two-factor theory, 83
environment and, 86
gender, culture, and lifespan issues,
91–92
individual differences and sensitivity
to, 85–86
inflammatory diseases and, 80
pain and treatment history and, 105
postoperative, 82
predictability and controllability and,
88–91, 92
Dental personnel
gender and cultural status of, 92
as relief stimuli, 91
as threatening stimuli, 91
Dental phobias
self-efficacy and, 204
uncovering and, 74
Dental prevention, medical model of, 237
Dental professionals, diabetic patients
and recommendations to, 250–251
Dental providers, communication and
relationship with, 86–87
Dental schools, geriatric dentistry and,
223
Dental self-efficacy, sources of, in oral
health behavior, 206–208
Dental trauma, community oral disease
and, 268
Dental visits
diabetic patients and, 245, 246*t*, 251
older patients and rates of, 222
self-efficacy and, 205
Dentistry
anxiety and fear of pain models in,
82–83
communication curriculum and, 256
hypnosis in, 65–75
importance of behavior change to,
149–150
quality of life issues and, 21

Dentists
  as biobehavioral clinicians, 109–111
  chairside manner of, 79
  effective communication between
      children and, 179–180, 184
  effective communication between
      patients and, 255–256
  gender and cultural status of, 92
  hypnosis and recommendations for,
      74–75
  improvements in patient's self-efficacy
      and, 210–211
  older patients, and attitudes of, 214
  patient death and bereavement and,
      215
  patient involvement and, 149
  pediatric, 178
Dentofacial asymmetry, detractions asso-
      ciated with, 6
Denture wearers
  food consumption and, 5
  quality of life for, 24
Depressed patients, cosmetic surgery
      and, 13
Depression, 29, 30
  aging and, 219–220
  chronic orofacial pain and assessment
      of, 105, 106
  dental pain and, 82
  dry mouth and, 40
  poor sense of social efficacy and, 204
  salivary gland hypofunction and, 42
Depth periodontal pockets, in diabetic
      patients, 244
Desired control, dental pain and, 90
DFA. See Dental-facial attractiveness
      rating
Diabetes, 272
  health behavior models and, 248–249
  oral health behavior and, 245, 247
  salivary biomarkers for, 47
  salivary gland hypofunction and, 42
  two-way relationship between dental
      health and, 250
Diabetes Control and Complications
      Trial Research Group, 247
Diabetes health behaviors, 247–248
  self-efficacy and, 248–249
  self-empowerment and, 208

Diabetes mellitus, 34
  oral diseases and, 244–245
  prevalence of, 243
Diabetes mellitus patients, oral health
      behaviors among, and possible
      controls, 246t
Diabetes-related emergencies, 249–250
Diabetes self-care practices
  components of, 247
  good adherence to, 248t
Diabetes self-efficacy, oral health habits
      and, 205, 206
Diabetics
  as dental patients, 249–250
      emergency situations with, 249–250
      special features of treatment for, 250
  recommendations to dental profes-
      sionals about, 250–251
DiAngelis, A. J., 214
Diaphragmatic breathing, relaxation
      and, 52, 53
Dickson, D., 257
DiClemente, C. C., 152, 208
Diet
  community health and, 266
  community practice action plans and,
      272–273
  diabetes self-care and, 247, 248t
  people with special needs and, 238
  self-efficacy and, 204
Differential signal, surface EMG sensors
      and, 58
Disabilities. See People with special
      needs
Discomfort
  pain response thresholds and, 196t,
      197
  reduction of, in dental procedures for
      children, 178–179, 184
Discrimination, age and, 213
Disruptive child behavior. See Children
Distraction
  with children in dental settings,
      180–181, 184
  dental fear management and, 116,
      118–119
  dental pain and, 87–88, 92
  raising pain response thresholds and,
      198

Distractive coping style, periodontal disease and, 141, 142
Divided attention, in older adults, 215
Dohrman, R. S., 55
Domestic violence, chronic orofacial pain and, 109, 111
Drug abuse
  chronic orofacial pain and, 108
  periodontal disease and, 145, 146
Drug addicts, oral parafunctions among, 132
Drug use, coping style, periodontal disease, and, 144
Dry mouth, 37
  in people with special needs, fluoride products, and, 239
  subjective, psychological origin of, 40
Dual-channel capability, sEMG instruments and, 60, 61
Dual pain fiber pathways, pain stimuli and, 195
Ductal cells, saliva and, 38
Durkheim, E., 265
Dying patients, dentists and, 215
Dysmorphic appearance, diagnosis and treatment paradoxes around, 8
Dystonias, bruxism and, 132

E. *See* Epinephrine
Eastman Esthetic Index, 8
Eating disorders, 209
Edentulism, community oral disease and, 270
Education. *See also* Dental education
  role of, in facilitation of change, 154
Educational strategies, pain management and, 191*t*
Edwards, R. R., 220
EEG. *See* Electroencephalography
Efficacy expectation, 203
Ekman, P., 10
Elderly. *See also* Aging; Geriatric dentistry
  dry mouth in, 41
Electrical interference, laptops, EMG units and, 61
Electroencephalography, 52
Electromyographic recordings, bruxism and, 127

Electromyography
  as measure of muscle activity, 57–58
  quantifiying activity with, 60
Electromyography signal, detecting, 58
Eli, I., 5, 8
Ellingson, S. A., 166, 170
Emergencies, diabetes-related, 245, 249–250
EMG. *See* Electromyography
Emotion, dental pain and, 79, 92
Enamel fluorosis, community oral disease and, 269–270
Engel, G. L., 21
Environment
  community health and, 266
  dental pain and, 79, 86, 92
  Mowrer's two-factor theory and, 83
Environmental enrichment, thumb sucking and, 171
Epinephrine, 31
Erickson, Carol, 68
Erickson, Milton, 66, 68, 69
Erikson, Erik, 218
Erosion, community oral disease and, 269
Escape motivation, children's control over dental routine and, 183
Ethnicity
  dental caries and, 268
  dental pain and, 93
  malocclusion and, 269
  oral health disparities and, 266
  orofacial pain and, 92
  tooth loss, edentulism, and, 270
Europe, oral cancer in, 269
Ewin, D., 65
Exercise, diabetes self-care and, 247, 248*t*, 249
Expectancy model of fear, 85
External locus of control, 90, 200
Extractions, pain management and, 190

Face
  perception of, 5–6
  socialization and, 3, 4
Facial Action Coding System, 10
Facial changes, patient-dentist communication, aging and, 221
Facial chimeras, studies of, 6–7

Facial expressions
    nonverbal communication and, 10–12
    universal, 10, *11*
Facial symmetry, importance of, 6
FACS. *See* Facial Action Coding System
Faculty development, in successful train-
        ing programs, 261
Family support, aging and, 221
Fear. *See also* Anxiety; Dental anxiety;
        Dental fear
    in children, during dental treatment,
        177
    dental pain and, 81, 92
    effective communication and reduc-
        tion in, 256
    expectancy model of, 85
    facial expression and recognition of,
        10
    pain, anxiety, and, 194
    pain affected by, 79
    predictability and, 88
Fear-avoidance model, 83, 84–85
Fear of pain models, in dentistry, 82–83
Felt control, dental pain and, 90
Fere, Charles, 54
Fernandez, E., 55
Fields, H. W., Jr., 269
"Fight-flight" reaction, pain and, 193
Filcheck, H., 181
Fillingim, R. B., 220
Finger sucking. *See* Thumb sucking
First impressions, facial appearance and,
        9
Fissured tongue, in diabetic patients,
        244
Flamenbaum, M. H., 24
Fleck-Kandath, C., 204
Flooding, dental fear management and,
        116
Flor, H., 55
Floss holders, for people with special
        needs, 233
Flossing
    behavior change linked to patient's
        values and, 156
    interventions in self-efficacy and, 208
    readiness for change and, 153
    self-efficacy analyses and, 204–205
    theory of planned action and, 151–152

Fluoridated water, 266
Fluoride
    community practice action plans and,
        273
    topical, 238
Fluoride-containing rinses, people with
        special needs and, 238–239
Fluoride toothpaste, people with special
        needs and, 239
Fluoride varnish, people with special
        needs and, 238, 239
Fluorosis, community oral disease and,
        269–270
Foot care, diabetes self-care and, 247
Forgione, A. G., 131
Frankl, S., 179
Franklin, Benjamin, 66
Franklin, M., 8
Frequency range, sEMG instruments
        and, 61–62
Freud, Sigmund, 66
Friesen, W. V., 10
Friman, P. C., 166, 167, 168
Fruits and vegetables, advocating diet
        rich in, 272
Functional analysis, of thumb sucking,
        165

Gale, E. N., 54, 55
Galsworthy, J., 3
Galvanic skin response, 52
Gangrene, diabetes and, 247
Gardea, M. A., 55
Gastrointestinal allergies, 34
Gatchel, R. J., 55
Gating mechanisms, role of, pain man-
        agement studies about, 191
Geboy, M. J., 123
Gel, electrode, 59
Gender
    dental pain and, 91–92, 93
    oral health disparities and, 266
Gene mapping, saliva and, 47
General adaptation syndrome, 30
General anesthesia, 178
Generality, efficacy expectations and,
        203
Generalization, people with special
        needs and, 237

Gene therapy
  saliva and, 47
  salivary gland dysfunction and, 46
Geriatric dentistry
  behavioral issues in, 213–223
  dental care issues in, 221–222
  practitioner-related issues in, 213–215
    ageism and stereotypes, 213–214
    dentist's attitudes toward older
        patients, 214
    patient death and bereavement, 215
  psychosocial issues in, 218–221
    depression, 219–220
    pain response/somatization,
        220–221
    personality, 218–219
    social/family support, 221
  understanding aging process in,
      215–218
    cognition, 215–216
    dementia, 216–271
    oral physical senses, 217
    sensory changes, 218
Giddon, D. B., 19, 139, 209
Gift, H. D., 21
Gilbert, G. H., 87, 92
Gingival bleeding, in diabetic patients,
    244
Girls, dental trauma in, 268
Glands, salivary, 38
Glaros, A. G., 54
Glasgow, R. E., 204
Global self-ratings, of oral-health-related
    quality of life, 22
Gloves, as thumb sucking deterrent, 166
Glucagon, 31, 32
Glucometers, 250, 251
Glucose testing, diabetes self-care and,
    247, 248t
Glycemic control, diabetic patients and,
    247
Gnashing of teeth, 127
Goldfarb, M. M., 222
"Good genes theory," 6
Graded chronic pain scale, 107t
Graded Pain Scale, RDC/TMD Axis 2
    Graded scale, 106–107
Graduated exposure, dental fear man-
    agement and, 116

Gray, S. A., 24
Grief, older patients and, 220
Grinding (bruxism), 105, 127, 133
  effects of, 128
  evidence of, 132
  prevalence of, 128
Gross, P. R., 85
Ground, 59
Growth factors, 31
Growth hormone, 31, 32
Gryll, S. L., 87
GSR. *See* Galvanic skin response
Guided imagery, 123
  cognitive anxiety and, 121–122
  dental fear management and, 116,
      120
Guillotin, Joseph, 66
Gustafson, C., 204
Gustatory system, socialization and, 5

Habit behavior modification, 110
Habit reversal, thumb sucking and, 169
Hair pulling, thumb sucking and, 167,
    168, 169
Halitophobia, 5
"Halo effect," 6
Hand-over-mouth procedure, 178
Hanson, B. S., 221
Happiness, facial expression and recog-
    nition of, 10
HCV. *See* Hepatitis C virus
Health
  biopsychosocial model of, 21
  community and, 265–267
  inappropriate coping styles and risk
      to, 143
  WHO definition of, 265
Health behavior, model of, 150–152
Health behavior models, diabetic
    patients and, 248–249
Health care, access to, 266
Health care costs, nocturnal parafunc-
    tions and, 129
Health care organization, 266
Health-promoting schools, 271
Health-promoting workplaces, 271
Health promotion, whole-population
    based approach to, 266
Healthy Cities project, 271

Hearing
   aging and, 218
   physical disorders, mental illness, and,
      11–12
Heart disease, 270, 272
Heavy trance states, 69
Heft, M. W., 87, 92
Henry, R. G., 215
Hepatitis C virus, salivary gland disor-
      ders and, 42
High-pass filtering, 62
Hill, K., 7
Hippocampus
   pain response thresholds and, 197
   pain-stimulus awareness and, 192
Hispanic children, dental caries in, 268
HIV-infected patients, dry mouth in, 41
Holland, G. R., 80
Holloway, P. J., 214
Hölund, U., 207
Homeostasis, survival and, 30
Hove, G., 167, 168
Howitt, J., 8
Hunger, 272
Hydrotherapy, relaxation and, 53
Hygienists
   gender and cultural status of, 92
   patient involvement and, 149
Hyperglycemia, 249–250
Hypersensitive patients, pain manage-
      ment and, 194
Hypnosis
   anxiety control and, 121, 122
   clinical, brief history of, 65–66
   clinical, map of, 68t
   defining and using, 67–69
   dental fear management and, 116, 120
   in dentistry, 65–75
   forms of, 68–74
      indirect suggestion, 70–71
      language, 70
      modeling, 71–72
      nontrance, 69–70
      stories, 71
      trance, 68–69
   nature of, 66–67
   raising pain response thresholds and,
      198t, 199
   recommendations for dentists, 74–75

recommended readings on, 76
relaxation and, 52, 53
styles of communication
   authoritarian, 72
   permissive, 72
   uses, 72–74
Hypnotic suggestion, 57
Hypochondriasis, 13
Hypoglycemia, 249–250
Hypothalmic-pituitary-adrenal (HPA)
      axis, 30, 31, 192

Iatrosedation, raising pain response
      thresholds and, 198t
Illness, chronic, biopsychosocial model
      of, 102
Imagery, 57
   hypnosis and, 73
   pain response thresholds and, 198
Imaging techniques, facial perception
      and, 7
Immediate memory, aging and, 216
Immune function, neuroendocrine-
      immune (NEI) network and, 34
Immune system, 29
   surgical stress and, 33
Immunodeficiencies, oral cancer and,
      269
Implants, speech articulation and, 12
Implication, 70
Implosion, dental fear management and,
      116
Index of Orthodontic Treatment Need,
      Aesthetic Component of, 8
Indirect suggestion, 70–71
Individual differences
   pain sensitivity and, 85–86
   predictability, controllability, and, 89
Infants, facial expressions in, 10
Infections, prophylactic, diabetic patients
      and, 251
Inflammation
   stress and: bidrectional relationship in,
      29–34
   stress response and, 31–33
Inflammatory diseases, dental pain and,
      80
Informational barriers, people with
      special needs and, 232–233

Information giving, predictability enhanced through, 89
Inglehart, M. R., 24, 25, 26, 150
Inhibitory stimulus control, thumb sucking and, 171
Injections, pain management and, 194–195
Injection time, prolonged, 178
Institute of Medicine, 25
Insulin, 31
  dental appointments and administration of, 250
  diabetes self-care and, 247, 248*t*
Insulin dependent diabetes mellitus (IDDM) patients
  dental visits and, 245
  self-efficacy scale for, 205
Insurance companies, salivary level screening and, 47
Interdental cleaning, diabetics and, 245, 246*t*
Interleukin-1 (IL-1), 29
Interleukin-6 (IL-6), 32
Internal locus of control, dental pain and, 90
International Association for the Study of Pain, 80
International Consortium for TMD Research, 104
Interocclusal appliances, 132, 134
Interpersonal attraction, visual perception and, 5–10
Interpersonal communication, simulated/standardized patients and evaluation of, 261–262
Interpersonal communication training in dental education, 256–259
  factors influencing design of, 257
  performance-based methodologies and, 258
Interpersonal strategies, pain management and, 191*t*
Interventions, community group-based, 266–267
Involving the individual technique, 236
IOTN. *See* Index of Orthodontic Treatment Need
Irritation fibromas, in diabetic patients, 244

Jacobsonian progressive muscle relaxation, 52, *53*
Janet, Pierre-Marie-Félix, 66
Japan
  communication education in, 256
  oral cancer in, 269
  simulated/standardized patient and dental education in, 259, 260
Jenny, J., 8
Johnston, V., 8
Jones, D., 7

Kasman, G. S., 60
Katahn, M., 87
Keffer, M. A., 204
Kisnisci, R. S., 11
Kiyak, H. A., 9, 214, 222
Klages, U., 255
Kneckt, M. C., 205
Knjuuttila, M. L. E., 206
Knowledge
  health behavior and, *150*, 151
  poor self-efficacy and lack of, 206
Kohout, F. J., 8
Kressin, N. R., 21
Kupffer cells, 32

Lactobacillus acidophilus, salivary levels of, 47
Lactoferrin, in saliva, 39
Lang, P. J., 81
Language, hypnotic quality of, 70
Laptops, EMG units, electrical interference and, 61
Lashley cup, 46
Laskin, D. M., 55
Latin American children, dental trauma in, 268
Lavoisier, Antoine, 66
Law enforcement agencies, salivary level screening and, 47
Leukoplakia, in diabetic patients, 244
Lichen planus, in diabetic patients, 244
Life expectancy, dental care and, 223
Lifespan issues, dental pain and, 91–92
Lifestyle, community health and, 266
Light trance states, 69
Lip cancers, 269
Lipids, stress and increase in, 32

Lipopolysaccharide, 32
Lipton, J. A., 92
Live-patient simulations, in communication training, 257, 258
Local injections, pain management and, 195
Locus coeruleus, corticotropin-releasing factor and, 31
Long, E. S., 169
Lorenz, K., 7
Loupe, M. J., 214
Low-pass filtering, 62
Lupus, 34
Lynn, S., 68
Lysozyme, in saliva, 39

Macek, M. D., 222
Magnitude, efficacy expectations and, 203
Mahalski, P. A., 166
Maintenance stage, in *Trans-Theoretical Model of Behavior Change,* 153, *153*
Maizels, A., 21
Maizels, J., 21
Malnutrition, kinds of, 272
Malocclusion, 8, 9
   community oral disease and, 269–270
   thumb sucking and, 163
Malpractice complaints, poor patient-dentist communication and, 256
Mandibulofacial dysostosis, speech apparatus and, 12
Manski, R. J., 222
Marback, J. J., 92
Massage, relaxation and, 52, *53*
Masseter muscle
   biofeedback training and, 55
   selection of, 62
Mast cells, 31
Masticatory muscles
   bruxism and pain in, 128–129
   chronic pain in, 100
Mating behavior, physical attractiveness and, 8
Maxwell, R., 9
McCaul, K. D., 204
McGill Pain Questionnaire, 80
McNeil, D. W., 83

Medial orbitofrontal cortex, attractive faces and, 7
Medical education
   background history of simulated/standardized patient in, 258–259
   simulated/standardized patient utilization in, 260
Medical model of dental prevention, 237
Medications, bruxism and, 132
Meditation, 54
   dental fear management and, 116
   relaxation and, 52, *53*
Mellor, A. C., 256
Memory, aging and, 216
Men
   dental pain and, 92
   oral cancer in, 269
Mercury (Hg) release, from dental fillings, grinding and, 129
Mesmer, Anton, 66
Metabolic balance, diabetic patients and, 247
Methylphenidate, bruxism and, 132
Mexican-Americans
   dental caries in children, 268
   tooth loss and, 270
Microarray chip technology, saliva and, 47
Microbial plaque, diabetics, dental caries, and, 245
Microorganisms, salivary levels of, 47
Middle Eastern children, dental trauma in, 268
Milgrom, P., 256
Miller, R. R., 214
Miller, S. M., 89
Miller, W. R., 153, 157
Minnesota Multiphasic Personality Inventory, 130
Minorities. *See also* African Americans; Hispanic children; Mexican Americans; Race
   older, dental care and, 222
   oral cancer among, 269
Mishra, K. D., 55
Model for the New Century, for oral health behavior, 150

Modeling
  dental fear management and, 116
  hypnosis and, 71–72
Monozygotic twins, oral parafunctions
      and, 128
Moore, A. W., 9
Moray, L. J., 269
Mother infant attachments, infant's facial
      expressions and, 10
Motivational Interviewing, 156–158
  evidence basis of, 157–158
  principles of, 156–157, 157t
  uses of, in oral health settings, 158
Mouth
  importance of, 3
  nonverbal communication and, 10
  physical attractiveness, self-concept
      and, 9
  as target of suffering and pleasure, 12
Mouth cancer, in United States, 269
Mouth guards, 132
Mouth odors, socialization and, 5
Mouth props, 234, *234, 235*
Mowrer, O. H., two-factory theory of, 83,
      84
MPD. *See* Myofascial pain disorder
MPI. *See* Multidimensional Pain
      Inventory
Multichannel computer-based sEMG
      systems, 61
Multidimensional health behaviors,
      diabetes and, 248
Multidimensional Pain Inventory,
      107–108
Multiple item surveys, of oral-health-
      related quality of life, 22
Muscle activity
  biofeedback and objective monitoring
      of, 51
  electromyography as measure of,
      57–58
Muscle pain, referred, 62
Muscles, selection of, for biofeedback
      training, 62
Musculoskeletal pain, chronic orofacial
      pain and, 100
Musculoskeletal pain literature, fear-
      avoidance model in, 84
Myalgia, 100

Myocardial infarction, diabetes and, 247
Myofascial pain disorder
  biofeedback and, 55
  causes/functional symptoms of, 51
MZ. *See* Monozygotic twins

Narcotics abuse, chronic orofacial pain
      and, 108
National Health and Nutrition
      Examination Survey, 22
National Health Interview Survey, 222
National Institute of Dental and
      Craniofacial Research, 21
National Institute on Aging, 213
NE. *See* Norepinephrine
Negative emotions, dental self-efficacy
      and, 207
Nerve cells, role of, pain management
      studies about, 191
Nervous system, low arousal states and
      avenues of entry to, 52
Neuralgias, 80
Neuroendocrine-immune (NEI) network,
      31
  immune function and, 34
Neuromatrices, subjective pain experi-
      ence and, 100
Neuropathic pain conditions, chronic
      orofacial pain and, 100
Neuropathy, diabetes and, 247
Neuropeptides, 34
NF-κB activity, stress, inflammation,
      and, 33, 34
NHANES. *See* National Health and
      Nutrition Examination Survey
Nicotine use, periodontal disease and,
      145
NIDCR. *See* National Institute of Dental
      and Craniofacial Research
Nitrous oxide sedation, informing
      patient about, 89
Nociception, chronic pain and, 102
Nociceptive sensation, pain factors and
      quality of, 192t
Nociperceptive activity, pain behavior
      and, 194
Nociperceptive signal, pain response
      thresholds and, 197
Nocturnal alarms, 133

Nocturnal grinding, effects of, 129
Nocturnal parafunctions, prevalence of, 128
Noise, 58
Nonconfronting stress-coping style, periodontal disease and, 144
Nontrance hypnosis, 69–70
Nonverbal communication, facial expression and, 10–12
Norepinephrine, 31
Norton, P. J., 85
Notch filter set, 62
NTI clenching suppression device, 133
Nutritional counseling, 272
Nutritional deficiencies, oral cancer and, 269

Obesity, 272
Objective signs, motivation for orthodontic treatment and, 9
Objective Structured Clinical Examination, 256, 258, 259, 260, 262
Occlusal disharmonies, bruxism and, 130
Occlusal equilibration, 132
Occlusal wear, bruxism and, 128
O'Doherty, J., 7
Odors in mouth, socialization and, 5
OHIP. See Oral Health Impact Profile
Ohman, A., 54
OHRQoL. See Oral-health-related quality of life
Older patients. See also Aging; Geriatric dentistry
  ageism and, 213–214
  dentists and, 214
Olfaction/olfactory sense
  aging and, 217
  socialization and, 5
Onder, E. M., 11
O'Neill, H. K., 205
Oral cancer
  community oral disease and, 269
  salivary biomarkers for, 47
Oral diseases
  assessing impact of, 22
  as community health problems, 267
  with diabetes, 243, 244–245

Oral health
  importance of behavior change to, 149–150
  older patients and, 219
  people with special needs and, 231–240
Oral health behaviors
  among diabetes mellitus patients, 246t
  dental self-efficacy and, 204–206
  diabetes and, 245, 247
  self-efficacy perceptions in, 203–204
  sources of dental efficacy in, 206–208
Oral health care plan, for people with special needs, 240, 241
Oral Health Impact Profile, 22
Oral Health in America (2000), 213
Oral-health-related quality of life
  assessment of, 22–23
  behavioral scientists and, 26
  clinical practice and, 24–25
  definition and historical reflection on, 20–22
  dental/dental hygiene education and, 25–26
  original conceptualization of, 19
  role of, in research, 23–24
Oral health settings, Motivational Interviewing used in, 158
Oral health status, dental self-efficacy and, 204–206
Oral leukoplakia, in diabetic patients, 244
Oral physical senses, aging and, 217
Orofacial pain. See also Chronic orofacial pain
  definition of, 80
  dual-axis approach to assessment of, 103–104
  ethnic and racial differences in, 92
Orthodontic treatment
  motivation for, 9
  perceptions of appearance and, 8, 9
  verbal/nonverbal communication and, 12
OSCE. See Objective Structured Clinical Examination
Osteoporosis, 272
Oster, H., 10
Ottawa Charter, 271

Outcome expectancy, 203
   brushing and flossing by college
      students and, 204–205
Ovarian cancer, salivary biomarkers for,
   47
Overcoming Obstacles to Dental Health,
   232, 233, 236, 237, 240
Overjets, bruxism and, 130
Overweight population, 272

Paced breathing
   anxiety control and, 121
   dental fear management and, 116, 119
Pacific Center for Special Care
      (University of the Pacific School
      of Dentistry), 232, 237
Pain. *See also* Dental pain
   acute, control of, 200
   aging and perception of, 220–221
   associated with oral cavity, 79
   biopsychosocial model for, 9
   chronic, biopsychosocial model of, *102*
   with clenching and grinding, 128, 129
   contemporary definitions of, 80
   fear, anxiety, and, 194
   graded chronic pain scale, *107t*
   individual differences and sensitivity
      to, 85–86
   Merskey and Bogduk's definition of,
      99
   pain response thresholds and, *196t,*
      197
   reduction of, in dental procedures for
      children, 178–179
   sociocultural meanings of, 81
Pain and treatment history, 105
Pain control
   for diabetic patients, 250
   treatment approaches to, *193t*
Pain factors, dental experience and
      affecting experiences around, *192t*
"Painless dentistry" solutions, 190
Pain management
   interpersonal, 199–200
   nonpharmacological approaches to,
      189–200
   strategies used in, *191t*
Pain pathways, role of, pain management studies about, 191

Pain response thresholds, *196t*
   behavioral strategies and raising of,
      197–199, *198t*
   identification of, 195
Pain Sensitivity Index, 85
Pain stimuli, sensations from, 195
Panic
   dental pain and, 82
   pain response thresholds and decrease
      in, *198t*
Parafunctional jaw behaviors, 105
Parasomnias, bruxism and, 129
Parents, presence of, in operatory with
      child, 179, 184
Parotid salivary gland, 38
Parotid-sparing radiotherapy, 23
Partial participation
   by people with special needs, 233
   with positioning and tongue blade
      mouth prop, 234, *235*
Passive distraction activities, for children
      in dental settings, 181
Passive emotion-oriented coping style,
      periodontal disease and, 141
Patient-centered education, oral-
      health-related quality of life
      and, 26
Patient involvement, oral health,
      dentistry, and, 149
Patients, effective communication with,
      255–256
Patzer, G. L., 7
Pediatric dentists, 178
Pediatric oral diseases, social impact of,
      267
People with special needs
   chemotherapeutic agents use and,
      237–239
   oral health care plan for, 240
      document, *241*
   oral health promotion for, 231–240
   oral-health-related quality of life
      measurements for, 22
   overcoming barriers for, 232–234,
      236–237
   overcoming obstacles to oral health
      for, 232
Perceived control, pain-reducing effects
      and, 90

Perception
   chronic pain and, 102
   definition of, 5
Performance accomplishment, efficacy
   expectations and, 203–204
Performance-based methods, in communication training, 257, 258
Performance evaluations, in communication training, 257
Periodontal disease
   community oral disease and, 268
   coping with stress: influence on,
      140–143
   definition of, 139
   dental pain and, 80
   diabetics and, 243, 244, 247
   low saliva flow rate and, 43
   older patients and, 221–222
   stress, coping and, 139–146
Periodontal therapy, coping with stress:
   influence on, 143–146
Permissive style, in hypnotic communication, 72
Perrin, F. A., 7
Personal experiences, oral health, self-
   efficacy and, 206
Personality, aging and, 218–219
"Phantom tooth pain," 80
Pharmacologic strategies, pain manage-
   ment and, 191t
Phobias, dental, 83
Phobic patients
   emotional disturbances seen in, 106
   relaxation-based procedures for, 120
Phosphate buffer system, in saliva, 38
Phrenology, 6
Physical abuse, chronic orofacial pain
   and, 109, 111
Physical appearance, cues provided
   through, 6
Physical barriers, people with special
   needs and, 232, 233–234, 236
Physical environment, community
   health and, 266
Physiognomy, 6
Physiological states, efficacy expecta-
   tions and, 204
Pilocarpine hydrochloride, 46
Pit and fissure sealant programs, 266

Pit and fissure sealants, people with
   special needs and, 238
Pittsburgh Sleep Quality Inventory, 108
Pituitary-adrenal axis, corticotropin-
   releasing hormone and, 29
Plaque
   dental self-efficacy and, 205
   in diabetic patients, 245
   low saliva flow rate and, 43
   people with special needs and, 238
Plaque-control programs, 149
Pohjamo, L., 245
Policies, community health and, 266
Polypharmacy, xerostomia and, 41
Polysomnography, bruxism and, 134
POMC. *See* Proopiomelanocortin
Positive reinforcement and feedback, for
   children in dental setting,
   181–182, 184
Postoperative complications, 33
Postoperative dental pain, 82
Post-traumatic stress disorder, chronic
   orofacial pain and, 108–109, 111
*Practical Preventive Protocols for Prevention
   of Dental Disease in People with
   Special Needs in Community
   Settings,* 237, 240
Prahl-Anderson, B., 9
Pranayama autogenics, relaxation and,
   52, *53*
Preamplified sensors, with EMG
   systems, 59
Precontemplation stage, in *Trans-
   Theoretical Model of Behavior
   Change,* 153, *153*
Predictability
   definition of, 88
   dental pain and, 88–91, 92
Pregelled electrodes, 59
Preparation stage, in *Trans-Theoretical
   Model of Behavior Change,* 153, *153*
Prevention
   importance of, in oral diseases, 149
   people with special needs and chal-
      lenges with, 232
Problem-oriented coping strategies, 141
Problem solving, aging and, 216
Prochaska, J. O., 152, 208
Proffit, W. R., 269

Progressive muscle relaxation, 57
  dental fear management and, 116,
    120–124
  Jacobsonian, 52, *53*
  raising pain response thresholds and,
    198
Prolonged injection time, children and,
  178
Proopiomelanocortin, 31
Prostheses, speech articulation and, 12
Protein buffer system, in saliva, 38
Pseudocholinesterase, 39
PSI. *See* Pain Sensitivity Index
Psychological factors, pain factors and,
  192*t*
Psychological status, chronic orofacial
    pain and assessment of, 105–106
Psychological stress, 31
Psychosocial issues, aging and,
    218–221
Psychosocial status, chronic orofacial
    pain and assessment of,
    106–107
PTSD. *See* Post-traumatic stress disorder
PTSD Checklist, 109
Public health research, role of oral-
    health-related quality of life in,
    23, 24
Pulpal origin, of dental pain, 80

Quality assurance
  case development and, 260–261
  in successful training programs, 261
Quality of life. *See also* Oral-health-
    related quality of life
  as crucial factor in treatment decision
    making, 21

Race. *See also* African Americans;
    Minorities
  dental caries and, 268
  dental pain and, 93
  malocclusion and, 269
  oral cancer and, 269
  orofacial pain and, 92
  tooth loss, edentulism, and, 270
Radiation therapy, salivary glands and,
    41, 46
Rapp, J. T., 165, 169

RDC/TMD. *See* Research Diagnostic
    Criteria for Temporomandibular
    Disorders
Reasoned action theory, brushing and
    flossing by college students and,
    204–205
Reference, 59
Referred muscle pain, biofeedback and,
    62
Reframing, raising pain response thresh-
    olds and, 198*t*
Reinforcers, for people with special
    needs, 236, 237
Reis, V. A., 7
Reisine, S., 21
Relationships, with dental providers,
    86–87
Relaxation
  chronic pain management and,
    110–111
  hypnosis and, 72–73
  methods of, 52, *53*
  phases in brief procedure of, 122
  raising pain response thresholds and,
    198*t*
  saliva levels and, 40
  somatic and cognitive orientation of
    methods of, *122*
Relaxation training
  approaches to, 57
  masseter feedback with, 55
Renin, 31, 32
Repression-sensitization stress concept,
    142
Reprimands, thumb sucking and, 169,
    170
Research, role of oral-health-related
    quality of life in, 23–24
Research Diagnostic Criteria for
    Temporomandibular Disorders,
    104, 111
Resigned coping style, periodontal
    disease and, 141
Resistance
  minimizing, advice-giving and, 153,
    154
  statements linked to arousal of, 155*t*
Response covariation, thumb sucking
    and, 166–167

Response prevention, for thumb suck-
    ing, 166
Restorations
    older patients and, 219
    pain management and, 190
Retinopathy, diabetes and, 247
Rett syndrome, bruxism and, 132
Reward systems, for people with special
    needs, 236
Rheumatoid arthritis, 29, 30, 34
Rhue, J., 68
Rice Test, 37
Rickardsson, B., 221
Riley, J. L., 87, 92
Rinses, fluoride-containing, 238–239
RMS. *See* Root mean square
Role-playing
    in communication training, 257, 258
    by simulated/standardized patients,
        260
Rollnick, S., 153, 154, 157
Root canal therapy
    dental pain and, 91–92
    fear-avoidance model and, 84–85
Root mean square, 60

Sadness, facial expression and recogni-
    tion of, 10
Saliva
    clinical significance of, 43–46
    complications in functioning of,
        42–43
    current diagnostic values and, 47
    dysfunction with, 39–42
    formation of, 38
    function of, 38–39, 39t
    role of, in health and disease, 37
Saliva collection, setting for, 45
Salivary flow, depression and, 220
Salivary gland hypofunction, 41
    chronic conditions associated with, 40t
    clinical/radiographic evidence of den-
        tal caries and dry lips and tongue
        in patient with, 43
    common signs/symptoms associated
        with, 42t
    identifying patients with or at risk for,
        44
    management of patient with, 46

Salivary glands, 38
Salivary output, preserving in head and
    neck cancer patients, 23
Saliva tests, 37–38
Sandell, R., 255
Sanders, M. R., 169
Sarhed, G., 255
Sarll, D. W., 214
Sarment, D., 24
SARS. *See* Severe acute respiratory
    syndrome
Scheduled breaks, for children in dental
    settings, 182–183, 184
Schools, health-promoting, 271
Schwartz, G. E., 121
Schwartz, M. S., 52, 56
Science research, role of oral-health-
    related quality of life in, 23
SCL-90, 105
    Anxiety Scale items, *106*
    Depression Scale items, *106*
    Somatization Scale items, *107*
Seattle Longitudinal Studies, 216
Selective attention, in older adults, 215
Self-actualization, mouth and, 3
Self-care practices
    among diabetics, 245, 247
    purpose of, for diabetics, 247
Self-efficacy
    brushing and flossing by college
        students and, 204–205
    childhood model and, 207
    cognitive dimension behind, 206
    dental visits and, 205
    dentist's role in patient's perception
        of, 210–211
    experiential dimension behind, 206
    formation of, 206
    improving oral health behavior and
        interventions in, 207–208
    knowledge, *150*, 151, 152
    negative emotions and, 207
    oral and diabetes health behaviors
        and, 248–249
    oral health behavior, oral health status,
        and, 204–206
    readiness to change and, 153–154
    self-empowerment and, 208–209
    sources of, 203–204

supportive dimension with, 207
  theory of, 203
Self-empowerment
  for changing behavior, 209–210
  self-efficacy and, 208–209
Self-esteem
  diabetes health behaviors and, 249
  older patients and, 219
  physical attractiveness and, 8
Self-regulation, historical development
    behind, 54
sEMG. *See* Surface electromyography
Seniors, dental care issues and, 221–222.
    See also Geriatric dentistry
Sensor placement, surface EMG and,
    58–59
Sensory changes, aging and, 218
Sensory detection theory, 195
Sensory qualities, of pain experience, 102
Separation anxiety, child disruptiveness
    in dental setting and, 179
Sergl, H. G., 255
Serotonin, 31
SES differences. *See* Sex-differentiated
    socioeconomic differences
Severe acute respiratory syndrome,
    salivary biomarkers for, 47
Sex-differentiated socioeconomic (SES)
    differences, 92
Sexual abuse, chronic orofacial pain and,
    109, 111
Shalala, Donna, 20
Shaping procedures, for people with
    special needs, 236
Sheiham, A., 21
Short-term memory, aging and, 216
Sialadenosis, bulimia nervosa and, 41
Sialometric evaluation, 45
Sick role, chronic pain and, 103
Simulated/standardized patient
  background history of, as tool in
    medical and dental education,
    258–259
  evaluating interpersonal communica-
    tion training with, 261–262
  faculty development, quality assur-
    ance, and, 261
Simulated/standardized patient
  methodology, benefits of, 259

Sjögren's syndrome
  dry mouth in, 41
  gene therapy and, 46
Skin preparation, surface EMG sensors
    and, 59–60
Slade, G. D., 21, 22
Sleep apnea, nocturnal parafunctions
    and, 128
Sleep bruxism, prevalence of, 128
Sleep disturbance, chronic orofacial pain
    and, 108
Sleep polysomnography, bruxism and,
    131
Sleep stages, nocturnal parafunctions
    and, 129
Smokeless-tobacco use, 272
Smoking
  oral cancer and, 269
  periodontal disease and, 139, 145, 146
Smoking avoidance
  dentists, diabetic patients, and, 251
  diabetes self-care and, 247, 248*t*
  self-efficacy and, 204
Smoking cessation
  counseling about, 145–146
  patient stages in, 153
  people with special needs and, 238
Smoking cessation programs
  community practice action plans and,
    272
  older patients and, 217
Snoring, nocturnal parafunctions and,
    128
SNS. *See* Sympathetic nervous system
Social cognitive theory, 204
Social contingencies, thumb sucking
    and, 169–170
Social efficacy, depression and poor
    sense of, 204
Social environment
  community health and, 266
  dental pain and, 91–92
Social indicators, of oral-health-related
    quality of life, 22
Socialization
  mouth and, 3, 4
  olfactory and gustatory system and, 5
Social norms, health behavior and, 150,
    150, 151–152

Social sufficiency, motivation for orthodontic treatment and, 9
Social support, aging and, 221
Socioeconomic status
dental caries and, 268
dental pain and, 92, 93
dental trauma and, 268
oral health disparities and, 266, 267
periodontal disease and, 268
Soft drinks, decreasing consumption of,
272
Somatic anxiety, 121
Somatic-motor system, low arousal
states and avenues of entry to, 52
Somatization
aging and, 220–221
chronic orofacial pain and assessment
of, 105
Somerman, M. J., 23
Sorrell, J. T., 83
South Central Asia, oral cancer in, 269
SP. *See* Simulated/standardized patient;
Substance P
"Spa dentistry," 72
Spatial qualities, of pain experience, 102
Special needs patients. *See* People with
special needs
Speech, impact of physical disorders and
mental illness on, 11–12
Speech patterns, in craniofacially
deformed individuals, 10
Splints, 132
for thumb sucking, 166
Sports, dental trauma and, 269
Stand-alone surface EMG instruments,
60
Standardized patient, 258
"Startle reactions," preventing, 197
Stereotypes
ageism and, 213–214
facial appearance and, 6
Stewart, J. E., 205, 208
Stimulated saliva, collecting, 46
Stimulus experience, pain factors and
onset of, 192, 192*t*
Stop-zit, thumb sucking reduction and,
167–168
Stories, hypnosis and, 71
Stoyva, J., 54

Strauss, R. P., 21
Strayer, M. S., 214
Street, R. L., Jr., 255
Strength, efficacy expectations and, 203
Streptococcus mutants, salivary levels of,
47
Stress
dry mouth and, 40
inflammation and: bidrectional relationship with, 29–34
management of, 34
molecular implications of, 33–34
neurobiology of, 31
surgical, 33
Stress coping
studies on, 140–146
about influence on periodontal
disease, 140–143
about influence on periodontal
therapy, 143–146
extracted factors after factor
analysis, 141*t*
Stress-coping questionnaire, 140, 144
Stress education, 110
Stress inoculation, dental fear management and, 116
Stressors, homeostasis and, 30
Stress reduction, for diabetic patients,
250
Stress response, inflammation and,
31–33
Stress syndrome, 30
Stricker, G., 8
Stricker, J. M., 168
Stroke, diabetes and, 247
Structuring the environment technique,
236
Subjective symptoms, motivation for
orthodontic treatment and, 9
Sublingual salivary gland, 38
Submandibular salivary gland, 38
Substance abuse, chronic orofacial pain
and, 108
Substance P, 31, 32
Substitute gratification, periodontal
disease and, 145
Sucking, 4
Suffering, pain response thresholds and
sense of, 196*t*, 197, 199

Sugar in diet, diabetics, dental caries, and, 245
Suggestion
    hypnosis and, 73
    raising pain response thresholds and, 198, 199
Supportive experiences, dental self-efficacy and, 207
Surface electromyography, 51, 52
    meta-analysis, 54–55
    reliability of, 57
Surface electromyography instruments
    selecting, 60–62
        frequency range, 61–62
        laptops and electrical interference, 61
Surface electromyography sensors and recording techniques, 58–60
    preamplified sensors, 59
    sensor placement, 58–59
    skin preparation, 59–60
    types of electrodes, 59
Surgeon General's Report on Oral Health (2000), 19
Surgical stress, 33
Survival
    homeostasis and, 30
    mouth and, 3, 4
Sustained attention, in older adults, 215, 216
SVF. *See* Stress-coping questionnaire
Sympathetic nervous system, 31
Syrjälä, A. -M. H., 205, 206
Syrjälä, L. K., 206
Systematic desensitization
    anxiety control and, 121, 122
    dental fear management and, 116, 120
Systemic lupus erythematosus, 34

Tarlov, A. R., 265
Taste, aging and, 217
Tedesco, L. A., 8, 25, 150, 204
Teeth, signs and symbols for in early civilizations, 4
Tell-Show-Do technique, 180
    raising pain response thresholds and, 198*t*, 199
Temporal qualities, of pain experience, 102

Temporomandibular joint disorder
    biobehavioral treatments and, 110–111
    catastrophizing and, 86
    causes/functional symptoms of, 51
    chronic orofacial pain and, 100
    with clenching and grinding, 128
    otologic complaints with, 11–12
    physical and sexual abuse and, 109, 111
    post-traumatic stress disorder and, 109, 111
    thumb sucking and, 163
Temporomandibular joint pain, biofeedback and relief of, 55
Terminally ill, dental support for, 215
Theory of Planned Action, with modifications, 150, *150*
Theory of Planned Behavior, 204
Theory of Protection Motivation, 204
Thermal feedback, 52
Th1 cells, immune function and, 34
"Three A's of Anxiety," 117
Throat cancer, in United States, 269
Th2 cells, immune function and, 34
Thumb sucking, 163–171
    assessment of, 164
    consequences of, 163
    functional assessment of, 164–165
    future research on, 170–171
    treatment for, 165–170
        antecedent interventions, 165
        combination interventions, 169–170
        consequent interventions, 167–168
        response covariation, 166–167
        response prevention, 166
TICS. *See* Two-item conjoint screening test
Time factors, pain factors and, 192*t*
Tissue engineering, 23
Tobacco chewing, oral cancer and, 269
Tobacco use, community practice action plans and, 272
Tolle, S. W., 215
Tongue, parafunctional displays of, 4
Tongue blade mouth prop, 234, *234*
    partial participation with positioning and, 234, *235*
Tongue cleaning, for older patients, 217
Toothache, pain syndromes and, 80

Toothbrush choices, theory of planned action and, 151
Toothbrushes, adaptive, 233, *233, 234*
Tooth brushing
  diabetics and, 245, 246*t*, 249
  interventions in self-efficacy and, 208
  self-efficacy analyses and, 204–205
Toothettes, 239
Tooth loss
  aging and, 219
  rates of, 270
  social/family support and, 221
Toothpaste, fluoride, 239, 273
Topical anesthesia, for children, 178, 184
Topical fluorides, people with special needs and, 238
Touch, raising pain response thresholds and, 198*t*
Training programs
  case development and, 260–261
  faculty development and quality assurance in, 261
  successful, 259–261
Trance, 66, 67, 68–69
Trans-Theoretical Model of Behavior Change, 152–153, *153*
Trigeminal neuralgia, 100
Turk, D. C., 55
Tuz, H. H., 11
Twins, oral parafunctions and, 128
Two-factory theory (Mowrer), 83, 84
Two-item conjoint screening test, 108
Type A behavior patterns, nocturnal parafunctions and, 130–131
Type 2 diabetes, rise in, 243

UCS. *See* Unconditioned response
Ultraviolet light exposure, oral cancer and, 269
Unconditioned response, 83
Uncovering, hypnosis and, 74
Underweight population, 272
Unidimensional health behaviors, diabetes and, 248, 249
United Kingdom
  dental erosion in children in, 269
  dental trauma in children in, 268

United States
  dental caries in, 267, 268
  oral cancer in, 269
United States Medical Licensing Examination, 256, 258
Unstimulated saliva, collecting, 46
Urinary catecholamines, bruxism in children and, 130

Valacovic, R. W., 25
Values, patient, linking requested behavior change to, 155–156
Van der Linden, F. P. G. M., 9
Vasoactive intestinal peptide, 31
Vegetables and fruits, advocating diet rich in, 272
Velocardiofacial syndrome, speech apparatus and, 12
Verbal communication, facial expression and, 10–12
Verbal persuasion, efficacy expectations and, 204
Vicarious experiences, efficacy expectations and, 203–204
Videotaped interviews, in communication training, 257
Violence
  community practice action plans and, 273
  dental trauma and, 269
Viral infections, oral cancer and, 269
Virtual reality, 87
Visual impairments, aging and, 218
Visual perception, interpersonal attraction and, 5–10
Visual signals, from craniofacial area, 10
Voice control technique, with children in dental settings, 180
Volunteers, as simulated/standardized patients, 260

Walker, J., 89
Water, fluoridated, 238, 266
  people with special needs and, 238
Watson, T. S., 167
Weight regulation, diabetes self-care and, 248*t*

Weinstein, 158
Weisenberg, M., 92
"White coat effect," 91
Whole saliva, 38
Willard, R., 65
Wilson, M. C., 214
Wolf, S. L., 60
Wolfe, G. R., 208
Women
   dental pain and, 92
   tobacco use by, 272
Work absence, oral diseases and, 266, 267
Workplaces, health-promoting, 271
World Health Organization, 268
   health defined by, 20, 21

Xerostomia, 220
   common signs/symptoms associated with, 42t
   in diabetic patients, 243, 244
   in elderly patients, 42
   medications and, 41
   in people with special needs, 232
      fluoride products and, 239
Xerostomia Related Quality of Life Scale, 22
Xylitol, 238

Yoga, relaxation and, 52, 53
Yoga meditation, 54

Zaidel, D. W., 7
Zen meditation, 54